Hip Preservation Techniques

T0203994

Hip Preservation Techniques

Edited by
Dr. K. Mohan Iyer
Senior Consultant Orthopedic Surgeon
Bengaluru, Karnataka, India

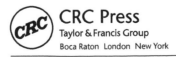

CRC Press is an imprint of the
Taylor & Francis Group, an **informa** business

CRC Press
Taylor & Francis Group
6000 Broken Sound Parkway NW, Suite 300
Boca Raton, FL 33487-2742

First issued in paperback 2020

© 2019 by Taylor & Francis Group, LLC
CRC Press is an imprint of Taylor & Francis Group, an Informa business

No claim to original U.S. Government works

ISBN 13: 978-0-367-72989-9 (pbk)
ISBN 13: 978-0-367-03099-5 (hbk)

This book contains information obtained from authentic and highly regarded sources. While all reasonable efforts have been made to publish reliable data and information, neither the author[s] nor the publisher can accept any legal responsibility or liability for any errors or omissions that may be made. The publishers wish to make clear that any views or opinions expressed in this book by individual editors, authors or contributors are personal to them and do not necessarily reflect the views/ opinions of the publishers. The information or guidance contained in this book is intended for use by medical, scientific or health-care professionals and is provided strictly as a supplement to the medical or other professional's own judgement, their knowledge of the patient's medical history, relevant manufacturer's instructions and the appropriate best practice guidelines. Because of the rapid advances in medical science, any information or advice on dosages, procedures or diagnoses should be independently verified. The reader is strongly urged to consult the relevant national drug formulary and the drug companies' and device or material manufacturers' printed instructions, and their websites, before administering or utilizing any of the drugs, devices or materials mentioned in this book. This book does not indicate whether a particular treatment is appropriate or suitable for a particular individual. Ultimately it is the sole responsibility of the medical professional to make his or her own professional judgements, so as to advise and treat patients appropriately. The authors and publishers have also attempted to trace the copyright holders of all material reproduced in this publication and apologize to copyright holders if permission to publish in this form has not been obtained. If any copyright material has not been acknowledged please write and let us know so we may rectify in any future reprint.

Except as permitted under U.S. Copyright Law, no part of this book may be reprinted, reproduced, transmitted, or utilized in any form by any electronic, mechanical, or other means, now known or hereafter invented, including photocopying, micro-filming, and recording, or in any information storage or retrieval system, without written permission from the publishers.

For permission to photocopy or use material electronically from this work, please access www.copyright.com (http://www.copyright.com/) or contact the Copyright Clearance Center, Inc. (CCC), 222 Rosewood Drive, Danvers, MA 01923, 978-750-8400. CCC is a not-for-profit organization that provides licenses and registration for a variety of users. For organizations that have been granted a photocopy license by the CCC, a separate system of payment has been arranged.

Trademark Notice: Product or corporate names may be trademarks or registered trademarks, and are used only for identification and explanation without intent to infringe.

Visit the Taylor & Francis Web site at
http://www.taylorandfrancis.com

and the CRC Press Web site at
http://www.crcpress.com

Dedication

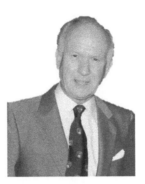

I have written this dedication with a very heavy mind full of fond memories for my late respected teacher, Mr. Geoffrey V. Osborne, without whose constant encouragement and freedom I could not have written this book. These teachers are extremely rare to spot these days where the turmoil of daily life overtakes one's ambitions, duties, and career aspirations. I have a remarkable store of personal and academic memories of him, with whom I spent 4 long years at the University of Liverpool, UK, during which I rarely looked upon him as my teacher, as he was more of a close friend and father to me during all those years.

And loving thanks to
My wife, Mrs. Nalini K. Mohan
My daughter, Deepa Iyer, MBBS, MRCP (UK)
My son, Rohit Iyer, BE (IT)
My grandsons, Vihaan & Kiaan

Contents

Foreword

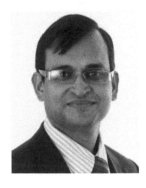

In life, you occasionally feel humbled by some requests, as I did when Dr. K. Mohan Iyer offered me the privilege of writing the foreword to his book on hip preservation surgery.

The readers might wonder what makes a good book: a good editor, an interesting title, a comprehensive coverage of the topic, a renowned author list, or the content.

Dr. Iyer has clearly been a prolific publisher, with more than 10 textbooks under his name, apart from the numerous papers and presentations ranging from his research on trapeziectomy to modifications in posterior approach to the hip, and even as recently as 2017, being open to evolving the anterior approach to the hip. He has spent a substantial period of his life in the United Kingdom, starting his career in the northeast of England, not far from where I work, in India practicing his skills, and also a few years in Riyadh and Sharjah. He clearly has experience and has dealt with health problems over a large part of the globe, developing an international perspective. Dr. Iyer's publication profile is wide-ranging, so he is particularly qualified to assemble the prestigious authors from diverse backgrounds and edit their work for this important book.

Hip preservation surgery is one of the fastest-growing streams in orthopedics demonstrated by its astronomical development over the last 10 years. Clearly, the evolution of techniques has allowed surgeons to deal with hip impingement and dysplasia, the two common conditions that lead to osteoarthritis in young adults in the Western world. These conditions have traditionally been underdiagnosed and perhaps suffered from treatment delays. In the developing world, proximal femoral nonunion after fractured neck of femur, sequelae of Perthes, and other developmental conditions form a significant proportion of work. With the ability to potentially modify the course of disease and delay hip replacement, surgeons and patients worldwide have found hip preservation an attractive proposition. So, clearly, the topic of this book is contemporary and of wide interest to surgeons.

Traditionally, surgeons have suffered from tunnel vision, and we often select interventions that work well in our hands, but while this approach may work for the majority, it will not work for all. We need to therefore broaden our spectrum. This book covers an impressive range of topics including open and arthroscopic impingement surgery, a variety of traditional pelvic and femoral osteotomies, novel procedures such as endoscopic shelf osteotomies, and cartilage regeneration. The readership will get an opportunity to gain more in-depth knowledge about surgeries they may not have been exposed to in their practice, and it will certainly help change their outlook.

Global experts in the field have contributed to this book. Without randomly choosing some names, which would be disrespectful to the rest, readers can themselves judge how esteemed authorities have taken time out from their busy practices and agreed to share their wisdom and experience. The techniques mentioned have evolved over time, some being novel, and the contributing authors have been instrumental in leading this evolution and development. To be able to procure such an impressive line of authors requires dedication, perseverance, and credibility. Dr. Iyer should be congratulated for being able to succeed in this.

While reading a book or a chapter, I always wonder if anything else could have been done to improve it. If in looking at the content one feels that in reality the authors have far exceeded the quality, one can only acknowledge that excellence has been achieved. This is what I feel when reading through this book. A substantial amount of time and effort has been spent in the background by the authors in constructing, writing, and presenting the content. It makes for easy reading, and the illustrations help in understanding the written material. However, the proof is in the readers, and the success will be determined by whether or not they have learned something new and whether they can apply it in their clinical practice.

This book is therefore a comprehensive package and possesses all the qualities of a great book; I would recommend it to everyone interested in hip preservation surgery.

My congratulations and best wishes to the team led by Dr. Iyer.

Ajay Malviya PhD, FRCS
T&O, MSc, MRCS Ed
Consultant Orthopaedic Surgeon—
Northumbria Healthcare
Senior Lecturer, Regenerative Medicine—ICM,
Newcastle University, United Kingdom

Acknowledgments

I am grateful for the thoughtful foreword by Ajay Malviya, PhD, FRCS T&O, MSc, MRCS Ed, a consultant orthopedic surgeon at Northumbria Healthcare NHS Foundation Trust. He trained in the Northern Deanery and has done specialist fellowships in hip preservation and joint replacement surgery in Cambridge, London, and Switzerland. Dr. Malviya is an expert in hip arthroscopy for femoroacetabular impingement, trochanteric pain syndrome, and periacetabular osteotomy for hip dysplasia using a minimally invasive approach. He deals with sports injuries of the hip, and has completed a PhD on the role of hip arthroscopy in femoroacetabular impingement. Preservation of the hip joint is his principal philosophy, but he has a wide experience in joint replacement surgery catering to the young. He was awarded the prestigious ABC (American–British–Canadian) Traveling Fellowship in 2016 by the British Orthopaedic Association, which involved visits to various high-profile centers in the United States and Canada. He is the editorial correspondent for *Journal of Hip Preservation Surgery* and is on the steering committee for the Non-Arthroplasty Hip Registry. He is a member of the British Orthopaedic Association's educational committee as the national lead of UK and Ireland In-Training Examination (UKITE) for orthopedic trainees.

I am honored by and indebted to all the distinguished authors who participated in the creation of this book. Their contributions are invaluable and for that I offer my sincere thanks.

I would especially like to thank Mohan Kumar, graphics designer, Bengaluru, Karnataka, India, for the line diagrams used in this book. Also, my thanks to my son, Rohit Iyer, in the presentation and publication of this book.

I am very thankful to Shivangi Pramanik, commissioning editor—medical, CRC Press, and Mouli Sharma, editorial assistant, CRC Press/Taylor & Francis Group, for taking an active interest in guiding me throughout the publishing process and for their invaluable help while preparing the manuscript.

Above all, I am extremely thankful to Victoria Balque-Burns, Project Manager, Nova Techset and Marsha Hecht, Project Editor, Taylor & Francis Group, LLC for their patience and support during the final stages of publishing of this book.

K. Mohan Iyer, MBBS (Mumbai),
MCh Orth. (Liverpool), MS Orth. (Mumbai),
FCPS Orth. (Mumbai), D'Orth. (Mumbai)
Bengaluru, Karnataka, India

Editor

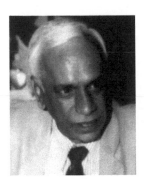

Dr. K. Mohan Iyer did his undergraduate and postgraduate in orthopedics at the Seth G.S. Medical College and K.E.M. Hospital, which is affiliated with the University of Mumbai, and MCh. Orth. (1981) at the University of Liverpool, UK. During this time, he wrote three theses on fractures of the patella, excision arthroplasty of the elbow, and excision of the trapezium for carpometacarpal arthritis of the thumb.

Dr. Iyer has presented numerous papers at state, national, and international conferences in Singapore and Bangkok. He was in charge of the teaching program in orthopedics for undergraduate students and an examiner for the MBBS degree at the University of Bangalore, India. He has also carried out a wide range of operative work on all kinds of major fractures, as well as arthroscopy of the knee, spinal surgery, and elbow and total hip replacements, and has published numerous articles and book chapters. He has done original research work, as can be seen on his website, http://kmohaniyer.com, and has been instrumental in devising a modified posterior approach to the hip joint, which he has followed since 1981.

Contributors

Mandar Agashe MBBS, MS
Consultant Paediatric Orthopaedic
  Surgeon
Agashe's Paediatric SuperSpeciality Care
Mumbai
and
Assistant Honorary Consultant
BJ Wadia Hospital for Children
Parel, Mumbai
and
Visiting Paediatric Orthopaedic Consultant
SRCC Hospital (managed by
  Narayana Health)
and
Surya Childcare
and
Fortis Healthcare
Mumbai

Mehmet Bülent Balioğlu MD
Department of Orthopaedics and
  Traumatology
Baltalimani Bone Diseases Research and Training
  Hospital
Istanbul, Turkey

Sanjeev Bhatia MD
Department of Orthopaedic Surgery
Northwestern Medicine
Warrenville, Illinois

Prakash Chandran MBBS, MS, FRCS
Warrington and Halton Hospitals
NHS Foundation Trust
Warrington, United Kingdom

Milind M. Chaudhary MS
Centre for Ilizarov Techniques
Akola, India
and
Hon Prof. RISC RTO "Ilizarov" Institute
Kurgan, Russia

Victoria Das BS
Cincinnati SportsMedicine & Orthopaedic Center
Mercy Health
Cincinnati, Ohio

Michael B. Ellman MD
Hip Arthroscopy Center
Panorama Orthopedics & Spine Center
Denver, Colorado

Mohamed M. H. El-Sayed MD, PhD
Professor and Consultant of Pediatric
  Orthopedics and Limb Reconstructive
  Surgeries
Faculty of Medicine
Tanta University
Gharbia, Egypt

Ashok S. Gavaskar MS Orth, FACS
Rela Institute of Orthopedics
Tamil Nadu, India

Alessandro Geraci MD, PhD
Orthopaedic Department
San Giacomo Apostolo Hospital
Castelfranco Veneto
Treviso, Italy

K. Mohan Iyer MCh Orth (Liverpool, UK), MS Orth (Bom),
  FCPS Orth (Bom), D'Orth (Bom), MBBS (Bom)
Senior Consultant Orthopedic Surgeon
Karnataka, India

Yasuhiko Kawaguchi MD
Department of Orthopaedic Surgery
The Jikei University Daisan Hospital
Tokyo, Japan

Swapnil M. Keny MS Orth
Sir JJ Group of Hospitals
Saifee Hospital
Mumbai, India

Wasim Khan MBChB, MRCS, Dip Clin Ed, MSc, PhD,
    FRCS (Tr&Orth)
Addenbrooke's Hospital
University of Cambridge
Cambridge, United Kingdom

Catalina Larrain MD
Orthopedics Department
Clínica Las Condes
Santiago, Chile

Dianzhong Luo MD
Joint Surgery & Sport Medicine
Orthopaedic Department
Beijing, China

Rodrigo Mardones MD
Orthopedics Department
Tissue Engineering Laboratory
Clínica Las Condes
Santiago, Chile

Dean K. Matsuda MD
DISC Sports and Spine Center
Marina Del Rey, California

Jose J. Minguell PhD
Centro de Terapia Regenerativa Celular
Clínica Las Condes
Santiago, Chile

Osman A. E. Mohamed MD
Department of Orthopaedics and Traumatology
Faculty of Medicine
Al-Azhar University–Damietta
Damietta, Egypt

Yasir Mohib MBBS, FCPS
Aga Khan University
Karachi, Pakistan

Takuya Otani MD, PhD
Department of Orthopaedic Surgery
The Jikei University Daisan Hospital
Tokyo, Japan

Talal Aqeel Qadri MBBS
Aga Khan University
Karachi, Pakistan

Haroon Rashid MBBS, FCPS
Aga Khan University
Karachi, Pakistan

Alberto Ricciardi MD
Orthopaedic Department
San Giacomo Apostolo Hospital
Castelfranco Veneto
Treviso, Italy

David Rojas MD
Denver Health Medical Center
University of Colorado
Denver, Colorado

Muhammad Zahid Saeed MBBS, MRCS, FEBOT
    (Tr & Ortho), FRCS (Tr & Ortho)
Royal Free Hospital
London, United Kingdom

Akinori Sakai MD
Department of Orthopaedic Surgery
Wakamatsu Hospital
University of Occupational and Environmental
    Health
Kitakyushu, Japan

Shalin Shaunak FRCS
Trauma and Orthopaedic Surgery
KSS Deanery
London, United Kingdom

Soshi Uchida MD, PhD
Wakamatsu Hospital
University of Occupational and Environmental
    Health
Kitakyushu, Japan

Masood Umer MBBS, FCPS
Aga Khan University
Karachi, Pakistan

Abhishek Vaish MS (Orth), MCh Orth (MIS), DNB (Orth),
  Dip SICOT, MNMAS
Central Institute of Orthopaedics
Safdarjung Hospital
New Delhi, India

Raju Vaishya MS Orth, MCh Orth, FRCS
Indraprastha Apollo Hospitals
New Delhi, India

Duan Wang MD
Department of Orthopedics
West China Hospital of Sichuan University
Chengdu, People's Republic of China

Hong Zhang MD
The First Affiliated Hospital of PLAGH
Beijing, China

Zong-ke Zhou MD, PhD
Department of Orthopedics
West China Hospital of Sichuan University
Chengdu, People's Republic of China

Hip preservation techniques

K. MOHAN IYER

INTRODUCTION

The hip joint is a unique joint. During the childhood years, pediatric doctors may place the hip back in the socket if it has come out or realign the socket if it is too shallow by osteotomies of the upper femur or the acetablum. Likewise, older patients with arthritis and hip pain are often treated with hip replacements once the smooth hip surface becomes degenerative. The field of nonarthroplasty surgical treatment of the adult hip is today being referred to as "hip preservation surgery," which may increase the survival of the original hip that we were born with or the affected hip and prevent or delay the need for arthroplasty. Basically, with respect to osteoarthritis (OA) of the hip joint, there are two definitions. The first one relates to various surgical procedures and techniques: (A) techniques such as (1) Periacetabular Osteotomy (PAO), (2) surgical dislocation of the hip, (3) proximal femoral osteotomies, and (4) hip arthroscopy, and (B) the most common surgical procedure within this field, femoroacetabular impingement (FAI), which includes (1) acetabular reorientation, (2) acetabuloplasty, (3) labral repair/reconstruction, (4) cartilage restoration, (5) femoroplasty, and (6) femoral reorientation. The second one relates to the conditions commonly treated in hip preservation surgery such as (1) hip dysplasias, (2) FAI, (3) other hip impingements, (4) sequelae of Legg–Calvé–Perthes, (5) hip cartilage injuries, and (6) coxa valga/vara.

The evolution of hip preservation surgery encompassed many years of growth in our understanding of pre-arthritic hip disorders seen and treated quite commonly in the east and has been described in detail. Some patients with borderline dysplasia may qualify for treatment with minimally invasive *hip arthroscopy*; others require advanced bone realignment procedures (PAO/DFO) Derotational Femoral Osteotomy to achieve a reasonable result. Determining whether a patient is fit and ideal for the minimally invasive approach is a complex process determined by various factors, even taking into consideration lifestyle-related factors.

Hip preservation surgery is a quickly expanding area of orthopedic surgery. Various new aspects of hip preservation surgeries are diverse and range from isolated arthroscopic or open procedures to hybrid procedures that combine the advantages of arthroscopy with open surgical dislocation, pelvic, and/or proximal femoral osteotomy and new treatments for cartilage restoration; hence, an understanding of the relationship between femoral and pelvic orientation, morphology, and the development of intra-articular abnormalities is necessary to formulate a patient-specific approach to treatment with the potential for a successful long-term result.

Several significant differences in the study, subject, and surgical technique conditions exist among various countries in the world. However, certain deficiencies in the use of the clinical outcome scores of various countries and certain definitions of treated pathologies, such as impingement, arthritis, and dysplasia, form a subject for future study quality improvements.

The rapid evolution of hip arthroscopy and advances in 3-D imaging, instrumentation, and surgical techniques are making it possible for surgeons now to perform procedures that were once typically performed by "open techniques" through arthroscopy. Various other extra-articular sources of pain, such as subspine impingement, ischiofemoral impingement, and trochanteric pelvic impingement, are identified arthroscopically in the evolution of hip preservation surgery. This particularly involves the sports medicine and orthopedic community.

Hip preservation is also a relatively new concept in pediatric and young-adult orthopedic surgery, mainly to delay or prevent the onset of end-stage *hip osteoarthritis*. Although a *hip replacement* has an excellent outcome and continues to remain a solution, there is concern for the longevity of the artificial joint, especially in the young and active patient; hence, it is ideal to avoid or postpone hip joint replacement surgery. Basically, hip preservation begins with a newborn child, with the diagnosis and treatment of hip dysplasia that was not done previously. Hip dysplasia in a skeletally immature child can be managed with a variety of bone surgical procedures on the pelvis and acetabulum, as described in this book, everywhere in the world. In adolescents and young adults, the following serve as the latest surgical techniques in hip preservation, such as *periacetabular osteotomy*, surgical dislocation of the hip, which allows complete visualization of the femoral head and acetablum, and *hip arthroscopy*, which has the ability to treat hip disorders in a minimally invasive fashion.

Procedures performed to correct anatomic variations and thus prevent or slow the progression of osteoarthritis are usually referred to as types of hip preservation surgery. Conditions that predispose individuals to femoroacetabular impingement include pincer- and cam-type morphology and hip dysplasia, where common surgical interventions include acetabuloplasty, osteochondroplasty, periacetabular osteotomy, and derotational femoral osteotomy. This plays an important role in postoperative imaging in the setting of hip preservation surgery done all around the world.

The use of joint-preserving surgery of the hip had been largely abandoned since the introduction of total hip replacement, which came as an immense help to the elderly population. But, with the modification of such techniques as pelvic osteotomy and the introduction of intracapsular procedures such as surgical hip dislocation and arthroscopy, previously unexpected options for the surgical treatment of sequelae of childhood conditions, including developmental dysplasia of the hip, slipped upper femoral epiphysis, and Perthes' disease, have become available.

The field of nonarthroplasty surgical treatment of the adult hip is increasingly being referred to as hip preservation surgery. Osteotomies of the hip joint may increase the longevity of the hip that we are born with and the affected hip and prevent or delay the need for arthroplasty.

Hip preservation surgery includes peri-acetabular osteotomies (PAO; Ganz osteotomy), proximal femoral osteotomies to change the shape of the femur to improve gait mechanics, and procedures such as acetabuloplasty and femoroplasty resulting in femoral reorientation. It also includes hip preservation surgery in conditions such as hip dysplasias, sequelae of Legg–Calvé–Perthes, and coxa valga/vara.

It is focused on helping patients postpone or even prevent the need for hip replacement later in life. Some common causes of hip pain are hip dysplasia, hip arthritis, fractures of the hip and pelvis, and nonunion of the femoral neck.

Hip preservation is mainly for hip problems affecting children, adolescents, young adults, and adults. Hip preservation surgery can be most accurately described as a hypothesis that surgery can preserve a hip and prevent the need for arthroplasty. Orthopedic surgeons have turned to joint preservation as a way to prevent or delay the onset of osteoarthritis or other degenerative conditions affecting the joints, particularly in young patients.

The *Journal of Hip Preservation Surgery* (JHPS) is not the only place where work in the field of hip preservation may be published.

Michael Leunig, MD, head of orthopedics at Schulthess Klinik in Zurich, has worked closely with Reinhold Ganz, MD, since Ganz pioneered the periacetabular osteotomy in 1984, a technique that has been a great asset in the field of joint preservation. Frequently, hip preservation can be achieved through arthroscopy. Once considered just a diagnostic tool used in conjunction with imaging, this keyhole surgery is now frequently employed to correct articular damage, impingement, and sequelae of impingement, such as labral or chondral tears in the hip joint. The techniques are being refined with every passing year; the technique is getting easier and more predictable.

In 1958, the AO group formulated four basic principles as guidelines for internal fixation: (1) anatomic reduction, (2) stable fixation, (3) early and active mobilization, and (4) preservation of blood supply.

This study seeks to define hip preservation surgery, then examines this premise critically in the context of treatment for its most commonly treated condition—femoroacetabular impingement.

There is strong evidence that surgical treatment results in a reduction or prevention of FAI and theoretically in preservation of the hip.

Hip preservation procedures are most often performed in young, active patients who are suffering from painful hip conditions like

1. Hip dysplasia
2. Femoroacetabular impingement
3. Residual effects of pediatric hip disorders like slipped capital femoral epiphysis (SCFE) and Legg–Calvé–Perthes disease (LCPD)

Surgical dislocation is ideal for cases of FAI that involve large cam bumps, especially when large, lateral cam bumps are suspected to be the major morphological culprit.

Another indication for surgical dislocation in the treatment of FAI is in the case of global pincer impingement, such as the case of coxa profunda, protrusio, or a circumferential ossified labrum.

The main advantages of surgical dislocation over other techniques are the (1) exposure of the entire femoral head and acetabulum, which gives unobstructed access to reshape both the acetabular rim and the femoral head; (2) ability to confirm sphericity of the femoral head–neck junction; and (3) ability to perform other procedures, such as cartilage restoration procedures.

In the second technique, arthroscopic hip surgery, arthroscopic instruments are used to reshape the acetabular rim and femoral head–neck junction and repair the labrum through several small incisions. This technique has dramatically increased in popularity over the past decade. Its main advantage is the reduced level of invasiveness compared with surgical dislocation and thus quicker rehabilitation. However, the major disadvantage is the limited region of access with arthroscopy. Specifically,

surgical access during hip arthroscopy is limited to the anterior and anterolateral regions of the extra-articular hip (referred to as the peripheral compartment). It is worth reiterating that this is the region where the vast majority of FAI pathology is found. It is also worth noting that some surgeons perform femoroplasty through a small "mini-open" direct anterior or anterolateral incision in combination with hip arthroscopy.

The third technique, reverse periacetabular osteotomy, can be used in cases of severe retroversion of the hip. This procedure allows the surgeon to reorient the acetabulum around the femoral head so that overcoverage on the anterior side can be rotated such that the anterior coverage is reduced while the posterior coverage is increased, removing an area of pincer conflict. In addition, an anterior capsulotomy can be performed, and a cam lesion—if present—can be reshaped as well. This procedure is exceptionally versatile because it allows for the removal of a pincer lesion without reducing acetabular coverage, and additionally provides an opportunity to address femoral-sided deformity. However, the disadvantage of reverse PAO is that it is an invasive procedure with a comparatively longer recovery and the potential for overcorrection, leading to posterior impingement.

The disorders hip preservation surgery commonly treats are: (1) hip dysplasias, (2) FAI, (3) other hip impingements, (4) sequelae of Legg–Calvé–Perthes, (5) hip cartilage injuries, and (6) coxa valga/vara.

The common procedures routinely done are: (1) acetabular reorientation, (2) acetabuloplasty, (3) labral repair/reconstruction, (4) cartilage restoration, and (5) femoroplasty.

Hip arthroscopy, arthroscopically assisted mini-open hip surgery, periacetabular osteotomy, and surgical hip dislocation (SHD) are used for the most complex cases. Surgical hip dislocation has been reported as safe and effective following acute traumatic hip instability in the adolescent.

Hip arthroscopy may be helpful in the following conditions in hip preservation:

1. Debridement of loose bodies
2. Repair of torn labrum
3. Removal of bone spurs
4. Restoration and reconstruction of joint surfaces
5. For evaluation and diagnosis

The current concepts in hip preservation surgery are extremely encouraging. Successful treatment of nonarthritic hip pain in young athletic individuals continues to remain a challenge. Often, a combination of open and arthroscopic techniques is necessary to treat more complex conditions. Hip preservation procedures and appropriate rehabilitation have allowed individuals to return to a physically active lifestyle. In short, effective postoperative rehabilitation must consider modifications and precautions specific to the particular surgical techniques used. Proper postoperative rehabilitation after hip preservation surgery may help optimize functional recovery and maximize clinical success and patient satisfaction.

Diagnosis and treatment of structural hip diseases such as FAI and acetabular dysplasia have improved dramatically over the past decade, with the goal of preservation of the hip joint.

Microinstability is a painful supraphysiological mobility of the hip. It results from the association of architectural and functional abnormalities impairing joint stability. Microinstability is distinguished from hyperlaxity by its painful nature and from traumatic (macro) instability by its progressive onset and chronicization following repeated microtrauma concerning at-risk patients.

There are a wide variety of symptomatic labral tears, chondral lesions, injuries of the ligamentum teres, femoroacetabular impingement, capsular laxity and instability, and various extra-articular disorders, including snapping hip syndrome. With a careful diagnostic evaluation and technical execution of well-indicated procedures, arthroscopic surgery of the hip can achieve successful clinical outcomes.

Hip preservation surgery has progressed to a stage where it is extremely useful in rehabilitation in sports medicine.

Hip preservation surgery aims at preserving the native (patient's own) hip. Minor anatomical factors (excess bone around the rim of the hip socket, hip region, or both) can predispose an individual to hip osteoarthritis by causing repetitive abutment or hip impingement, leading to early hip arthritis. Keyhole surgery of the hip (hip arthroscopy) such as repair of a torn labrum (soft cartilage of the hip) can improve hip symptoms if patients are carefully prepared and appropriately selected for surgery. It is a technically challenging procedure when the surgeon has appropriate training, interest, and sufficient operative volume to ensure that a good result is obtained from surgery.

Cartilage restoration can be achieved using different techniques, such as (1) microfracture surgery, (2) drilling, (3) abrasion arthroplasty, (4) autologous chondrocyte implantation, (5) osteochondral autograft transplantation, and (6) osteochondral allograft transplantation, and expanded mesenchymal stem cells seeded in a collagen membrane injected into hip chondral lesions were beneficial and showed promising results as reported in the *Journal of Hip Preserving Surgery* 2 years ago.

An emerging new concept in hip preservation surgery is a procedure called subchondroplasty in which a bone substitute material is injected into the joint, filling any voids or lesions. The procedure is also much less invasive than a total hip replacement, allowing patients to get back on their feet sooner.

Subchondroplasty is a minimally invasive surgical technique that targets and treats subchondral bone pathology associated with bone marrow lesions (BMLs), which in turn allows bone healing. It is usually performed along with arthroscopy for guided insertion and concurrent treatment of other pathology inside the joint. During subchondroplasty, a calcium phosphate bone substitute material (BSM) is injected into the trabeculae of cancellous bone in the subchondral region, and the flowable, synthetic calcium phosphate readily fills subchondral defects, crystallizing endothermically in approximately 10 minutes with a porosity and strength that mimic healthy cancellous bone. This provides a scaffold for endogenous osteoclasts and osteoblasts to grow into and repair the bone. Over time, the calcium phosphate is resorbed and replaced with new healthy bone.

Subchondroplastic treatment of subchondral defects can result in reduced pain and improved function in OA patients. OA can result in bone marrow lesions that progress to severe joint degeneration and the need for joint replacement. Joint-preserving treatments that reverse the progression of pain and immobility are limited for patients who have OA.

Also, certain reports from Australia indicate that low birth weight and preterm birth are linked to increased risk for osteoarthritis-related hip replacements in adulthood. The findings also indicate that low birth weight and preterm babies were not at greater risk of knee arthroplasty due to OA as adults.

Cartilage restoration techniques of the hip

RODRIGO MARDONES AND CATALINA LARRAIN

INTRODUCTION

Femoroacetabular impingement is frequently associated with chondral damage. The abnormal contact between the femoral neck and the acetabular rim results in labral detachment and acetabular chondral damage.[1]

In the hip, the types of chondral lesions differ from other joints; cam-type femoroacetabular impingement is frequently associated with chondrolabral junction damage with subsequent acetabular cartilage detachment.[2]

Delamination is a characteristic chondral lesion of the hip (wave sign) in which the cartilage detaches from the subchondral bone, leading to a "bag lesion" and chondral flaps. Outerbridge is the most-used chondral lesion classification system; although delamination was not originally described, it could be considered type III. Konan et al. recently described a new classification system for hip chondral lesions, including wave sign, delamination, and chondrolabral lesions considering extension and location.[3]

The frequency of chondral lesions in hip arthroscopy for femoroacetabular impingement is high, up to 67.3% of patients, as described by Nepple et al. Risk factors for the presence of a chondral lesion are: male, tonnis 1 or 2, and alpha angle over 50°.[4]

Standard treatment for chondral lesions

Arthroscopic treatment of chondral lesions of the hip is limited to excision (rim trimming and femoral neck osteoplasty), debridement, chondroplasty, and microfractures.[5] Rim trimming and femoral neck osteoplasty could lead to the complete excision of the chondral lesion if located in the overcoverage area. When chondral damage extends beyond the resection area, the treatment of choice will be according to Outerbridge or Konan classifications, as follows:

- *Type I or II*: The treatment of choice in this type of lesion is thermal chondroplasty. It has been shown to be a safe technique for closed chondral lesions, leading to morphological changes with better structural characteristics than mechanical debridement.[4,5,8,9]

- *Delamination*: Delamination represents a treatment challenge among chondral lesions. Excising such an area of chondral instability seems an unnecessary surgical maneuver, particularly if the articular cartilage itself may contain a significant number of viable chondrocytes.[10] The main objective is the reattachment of the cartilage to the underlying subchondral bone. This could be achieved with transchondral microfractures, forming an adherent retrolabral clot, or with the use of an adhesive such as fibrin glue. Tzaveas and Villar reported on a series of 19 patients treated with fibrin adhesive showing improvement in pain and function at 6 months and 1 year after surgery.[11]

- *Type III or IV (full thickness chondral lesion)*: The indications for microfracture of the hip are similar to the knee and include focal and contained lesions, typically less than 2–4 cm^2 in size (Outerbridge III or IV), including delamination. Microfracture is a marrow-stimulating procedure that brings undifferentiated stem cells from a subchondral perforation into the chondral defect.[12] A clot formed in the microfractured area provides an environment for both pluripotent marrow cells and mesenchymal stem cells to differentiate into stable fibrocartilaginous tissue.[13,14] Several studies have shown good midterm results with this technique; however, we know that this fibrocartilaginous tissue does not have the required mechanical properties and eventually will fail, leading to advanced chondral damage and osteoarthritis.[14,15]

Novel treatments for chondral lesions

As we mentioned before, the fibrocartilage newly formed at the microfractured area is a low-quality tissue; therefore, we will describe some techniques, based on stem cell therapy, that may lead to a better-quality hyalinelike cartilage. The use of these novel technologies has demonstrated promising results in animal and clinical studies.[16–19]

MONONUCLEAR CONCENTRATE IN A PLATELET-RICH PLASMA MATRIX

Hip chondral lesions have traditionally been handled as equal to other joints, with similar results to those obtained at the knee, but the spherical form of the hip, composition and anatomy of the cartilage, and unique types of chondral lesions (delamination) make the techniques and results obtained at other joints not replicable at the hip. Hip chondral lesion clinical studies are limited to treatment with microfractures and fibrin clot (fibrin glue) for delamination.[12,20] These, though they are small clinical series, showed some promising results in localized chondral lesions. Milano et al., in a study conducted in sheep, demonstrated that the use of a Platelet-Rich Plasma (PRP) clot associated with microfractures achieved a complete filling of the chondral lesion with macroscopic, biomechanic, and microscopic characteristics similar to normal hyaline cartilage.[22]

Currently, the PRP clot is used as a carrier or membrane carrier of mesenchymal stem cells, a technique that will be explained later.

In summary, the use of a PRP clot in hip chondral lesions has little published evidence; however, the minimal cost and risks of the procedure associated with the promising results obtained in both animal and preliminary clinical studies support its use in the clinical practice of arthroscopic hip surgery.

Surgical techniques

In our clinical practice, the treatment of choice for hip chondral lesions is the use of a platelet-rich plasma clot and mononuclear concentrate over the microfractured area (Figure 2.1).

After rim trimming and labrum refixation, cartilage assessment is made. If a chondral lesion exists, we proceed to harvest autologous bone marrow stem cells, which are centrifuged, obtaining 2–4 cc of autologous bone marrow–mesenchymal stem cell concentrate (average 14 million nucleated cells/cc3). At the same time, 50 cc of peripheral blood is taken and centrifuged twice in order to obtain 4 cc of PRP (6–9x), ready to be activated with autologous thrombin. Treatment of the chondral lesion is done as described by Steadman in the knee, with debridement of all remaining unstable cartilage, followed by removal of the calcified plate. After preparation of the bed, multiple holes in the exposed subchondral bone plate are made, leaving about 3–4 mm between each. Once microfracture is complete, traction is released and we focus on the femoral osteoplasty, obtaining free range of motion with no abnormal contact between the acetabular

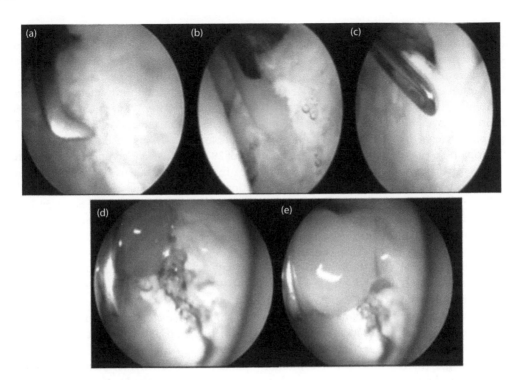

Figure 2.1 Hip chondral lesions: Surgical alternatives and novel technique with platelet-rich plasma and mononuclear cell concentrate. (a–c) Standard alternatives for hip chondral lesions. (a) Microfractures. (b) Thermal chondroplasty. (c) Chondral flap resection. (d) and (e) Novel surgical technique. The PRP clot is positioned over the microfractured area and mononuclear cell concentrate is instilled under it.

rim and femoral neck-head junction. At the end of the procedure, traction is reinstalled and we proceed to the final part of the procedure. After activation of platelet-rich plasma and clot formation, a slotted cannula is inserted via the anterior portal. A platelet-rich plasma clot is inserted through the cannula and positioned over the microfractured area. A 21-gauge trocar is then inserted, passing through the previously located clot, and autologous bone marrow–mesenchymal stem cell concentrate is instilled under the PRP clot. Traction is then released and the procedure is finished.

Rehabilitation protocol: A passive motion device is maintained for 8 hours. Two crutches with partial weight bearing are indicated for 6–8 weeks. Progressive physical activities are allowed.

INTRA-ARTICULAR INJECTIONS OF EXPANDED MESENCHYMAL STEM CELLS

As we mentioned before, in focal chondral lesions, mesenchymal stem cells represent a valid alternative for treatment, but multiple chondral lesions or established osteoarthritis are not suitable for focal treatment.

Adult mesenchymal stem cells were originally believed to differentiate only into tissue-specific cells. However, these cells have two major properties that could explain some of the results seen with intra-articular injections of expanded mesenchymal stem cells: *homing* and *response to specific signals*. Homing is a particular property of these cells meaning that they respond to systemic stimuli and "travel to the place that needs repair." The homing effect has been demonstrated in several animal studies using labeled mesenchymal stem cells administered via systemic intravascular route or by direct local implantation, showing the presence of the marker at the injury site.[23] Mesenchymal stem cells have the ability to differentiate into a different tissue in response to specific signals released by the injury site, such as chondrogenic lineage in an osteoarthritic joint.[24]

Intra-articular injections of expanded mesenchymal stem cells have not been described in the hip joint; however, there are some animal and clinical studies in other joints. Mokbel et al. labeled autologous adult stem cells suspended in hyaluronic acid that were injected intra-articularly into carpal joints in an experimental arthritis induced by intra-articular (IA) amphotericin-B in donkeys.[24] Significant improvement was noted in clinical and radiographic Osteoarthritis (OA), and significantly fewer histopathological changes of OA were seen in carpal joints that received stem cells compared to control contralateral joints. Importantly, injected stem cells were incorporated into the articular cartilage of the injected joint, as evident by their integration in the surface of the cartilage and also the interior of the cartilage.[24] Emadedin et al. injected expanded mesenchymal stem cells in six female patients with OA who required joint replacement. At 12 months follow-up, there was a significant decrease in mean pain, as well as improvements in joint functioning, walking distance, time to gelling, patellar crepitus, and knee flexion. Magnetic resonance images (MRIs) obtained at 6 months after treatment showed an increase in cartilage thickness and extension of the repair tissue over the subchondral bone in half of the patients, in addition to a decrease in subchondral bone edema.[25] McIlwraith et al. evaluated intra-articular injection of bone marrow–derived mesenchymal stem cells to augment healing with microfractures in horses. At 6 months, arthroscopic and gross evaluation confirmed a significant increase in repair tissue firmness and a trend toward better overall repair tissue quality in treated joints compared to microfractures alone. Immunohistochemical analysis showed significantly greater levels of aggrecan in repair tissue treated with stem cell injection.[17]

Our group has published two clinical series of 10 and 29 osteoarthritic hips treated with intra-articular injections of expanded mesenchymal stem cells, with a minimum of 2 years follow-up. Clinical evaluation showed great improvement in modified Harris hip score (mHHS), Western Ontario and McMaster universities OA index (WOMAC), and Vail scores. Radiological assessment showed regression of OA in 6 of 29 hips. No major complications occurred.[7,27]

In summary, the use of intra-articular injections of expanded mesenchymal stem cells in OA has little published evidence; however, in a young, active patient, it seems to be a promising nonarthroplasty treatment.

OUR TREATMENT OF CHOICE

In our clinical practice, the treatment of choice for hip diffuse chondral damage and mild osteoarthritis in an active patient seeking nonarthroplasty treatment are intra-articular injections of expanded mesenchymal stem cells. The surgical technique is described below.

Surgical technique

Patients were placed on an operating table in the prone position under general anesthesia. We proceeded to harvest 15 cc of bone marrow from the iliac crest and centrifuged, obtaining 2–4 cc of autologous bone marrow–mesenchymal stem cell concentrate (average 14 million nucleated cells/cc3) (Figure 2.2).

The bone marrow concentrate was then processed in our GMP laboratory, and over a 1-month period, mesenchymal stem cells expanded to 20×10^6 cells and were taken to the hospital in a

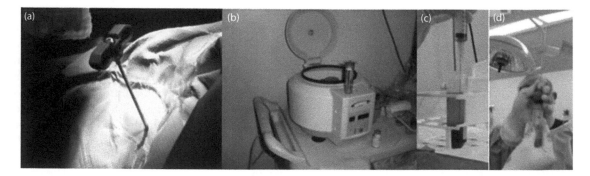

Figure 2.2 Autologous mesenchymal stem cell concentrate: (a) Autologous bone marrow autograft. (b) Centrifugation process with a single spin. (c) Layer separation by a density filter and identification of mononuclear cell layer. (d) Autologous mononuclear cell concentrate—final view.

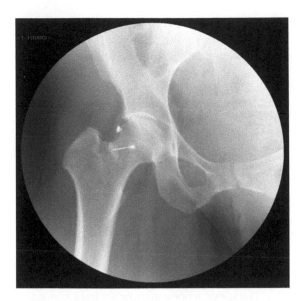

Figure 2.3 Intra-articular injection of expanded mesenchymal stem cells. Fluoroscopic image.

portable incubator. Under fluoroscopy, cells were injected into the patients' hips (Figure 2.3).

EXPANDED MESENCHYMAL STEM CELLS SEEDED IN A COLLAGEN MEMBRANE

When chondral lesions are larger than 2 cm^2, microfractures will be an insufficient treatment. In these cases, bone marrow concentrate in a PRP clot seems to be a good alternative. Other treatment options include autologous chondrocyte implantation (ACI), matrix-induced ACI (MACI), autologous matrix-induced chondrogenesis (AMIC), and membrane seeded with expanded mesenchymal stem cells.

ACI has been used increasingly for the repair of larger chondral lesions in the knee. For hip chondral lesion management, only two reports were found. Fontana et al. described a case control study in 30 patients with hip chondral lesions, 15 treated with ACI and 15 with debridement alone.[21] At 74 months follow-up, the Harris Hip Score was significantly better in the ACI group compared to the debridement group.[12] Akimau et al. described a case of severe chondrolysis and osteonecrosis of the femoral head after a severe fracture dislocation in a 31-year old man. Twenty-one months after the injury, they performed a MACI technique. At 1 year follow-up, the subjective hip score and range

of motion had increased compared to preoperative values. At 15 months follow-up, biopsy demonstrated a 2-mm-thickness cartilage, well populated with viable cells and integrated with the underlying bone.[6]

Fontana described a fully arthroscopic technique for the hip for AMIC. This is a low-cost, single procedure and arthroscopic technique in which the author used a collagen matrix (Chondro-gide, Geistlich Pharma AG, Wolhusen, Switzerland) over the microfractured area, containing the blood and bone marrow for a better-quality reparative tissue.[26]

The use of membranes seeded with expanded mesenchymal stem cells has risen in response to some problems observed with the use of MACI, such as the morbility of the donor site and insufficient coverage of the defect area due to some shrinkage effect. This technique has shown good results in other joints, but it has not been described in the hip joint.

SUMMARY

Hip chondral lesions are a frequent finding in hip arthroscopy for femoroacetabular impingement. Treatment is often difficult and insufficient. Novel strategies based on cell regenerative therapy represent an interesting treatment alternative. We reviewed the alternatives for hip chondral lesion treatment and described our surgical techniques.

REFERENCES

1. Bedi A et al. Elevation in circulating biomarkers of cartilage damage and inflammation in athletes with femoroacetabular impingement. *Am J Sports Med* 2013; 41(11): 2585–90.
2. Johnston TL, Schenker ML, Briggs KK, Philippon MJ. Relationship between offset angle alpha and hip chondral injury in femoroacetabular impingement. *Arthroscopy* 2008; 24(6): 669–75.
3. Konan S, Rayan F, Meermans G, Witt J, Haddad FS. Validation of the classification system for acetabular chondral lesions identified at arthroscopy in patients with femoroacetabular impingement. *J Bone Joint Surg Br* 2011; 93(3): 332–6.

4. Nepple JJ, Carlisle JC, Nunley RM, Clohisy JC. Clinical and radiographic predictors of intra-articular hip disease in arthroscopy. *Am J Sports Med* 2011; 39(2): 296–303.

5. Yen YM, Kocher MS. Chondral lesions of the hip: Microfracture and chondroplasty. *Sports Med Arthrosc* 2010; 18(2): 83–9.

6. Akimau P et al. Autologous chondrocyte implantation with bone grafting for osteochondral defect due to posttraumatic osteonecrosis of the hip—A case report. *Acta Orthop* 2006; 77(2): 333–6.

7. Mardones R, Via AG, Jofré C, Minguell J, Rodríguez C, Tomic A, Salineros M. Cell therapy for cartilage defects of the hip. *Muscle Ligaments Tendons J* 2016; 6(3): 361–6.

8. Kaplan LD, Chu CR, Bradley JP, Fu FH, Studer RK. Recovery of chondrocyte metabolic activity after thermal exposure. *Am J Sports Med* 2003; 31(3): 392–8.

9. Lotto ML, Wright EJ, Appleby D, Zelicof SB, Lemos MJ, Lubowitz JH. *Ex vivo* comparison of mechanical versus thermal chondroplasty: Assessment of tissue effect at the surgical endpoint. *Arthroscopy* 2008; 24(4): 410–5.

10. Edwards RB, Lu Y, Cole BJ, Muir P, Markel MD. Comparison of radiofrequency treatment and mechanical debridement of fibrillated cartilage in an equine model. *Vet Comp Orthop Traumatol* 2008; 21(1): 41–8.

11. Voss JR, Lu Y, Edwards RB, Bogdanske JJ, Markel MD. Effects of thermal energy on chondrocyte viability. *Am J Vet Res* 2006; 67(10): 1708–12.

12. Tzaveas AP, Villar RN. Arthroscopic repair of acetabular chondral delamination with fibrin adhesive. *Hip Int* 2010; 20(1): 115–9.

13. Frisbie DD, Oxford JT, Southwood L, Trotter GW, Rodkey WG, Steadman JR, Goodnight JL, McIlwraith CW. Early events in cartilage repair after subchondral bone microfracture. *Clin Orthop Relat Res* 2003; 466(407): 215–27.

14. Steadman JR, Rodkey WG, Rodrigo JJ. Microfracture: Surgical technique and rehabilitation to treat chondral defects. *Clin Orthop Relat Res* 2001; 466(391 Suppl.): S362–9.

15. Steadman JR, Rodkey WG, Briggs KK. Microfracture to treat full-thickness chondral defects: Surgical technique, rehabilitation, and outcomes. *J Knee Surg* 2002; 15(3): 170–6.

16. Philippon MJ, Schenker ML, Briggs KK, Maxwell RB. Can microfracture produce repair tissue in acetabular chondral defects? *Arthroscopy* 2008; 24(1): 46–50.

17. McIlwraith CW, Frisbie DD, Rodkey WG, Kisiday JD, Werpy NM, Kawcak CE, Steadman JR. Evaluation of intra-articular mesenchymal stem cells to augment healing of microfractured chondral defects. *Arthroscopy* 2011; 27(11): 1552–61.

18. Gobbi A, Karnatzikos G, Scotti C, Mahajan V, Mazzucco L, Grigolo B. One-step cartilage repair with bone marrow aspirate concentrated cells and collagen matrix in full-thickness knee cartilage lesions: Results at 2-year follow-up. *Cartilage* 2011; 2(3): 286–99.

19. De Girolamo L, Bertolini G, Cervellin M, Sozzi G, Volpi P. Treatment of chondral defects of the knee with one step matrix-assisted technique enhanced by autologous concentrated bone marrow: *In vitro* characterization of mesenchymal stem cells from iliac crest and subchondral bone. *Injury* 2010; 41(11): 1172–7.

20. Philippon MJ, Schenker ML, Briggs KK, Maxwell RB. Can microfracture produce repair tissue in acetabular chondral defects? *Arthroscopy* 2008; 24(1): 46–50.

21. Fontana A et al. Arthroscopic treatment of hip chondral defects: Autologous chondrocyte transplantation versus simple debridement—A pilot study. *Arthroscopy* 2012; 28(3): 322–9.

22. Milano G, Sanna Passino E, Deriu L, Careddu G, Manunta L, Manunta A, Saccomanno MF, Fabbriciani C. The effect of platelet rich plasma combined with microfractures on the treatment of chondral defects: An experimental study in a sheep model. *Osteoarthritis Cartilage* 2010; 18(7): 971–80.

23. Chen A et al. Transplantation of magnetically labeled mesenchymal stem cells in a model of perinatal injury. *Stem Cell Research* 2010; 5(3): 255–66.

24. Mokbel AN et al. Homing and reparative effect of intra-articular injection of autologous mesenchymal stem cells in osteoarthritic animal model. *BMC Musculoskelet Disord* 2011; 12: 259.

25. Emadedin M et al. Intra-articular injection of autologous mesenchymal stem cells in six patients with knee osteoarthritis. *Arch Iran Med* 2012; 15(7): 422–8.

26. Fontana A. A novel technique for treating cartilage defects in the hip: A fully arthroscopic approach to using autologous matrix–induced chondrogenesis. *Artrhoscopy Techniques* 2012; 1(1): e63–8.

27. Mardones R, Jofré C, Tobar L, Minguell JJ. Mesenchymal stem cell therapy in the treatment of hip osteoarthritis. *J Hip Preserv Surg* 2017; 4(2): 159–63.

3

Mesenchymal stem cell therapy logistics: A paradigm between quantity and/or quality of the "reparative" cell product

JOSE J. MINGUELL

CLINICAL USES OF MESENCHYMAL STEM CELLS

It is difficult to formulate a comprehensive explanation for the popularity of mesenchymal stem cells (MSCs) in the field of cell therapy. The above seems to be supported by their attractiveness associated with self-renewal, which in turn is associated with a pluripotency to commit, differentiate, and mature into specific phenotypes under the control of cell-intrinsic signaling mechanisms.

In addition, other distinctive reparative properties of MSCs are linked to various attributes, including trophic support to other cells, slowing of degenerative processes, and secretion of a large assortment of biochemical substances (growth factors, cytokines, neurotransmitters, and extracellular matrix compounds).

All these compelling issues are epitomized by: (a) the residence of MSCs in various fetal and adult tissues, among them bone marrow, umbilical cord blood, adipose tissue, and placenta-derived tissues;

(b) a privileged immunophenotype; and (c) the availability of straightforward techniques for their *ex vivo* expansion, cryopreservation, and long-term storage.

Accordingly, these relevant characteristics have been instrumental in the development of clinical trials intended to treat patients suffering from a vast group of diseases.

MANUFACTURE OF BONE MARROW–DERIVED MESENCHYMAL STEM CELLS FOR USE IN CLINICAL STUDIES

In an important number of clinical trials that are either completed or currently under development, the tissue source of MSCs has been adult bone marrow.

The frequency of human bone marrow–resident MSCs is rather low (one cell for each 10,000–250,000 bone marrow mononuclear cells) and dependent on the age of the donor. Accordingly, for their use in a clinical setting, the minute quantity of MSCs obtained after a bone marrow aspiration is further increased by *ex vivo* expansion procedures. Under these conditions, MSCs adhere to the plastic surface of the tissue culture vessel and start a rapid process of cell proliferation. As soon as the resulting primary monolayer of expanded MSCs becomes confluent, adherent cells are gently dislodged by using either enzymatic or nonenzymatic cell dissociation reagents. Subsequently, the expansion procedure is reinitiated several times until the achievement of the protocol's established number of cells.[1] Due to the scarcity of data on the attributes of bone marrow–resident ("native") MSCs,[2,3] it has been difficult to establish to what extent *ex vivo* expansion procedures modify MSCs biological traits.

Nonetheless, it is known that as the passage number increases (long-term *ex vivo* expansion), morphological and attachment attributes are maintained; however, functional markers are severely modified in conjunction with the onset of senescence indicators.[4] Consequently, to ensure optimal efficacy and safety of an *ex vivo*–expanded MSCs product, regulatory agencies (the Food and Drug Administration [FDA] and others) have recommended classifying *ex vivo*–expanded MSC products as "minimally" and "more than minimally" manipulated.[5,6]

Minimal manipulation of a cell product is defined as *ex vivo* processing that does not alter the original relevant characteristics that may affect the product's use for tissue reconstruction, repair, or replacement. In the case of MSC products, the above observations also include washing, long-term frozen storage, thawing, and other manipulations. In addition, the growth and processing of cells must be performed under conditions that do not involve combination with other products that may affect cell functionality, like growth factors and preserving and/or storage agents.[7–9]

The onset of senescence indicators resulting from extended *ex vivo* cultivation of bone marrow (BM) MSCs has been elegantly explored by using quantitative proteomics, which allowed comparison of the expression program of passage 3 (P3) cells, commonly used in clinical studies, with passage 7 (P7) expanded MSCs. While P3 cells are fully functional, P7 cells exhibit significant signs of culture-induced senescence.[10–12]

In this regard, it is important to mention that extended *ex vivo* cultivation is not the only factor that could affect the functional (reparative) attributes of MSCs. Several studies have shown that patient age and gender,[13–16] as well as comorbidities, medication use, and other factors,[17–22] may well modify the functional attributes of bone marrow–resident MSCs.

Despite abundant cellular and molecular tools being available to confirm the "reparative quality" of a MSC-based product, in most reported clinical studies, the attributes of the manufactured cell product are solely evaluated according to "minimal criteria for defining multipotent mesenchymal stromal cells."[23] Paradoxically, the latter evaluate the cellular but not functional attributes of the manufactured product. However, promising recommendations predicting stem cell activity to ensure safe and effective therapies have recently been proposed.[24]

FUTURE PERSPECTIVES FOR THE USE OF MESENCHYMAL STEM CELL–BASED THERAPY

MSCs have gained widespread use in regenerative medicine due to their demonstrated potency in a broad range of experimental animal models of disease and their excellent safety profile in human clinical trials. However, while MSC-based therapies have clearly shown benefits in patients with specific disorders, many trials completed to date have yielded suboptimal outcomes, and several have failed to meet their primary endpoints of efficacy.

The development of efficacious MSC-based therapies, manufactured under the concept that the clinical benefit will be solely sustained by the certainty that methods used for tissue-isolation and *ex vivo* expansion of MSCs consistently yield homogeneous populations, exhibits the highest growth rate, life span, differentiation potential, and functional (reparative) potency.

At present, more than 500 clinical trials using MSC-based therapy are under investigation for treating human diseases.[25] It is evident that the results of these studies will contribute to the redesign or design of new therapeutic options[26] and/or further strengthen the development of MSC-based tissue engineering approaches for tissue repair and/or regeneration.[27]

REFERENCES

1. Caplan AI. Adult mesenchymal stem cells for tissue engineering versus regenerative medicine. *J Cell Physiol* 2007; 213: 341–7.

2. Pereira RF et al. Cultured adherent cells from marrow can serve as long-lasting precursor cells for bone, cartilage, and lung in irradiated mice. *Proc Natl Acad Sci USA* 1995; 92: 4857–61.

3. Pontikoglou C, Delorme B, Charbord P. Human bone marrow native mesenchymal stem cells. *Regen Med* 2008; 3: 731–41.

4. Minguell JJ, Allers C, Lasala GP. Mesenchymal stem cells and the treatment of conditions and diseases: The less glittering side of a conspicuous stem cell for basic research. *Stem Cells Dev* 2013; 22: 193–203.

5. Murphy MB, Moncivais K, Caplan AI. Mesenchymal stem cells: Environmentally responsive therapeutics for regenerative medicine. *Exp Mol Med* 2013; 45: 54.

6. http://stemcellassays.com/2014/12/fda-clarification-minimal-manipulation

7. https://www.accessdata.fda.gov/scripts/cdrh/cfdocs/cfcfr/CFRSearch.fr=1271

8. Perez-Ilzarbe M et al. Comparison of *ex vivo* expansion culture conditions of mesenchymal stem cells for human cell therapy. *Transfusion* 2009; 49: 1901–10.

9. https://blogs.fda.gov/fdavoice/index.php/2018/03/predicting-stem-cell-activity-to-ensure-safe-and-effective-therapies/

10. Madeira A, da Silva CL, dos Santos F, Camafeita E, Cabral JMS, Sá-Correia I. Human mesenchymal stem cell expression program upon extended *ex-vivo* cultivation, as revealed by 2-DE-based quantitative proteomics. *PLoS One* 2012; 7: e43523.

11. Rinaldi S et al. Stem cell senescence. Effects of REAC technology on telomerase-independent and telomerase-dependent pathways. *Scientific Reports* 2014; 4: 6373.

12. Turinetto V, Vitale E, Giachino C. Senescence in human mesenchymal stem cells: Functional changes and implications in stem cell-based therapy. *Int J Mol Sci* 2016; 17: 1164.

13. Zhou S, Greenberger JS, Epperly MW, Goff JP, Adler C, Leboff MS, Glowacki J. Age-related intrinsic changes in human bone-marrow-derived mesenchymal stem cells and their differentiation to osteoblasts. *Aging Cell* 2008; 3: 335–43.

14. Maijenburg MW et al. The composition of the mesenchymal stromal cell compartment in human bone marrow changes during development and aging. *Haematologica* 2012; 97: 179e83.

15. Siegel G et al. Phenotype, donor age and gender affect function of human bone marrow-derived mesenchymal stromal cells. *BMC Medicine* 2013; 11: 146.

16. Schimke M, Marozin S, Lepperdinger G. Patient-specific age: The other side of the coin in advanced mesenchymal stem cell therapy. *Front Physiol* 2015; 6: 362.

17. Efimenko AY, Kochegura TN, Akopyan ZA, Parfyonova YV. Autologous stem cell therapy: How aging and chronic diseases affect stem and progenitor cells. *BioResearch Open Access* 2015; 4: 26–38.

18. Benvenuti S et al. Rosiglitazone stimulates adipogenesis and decreases osteoblastogenesis in human mesenchymal stem cells. *J Endocrinol Invest* 2007; 30(9): 26–30.

19. Randau TM, Schildberg FA, Alini M, Wimmer MD, Haddouti e-M, Gravius S, Ito K, Stoddart MJ. The effect of dexamethasone and triiodothyronine on terminal differentiation of primary bovine chondrocytes and chondrogenically differentiated mesenchymal stem cells. *PLoS One* 2013; 8: e72973.

20. Oh J et al. Differential cytotoxicity of corticosteroids on human mesenchymal stem cells. *Clin Orthop Relat Res* 2015; 473: 1155–64.

21. Almaawi A, Wang HT, Ciobanu O, Rowas SA, Rampersad S, Antoniou J, Mwale F. Effect of acetaminophen and nonsteroidal anti-inflammatory drugs on gene expression of mesenchymal stem cells. *Tissue Eng Part A* 2013; 19: 1039–46.

22. Allers C, Lasala GP, Minguell JJ. Presence of osteoclast precursor cells during *ex vivo* expansion of bone marrow-derived mesenchymal stem cells for autologous use in cell therapy. *Cytotherapy* 2014; 16: 454–9.

23. Dominici M et al. Minimal criteria for defining multipotent mesenchymal stromal cells. The International Society for Cellular Therapy position statement. *Cytotherapy* 2006; 8: 315–7.

24. Steven R. Bauer. Predicting Stem Cell Activity to Ensure Safe and Effective Therapies. March 7, 2018, by FDA Voice.

25. http://www.clinicaltrials.gov

26. Boregowda SV, Phinney DG. Quantifiable metrics for predicting MSC therapeutic efficacy. *J Stem Cell Res Ther* 2016; 6: 365.

27. Mardones R, Jofré CM, Minguell JJ. Cell therapy and tissue engineering approaches for cartilage repair and/or regeneration. *Int J Stem Cells* 2015; 8: 48–53.

4

Biomechanics of the hip

MOHAMED M. H. EL-SAYED

The human body is a well-engineered structure where bone and soft tissues interact in both static and dynamic situations to maintain balance and generate movement. Statics is a branch of mechanics that models and analyzes load on a physical system, where structures are motionless or moving at a constant velocity. Such models include the hip joint when standing still. During static standing, the combined forces acting on any component, measured in Newtons (N), must be zero in all axes. Torque, measured in units of Newton metres (Nm), at the hip joint is also experienced and is the consequence of a load acting at a distance. For rotational static equilibrium, the sum of the moments also needs to be zero.[1]

During walking, the leading leg leaves the ground to step forward; thus, the body is temporarily standing on one leg. The force from our body weight (BW) at this time acts downward, pulling the body to lean over; however, this is balanced by the action of the abductors. Thus, the hip behaves much like a lever (Figure 4.1), with a load/effort acting on either side of a fulcrum (the femoral head).

During standing, however, BW is supported by both hips; therefore, if the body were perfectly balanced, the abductor muscles would not be required and there would be an equal force of 1/2 BW on each hip. As it is unlikely that the body is ever perfectly balanced, the joint reaction force during standing likely varies from 1/2 BW to 3 BW, for the perfectly balanced case and single-leg-stance case, respectively. The abductor muscles are thus very

important in balance and pelvic stability, their role becoming more important as motion becomes more dynamic. It is worth noting that although 2D static analysis provides a realistic estimation of forces and moments, a number of assumptions are necessary.[2]

During gait, there are two distinctive phases: the stance phase, when the foot is in contact with the floor, and the swing phase, when the leg is returning. The role of the abductors is that of balance on the loaded side and managing limb motion on the unloaded side as the leg is brought forward. From the simplistic representation in Figure 4.1, the abductor muscle force (ABD) on the stance side is equal to body weight multiplied by the ratio of the moment arms of BW (b) and the abductors (a) measured from the hip joint center.[2]

The application of force by the abductor muscles means that the hip is never totally unloaded even when no BW is being applied, as movement of the mass of the leg during the swing phase requires muscles to control this motion. The moment (force of the abductor muscle – moment arm of the abductor muscle) applied by the abductors relative to the hip center during gait is shown in Figure 4.2. It is clear that during stance, the magnitude of the moment applied by the abductors is far greater than that during swing.

The understanding of these mechanics is important when understanding pathologies that might change the length of the muscle moment arms, because if moment arms shorten to achieve

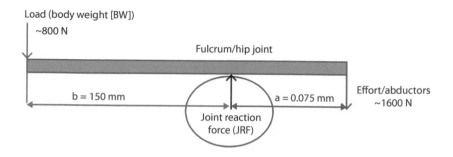

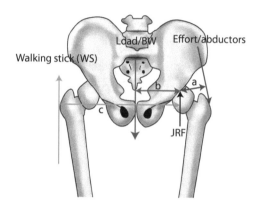

Using $\sum F = 0$ then; BW (0.15 mm) – Abductors (0.075 m) = 0, Abductors = 2 BW

Using $\sum F = 0$ then; JRF = Abductors + BW = 3 BW

Figure 4.1 A simple representation of walking, balancing load and effort with the load represented by body weight on one side of the lever and the effort being applied by the abductor force on the other side, acting around the fulcrum (hip joint center), and a schematic of the forces overlaid onto a hip model with the addition of a walking stick used as an aid to alleviate a painful joint.

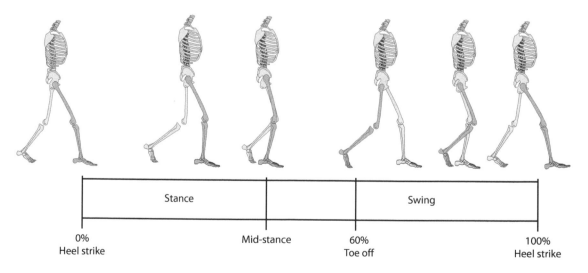

Figure 4.2 Gait cycle normalized to 100% showing heel strike to heel strike of the right limb (shaded limb) with toe off indicated at 60%, where the stance phase ends and the swing phase begins.

the same moment, the muscle force must increase. Thus, if the mechanics change considerably, the patient will have to adopt coping strategies to maintain balance and equilibrium.

If a hip becomes painful due to arthritis, the pain can be alleviated by reducing the joint reaction force if the patient leans toward the painful hip so that the abductor muscle can apply a reduced force to achieve stability. The same thing happens if we stand on one leg, as we tend to try to get our BW centered above the hip so it requires the least amount of force from the stabilizing musculature. An alternative method to alleviate hip pain is to use a walking stick on the opposite side from the painful hip (Figure 4.1); this reduces the hip abductor force and thus can reduce the joint contact force and pain in the affected limb.

Clinically, abductor weakness often leads to a characteristic drop in the pelvis during the stance phase of walking, to the non–weight-bearing side, referred to as a Trendelenburg gait. A similar tilt of the pelvis to the opposite side during a single-leg stance is referred to as a positive Trendelenburg sign.

This should not be confused with the Trendelenburg test (or Brodie–Trendelenburg test), which is a test of leg vein competency, although the terms *sign* and *test* are often used interchangeably in textbooks.

When weakness occurs on one side, compensating movement of the body may change the direction of the load, transferring forces further down the kinetic chain to other joints. For example, to compensate for pelvic drop during Trendelenburg gait, the knee of the contralateral limb may go into a valgus/rotated position. This is recognized as a risk for knee injury, as well as arthritis, due to excessive shear forces acting on the knee joint. Therefore, maintaining the balance of the pelvis is an important consideration for the clinician when protecting other joints as well as the affected joint.[2,3]

THE HIP DURING ACTIVITIES OF DAILY LIVING

Motion capture allows for a comprehensive analysis of the movements performed during gait that may subsequently be used to calculate muscle/joint forces. Motion capture is frequently performed in a lab, which generally contains a number of infrared cameras to capture movement and force plates to measure ground reaction forces. During gait analysis, one single gait cycle is typically normalized to 100%, with one cycle beginning with a heel strike and ending the next time the same heel makes contact with the ground, with a toe-off event at 60% of the gait cycle. The cycle can then be subsequently broken down into subsections and events such as stance and swing, heel strike and toe off; this can be seen in Figure 4.2.

When discussing hip movements, we refer to the femoral movement in relation to the pelvis around the hip joint center. The hip allows for a large range of motion (ROM) in all three planes, allowing for 120_flexion/10_extension, 70_abduction/adduction, and 50_rotation; these movements are depicted in the normal range of motion.

These ranges are the maximum angles that the hip can safely achieve; however, these ranges are rarely reached during activities of daily living. Hence, under normal activities, muscles are generally responsible for providing all of the rotational stability (Figure 4.3).[4]

During the gait cycle (Figure 4.2), the hip is flexed at the initial heel contact of the stance phase before the hip joint begins to extend until the end of the stance phase where flexion begins. This is coupled with hip abduction during midstance when the hip begins to abduct until the end of the stance phase prior to adduction until the end of the gait cycle.

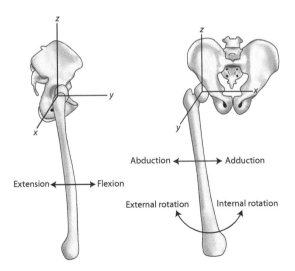

Figure 4.3 Axis of rotation around the hip joint center and movements produced by the hip joint. Flexion and extension occur in the sagittal plane around the frontal (*y*) axis. Abduction and adduction movement occur in the frontal plane around the sagittal (*x*) axis. Internal and external rotation occur in the transverse plane around the vertical (*z*) axis.

In the majority of past studies, gait has been used as the primary activity to analyze kinematics of the hip joint. However, studies involving total hip replacement have highlighted functional demand as an important outcome measure for patient satisfaction. Thus, there has recently been growing interest in activities of daily living (ADLs) to obtain a true representation of how the hip moves on a day-to-day basis.

The ADLs that are analyzed are often more demanding than gait and require increases in ranges of motion and/or joint moments. The typical activities of daily living that are often analyzed are increased walking speed, a sit-to-stand task, and ascending and descending stairs.[5]

REFERENCES

1. Beer FP, Johnston E, DeWolf J. *Mechanics of Materials*. New York: McGraw-Hill, 1992.

2. Trepczynski A, Kutzner I, Bergmann G, Taylor WR, Heller MO. Modulation of the relationship between external knee adduction moments and medial joint contact forces across subjects and activities. *Arthritis Rheumatol (Hoboken, NJ)* 2014; 66: 1218e27.

3. Powers CM. The influence of abnormal hip mechanics on knee injury: A biomechanical perspective. *J Orthop Sports Phys Ther* 2010; 40: 42e51.

4. Bowman Jr KF, Fox J, Sekiya JK. A clinically relevant review of hip biomechanics. *Arthroscopy: J Arthrosc Relat Surg* 2010; 26: 1118e29.

5. Bovi G, Rabuffetti M, Mazzoleni P, Ferrarin M. A multiple-task gait analysis approach: Kinematic, kinetic and EMG reference data for healthy young and adult subjects. *Gait Posture* 2011; 33: 6e13.

5

History of osteotomies around the hip joint and their classification

K. MOHAN IYER

References   27

The first femoral osteotomy was performed by John Rhea Barton in 1826 when he tried to secure the motion of an ankyloid hip. Osteotomy is one of the most common surgical procedures performed every day all over the world. This technique dates back to the first half of the nineteenth century and the fundamental contribution made by Pennsylvania hospital surgeon Barton (1794–1871), who can be considered the pioneer of modern osteotomies; this chapter focuses on his life and career highlights, with a description of the first corrective osteotomies for hip and knee ankylosis (documented in two fundamental papers whose original pictures are here reproduced). The success of osteotomy as a current surgical approach to treat several orthopedic conditions is confirmation of the importance of this procedure in the orthopedic discipline and prompted an investigation into the pioneering mind of the man who introduced it. In 1835, Sourvier performed the first subtrochanteric osteotomy for the treatment of congenital dislocation of hip (CDH). In 1854, Langenback introduced subcutaneous osteotomy of the femur. In 1918 and 1919, Von Baeyer and Lorenz described the bifurcation operation of upper femoral osteotomy to secure stability in old CDHs. In 1922, Schanz reported his low subtrochanteric abduction osteotomy. Thereafter, in 1935, Pauwels described osteotomy at an intertrochanteric level adduction deformity. In 1936, McMurray performed an oblique displacement osteotomy for osteoarthritis of hip and nonunion fracture of the neck of the femur. In 1955, Chiari did a pelvic osteotomy for stable coverage of the head. Blount and Moore described an excellent blade plate for fixation of high subtrochanteric osteotomy. The anterior approach remains a standard approach to the hip in pediatric orthopedic surgery for developmental hip dysplasia, whereas in adult orthopedic surgery, it is used mostly to expose the anterolateral aspect of the femoral head, femoral neck, and anterior aspect of the acetabulum to treat femoral head fractures, for biopsy, or for excision of ectopic bone. With increasing interest in femoroacetabular impingement, hip resurfacing, and minimally invasive total hip arthroplasty, the anterior approach has regained popularity as a versatile approach to the hip in adult orthopedic patients. Marius N. Smith-Petersen (1886–1953), a Norwegian-born American surgeon, is credited with spreading the use of the anterior approach in the English-speaking world, and today the approach is commonly referred to as the "Smith-Petersen approach" because of his prolific use of the approach throughout his career. The periacetabular osteotomy, as advocated by Ganz in 1988,[1] also takes advantage of the anterior approach. Additionally, the modified Smith-Petersen approach allows a simultaneous anterior capsulotomy to visualize the hip joint and labrum or to assess the hip dynamically before and after the osteotomy. With the advent of minimally invasive total hip arthroplasty, the anterior approach, as proposed by the Judet brothers[2] using an orthopedic traction table, has gained popularity through reports by Siguier and collegues[3] and Matta and colleagues.[4]

An osteotomy is a surgical corrective procedure used to obtain the correct biomechanical alignment of the lower extremity so as to achieve equivocal and uniform load transmission, which may be done with or without removal of a portion of the bone from either cortex calculated by radiological estimation.[5] A clear understanding is obtained by the appreciation of the imaging techniques available and their correct application. A number of indices give a good idea of its severity and of the degree of congruency, instability, and degenerative change that have been defined on these radiographs to facilitate surgical planning and to evaluate surgical outcomes. It is important to realize that plain radiographs or fluoroscopy are usually the only diagnostic means available pre-operatively. The imaging modalities of projection radiography, computerized tomography (CT), and magnetic resonance imaging (MRI), including direct magnetic resonance-arthrography, are discussed with regard to their diagnostic capability in the postoperative assessment of the hip joint.[6] Consolidation of osteotomies and position of implants should be assessed in postoperative radiography. MRI is useful for confirming correct articulation after treatment of congenital hip dislocation.

With the advent of total hip arthroplasty nearly three decades ago, the number of osteotomies about the hip for the treatment of adult hip disease has considerably decreased, but in spite of the advancements in joint replacement technology, the problems remain very much the same as they were before because of the survivorship of joint replacements in the lifetime in a healthy patient younger than 50 years, especially since life expectancy has increased compared to what it was about 50 years ago, with the survivorship of joint replacements in these younger adults being less than 10 years.

Many of these younger patients can be successfully treated with an osteotomy of the pelvis or proximal femur (or both) before they develop advanced arthritis. There is definite evidence that anatomically abnormal hips in childhood do not last a lifetime, since many of those who develop

osteoarthritis have preexisting pathology such as developmental dysplasia of the hip (DDH), Legg–Calvé–Perthes (or Perthes) disease, slipped capital femoral epiphysis (SCFE), osteonecrosis, and trauma, the most common being DDH. Usually, the disease was subclinical and went undiagnosed until the onset of adult hip pain, as many of these patients required hip replacement surgery before 50 years of age.

The treatment of dysplasia has considerably improved through the development and success of the Bernese periace-tabular osteotomy, since prior to this, most surgical procedures were of a salvage nature for moderate arthritis in the form of a valgus–extension intertrochanteric osteotomy or a Chiari osteotomy, which did not correct the primary abnormality. When an anatomic abnormality exists that exposes the joint cartilage to high stresses, and this situation is correctable by osteotomy, the long-term benefits of reorienting or realigning the joint must be considered. Salvage of a young patient's joint cartilage holds greater promise for a good lifelong result than does an early implant arthroplasty, while in other cases, an osteotomy may serve as a bridge of time to carry the patient safely into the age range appropriate for total joint replacement.

Osteotomies are extremely important and useful in the treatment of hip dysplasia, as they can address the underlying morphologic abnormality in the hip joint since they can reorient the articular surfaces of the hip joint and hence allow load transmission through a broader surface area, thus subjecting the joint to less force. Osteotomies can shift the center of hip rotation medially and thus decrease the reactive forces acting through the joint, which helps in decreasing pain by protecting the articular cartilage and can result in improving the range of movements at the hip joint.

These procedures are usually indicated in young patients with symptomatic hip dysplasia, without any proximal migration of the hip center of rotation, who have preserved their range of motion and have no more than a mild degenerative change.

Osteotomies about the hip joint can be carried out either at the acetabulum, at the proximal femur, or using some combination of both in some selected cases.

Pelvic osteotomies are usually indicated to address the location of the primary pathology when they correct any major anatomic abnormality and do not create a secondary deformity, which thus affects future reconstructive procedures.

Pelvic osteotomies can be divided into two types: (1) reconstructive and (2) salvage.

1. Reconstructive osteotomies are basically intended to restore normal hip anatomy and biomechanics and hence improve symptoms and prevent degenerative changes, resulting in a hip joint in which the femoral head and the acetabulum are congruent.
2. Salvage osteotomies are mainly carried out to relieve pain when the articular surface congruency cannot be restored to normal, and hence are performed in patients who have a hip joint in which the femoral head and the acetabulum are not the same shape.

Various periacetabular osteotomies have been undertaken to remodel the hyaline cartilage of the hip in mature patients. Salter's innominate osteotomy was first used in mature hips more than 50 years ago and proved useful in the treatment of mild dysplasia but was not indicated in major acetabular remodeling. More consistent major acetabular remodeling was introduced independently in Germany and Japan with spherical osteotomies, which allow excellent femoral head coverage, but medialization of the center of the hip joint can be difficult. Other complex osteotomies were later introduced by Tonnis and Steel.

In 1988, Ganz and colleagues introduced the Bernese periacetabular osteotomy. This procedure, which is also known as a "Ganz osteotomy," allows both remodeling of the acetabulum and medialization of the center of the hip joint. The basic and most important goal of this procedure is to correct the acetabular insufficiency and improve femoral head coverage by remodeling the weight-bearing surface laterally and anteriorly, while the secondary goals include improved hip stability and medialization of the center of hip rotation.

The ideal patient for these procedures is one with (1) a symptomatic structural abnormality, (2) a congruent joint, and (3) the absence of advanced secondary arthritis. These patients also need to have a well-maintained range of movement at the hip joint. These osteotomies are hence contraindicated in patients with excessive posterior wall coverage and require a surgical dislocation in order to adequately address their deformities.

Patients with advanced cartilage degeneration anteriorly also should not undergo this procedure, as the degenerative area will wind up in the weight-bearing zone after osteotomy and hence will not serve any purpose of pain relief.

Acetabular osteotomies are indicated in bony abnormalities, but most patients will have intra-articular pathology at the time of presentation that requires them to undergo an anterior arthrotomy performed in association with a periacetabular osteotomy (PAO), which allows resection of anterior labral tears and limited femoral neck osteoplasty. However, joint exposure is limited unless an extensive abductor dissection is performed or either simultaneous or staged hip arthroscopy to assess and treat the intra-articular pathology.

Femoral osteotomies: Proximal femoral osteotomies have been used in the treatment of hip dysplasia for approximately a century, with a varus osteotomy mainly indicated to correct the coax valga and a distal transfer of the greater trochanter to correct for trochanteric overgrowth. However, proximal femoral osteotomies alone are rarely useful in stabilizing hips with acetabular dysplasia in skeletally mature patients. They are useful when the femur is the primary source of deformity or when the pelvic osteotomy alone provides inadequate correction.

Patients with deformity of the proximal femur eventually develop arthritis in the long run because of abnormal joint wear from malalignment. These deformities include a varus or valgus neck-shaft angle, rotational malalignments, and leg-length discrepancy in any combination. These deformities may be acquired, as in the case of proximal femur fracture to include malunions and nonunions, or developmental, such as fibrous dysplasia, coxa vara, and developmental dysplasia.

Once arthritis has begun, it is further aggravated by mechanical malalignment from the femoral deformity, giving rise to the development of pain and arthritis in the affected hip, which is further aggravated by the mechanical malalignment from the femoral deformity.

Proximal femoral osteotomy was a technique used in adults for the treatment of hip dysplasia and osteoarthritis. Varus- and valgus-producing osteotomies were devised to maximize joint congruity and redistribute the weight-bearing load across the femoral head to a less affected area. Historically analyzing, the best results were obtained in patients with long-standing deformities, such as Perthes osteonecrosis, coxa vara, and developmental dysplasia.

Proximal femoral osteotomy is applicable even today in adults for the treatment of hip fracture nonunions and malunions and in cases of congenital and acquired hip deformities, though modern periacetabular osteotomies and joint arthroplasty techniques have narrowed the indications for this.

The benefits of early proximal femoral osteotomy to correct the deformity are as follows: (1) in the deformed hip prior to the onset of arthritic changes, the realignment often decreases the symptoms and also prevents further joint degeneration, as restoration of normal alignment can often decrease pain and improve function, and even if (2) the relief of symptoms is partially complete and the patient later requires hip replacement surgery, the arthroplasty procedure is simplified by restoration of the anatomy.

However, in young patients with symptomatic hip disease, total joint arthroplasty has universally been debatable as an option because problems with accelerated bearing wear and premature implant loosening leading to early revision surgery are well known. Intertrochanteric osteotomy has been of some use in providing temporary relief of pain in some patients, whereas the newer bearing materials with improved wear properties may improve the longevity of total joints in young patients, which is an assumption.

Indications:

1. Nonunion of a femoral neck fracture
2. Nonunion or malunion of an intertrochanteric hip fracture deformity, such as (1) *rotational* deformities caused by severe femoral anteversion or slipped capital femoral epiphysis and developmental dysplasia of the hip; (2) *frontal plane* such as varus/valgus deformities: (a) congenital coxa vara, (b) varus fracture malunion, and (c) shepherd's crook deformity from fibrous dysplasia; (3) sagittal deformities, such as flexion and extension deformity; and (4) significant shortening or bone loss of the distal femur, requiring a proximal lengthening
3. Combinations of the above, such as in intertrochanteric fracture malunion with varus, external rotation, and shortening deformity

4. Simultaneous femoral osteotomy and total hip arthroplasty
5. Hip osteoarthritis or osteonecrosis in the young, active patient

Contraindications:

1. The presence of infection may prevent the use of internal fixation; however, external fixation may be a viable option in such cases.
2. Limitations of hip movements that make realignment unsuccessful without soft-tissue release or compensation through the osteotomy.
3. Advanced osteoarthritis or osteonecrosis is a relative contraindication.
4. Inflammatory arthritis can also be a contraindication.

In order to perform an isolated proximal femoral osteotomy, certain criteria are required, such as: (1) the osteotomy must completely correct the pre-operative deformity, (2) the patient must have a functional range of movements, (3) the hip joint needs to be congruous on both sides, and (4) placing the hip in the position of proposed correction should relieve the patient of the pre-operative discomfort. This situation is usually found in patients with coax valga and mild acetabular dysplasia.

As regards the history, most patients do not have any proper childhood hip disorder, but eventually present with groin pain or trochanteric bursitis with some difficulty in playing sports when radiological evidence taken shows significant dysplasia.

A detailed clinical examination, including Trendelenburg's test, reveals evidence of labral pathology with some degree of hip dysplasia. The whole range of movement is then recorded in detail along with artgroscopy and MRI tests, which are mandatory before planning any osteotomy. An anteroposterior (AP) radiograph of the pelvis, as well as AP and frog-lateral views, is very helpful in arriving at a diagnosis. An AP view of the hip with the femur in abduction–internal rotation provides an idea of the potential advantages of coverage afforded by a rotational acetabular osteotomy. Views of the hip with the femur in abduction and adduction allow visualizing the joint space in planning any angular intertrochanteric osteotomy. If the overall alignment of the lower extremity will be benefited or changed by an osteotomy, a full-length standing radiograph for measuring the biomechanical axis can be done. This allows prediction of the effect of the surgery on the weight-bearing axis, especially since it may affect the knee. In cases of avascular necrosis (AVN), special radiographs are done to locate the necrotic area of the femoral head, or an MRI is much better than plain radiographs. A three-dimensional computed tomography scan is routinely done, as it helps tremendously in preoperative planning.

Certain other factors that play an important part are physiological age, chronological age, actual status of the joint cartilage, and lifestyle of the patient.

In general, all osteotomies have the best results when performed for clearly correctable biomechanical abnormalities in joints with at most mild arthrosis, just as a good range of motion also correlates with a better long-term outcome for hip osteotomies. The risks of increased stiffness, pain, or other modes of clinical failure increase with the degree of preoperative degenerative changes.

An osteotomy (either pelvis or hip or both) is a procedure that can circumvent the need for any definite treatment in a large proportion of patients, since anatomically abnormal hips do not last a lifetime. This is extremely helpful in conditions such as developmental dysplasia of the hip, Legg–Calvé–Perthes disease, slipped capital femoral epiphysis, osteonecrosis, and trauma, which lead to secondary arthritis of the hip joint, hence the importance of early diagnosis for these at-risk hips.

As knowledge has increased in this area, so has the importance of early diagnosis for these at-risk hips. When an anatomic abnormality exists that exposes the joint cartilage to high stresses and this situation is correctable by osteotomy, the potential long-term benefits of reorienting or realigning the joint must be considered.

Salvage of a young patient's joint cartilage holds more promise for a good life-long result than does an early implant arthroplasty. In other cases, an osteotomy acts as a bridge to carry the patient safely into the age range appropriate for total joint replacement.

The main ways in which osteotomies work or improve hip function are as follows:

1. Increase contact area, which increases congruency.
2. Improve coverage of the femoral head.
3. Move the normal articular cartilage into the weight-bearing zone.

4. Restore biomechanical advantage by decreasing joint reactive forces.
5. May stimulate cartilage repair.

The pre-operative evaluation must include the following:

1. Detailed physical examination to note the range of movements
2. Plain radiographic films to include standing AP, frog-leg lateral, anterior lip cover, and full abduction, along with full adduction films
3. Finally, a CT scan with 3D reconstruction

In short, hip mechanics have the following five features:

1. The hips are designed to support body weight in order to allow mobility.
2. There is a maximum range of mobility of flexion to 140° and 75° of abduction adduction.
3. The functional range of movements is 50/60° of flexion/extension.
4. About 1.8–4.3 times the body weight is transmitted through the hip.
5. The highest are while climbing stairs.

There are certain contraindications to osteotomy, as follows:

1. Neuropathic arthropathy
2. Inflammatory arthropathy
3. Active infections
4. Severe ostopenia
5. Advance arthritis or ankylosis
6. Advanced age
7. Smoking and obesity

There are five main types of classification of osteotomies.

A. Those done to obtain stability:
   1. Schanz low subtrochanteric osteotomy
   2. Lorenz bifurcation osteotomy
      Both are mainly used for old, unreduced dislocations.
      a. To obtain union, such as in nonunion of fractures of the femoral neck, where McMurray's osteotomy, Dickson's high geometric osteotomy, or Schanz angulation osteotomy is helpful.

b. For unstable intertrochanteric fractures, where either Dimon Hughston osteotomy or Sarmiento's osteotomy is helpful.

B. Classification based on location:
  1. Pelvic osteotomy: Salvage osteotomies like Chiari or shelf, or reconstructive osteotomies such as periacetabular and single, double, and triple innominate osteotomies.
  2. Femoral osteotomy, such as high cervical, intertrochanteric, subtrochanteric, or greater trochanteric osteotomies.

C. Classification based on relief of pain:
  1. In osteoarthritis, when either Pauwels type I varus or type II valgus osteotomy is used.
  2. To correct deformities, such as coxa vara or slipped upper femoral epiphysis, such as intracapsular cuneiform osteotomy of Dunn, compensatory basilar osteotomy of the femoral neck, extracapsular base-of-neck osteotomy, ball-and-socket trochanteric osteotomy, or Pauwels osteotomy (Y-shaped).

D. Classification based on neurologic conditions:
  1. Osteonecrosis of the femoral head with varus derotation osteotomy of Axer or Sugioka's transtrochanteric osteotomy.
  2. Paralytic disorders of the hip joint, when a varus osteotomy or rotational osteotomy may be helpful.

E. Osteotomies around the hip joint can be broadly classified into:
  1. Osteotomies of the proximal femur, which can be further subclassified into:
    a. Displacement of the distal fragment, which are further classified into:
      i. Transpositional osteotomy (Figure 5.1), where the longitudinal axis of the distal fragment remains parallel to the longitudinal axis of the proximal fragment. It is used in the fractured neck of the femur and osteoarthritis, such as McMurray's osteotomy, Pauwels osteotomy, and Putti osteotomy.
      ii. Angulation osteotomy (Figure 5.2), in which the longitudinal axis of the distal fragment forms an angle with the proximal fragment. It is done in the sagittal plane as an extension osteotomy of the proximal femoral defeciency (PFD), or in the coronal plane, such as adduction osteotomy/abduction osteotomy.
  2. Anatomical location such as high cervical, intertrochanteric, greater trochanteric, or subtrochanteric.

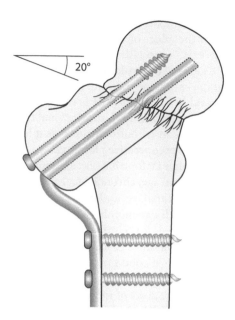

Figure 5.1 A transpositional osteotomy.

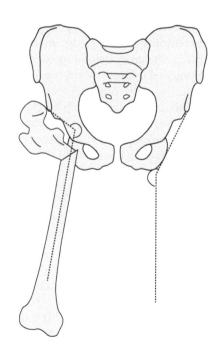

Figure 5.2 An angulation osteotomy.

3. Based on indication, which may be:
   a. Nonunion neck of femur, such as McMurray's, Pauwels, Putti, or Schanz osteotomies.
   b. Osteoarthritis, such as Pauwels varus/valgus osteotomies or McMurray's osteotomy.
   c. Unstable intertrochanteric fractures, such as Dimon and Hughston or Sarmiento osteotomy.
   d. Unreduced CDH, such as Lorenz bifurcation osteotomy, Schanz low subtrochanteric osteotomy, or Pemberton acetabuloplasty.
   e. Congenital coxa vara, such as cuneiform osteotomy of Fish, Pauwels Y osteotomy, and valgus or basilar osteotomy.
   f. Legg–Calvé–Perthes disease, such as varus derotation osteotomy, Salter osteotomy, and Shelf and Chiari osteotomy.
   g. AVN, such as Sugioka's transtrochanteic osteotomy, varus derotation osteotomy, and girdle stone osteotomy.
   h. Slipped capital femoral epiphyses:
      i. Closing wedge osteotomy, such as that of Fish, Dunn's technique just distal to the slip, the base-of-the-neck technique of Kramer et al., or the technique of Abraham et al.
      ii. Compensatory osteotomies, such as ball-and-socket osteotomy and Southwick's biplanar intertrochanteric (IT) osteotomy.
   i. Osteotomies in paralytic disorder of the hip, such as varus osteotomy, rotation osteotomy, and extension osteotomy.
4. Osteotomies of the pelvis are divided into:
   a. Single innominate, such as Salter's osteotomy.
   b. Double innominate, such as Sutherland.
   c. Triple innominate, such as Steel or Tonnis.
   d. Peracetabluar, such as Wagner or Ganz osteotomy.

There are certain complications that are extremely specific to osteotomies alone, such as:

1. Trochanteric bursitis with painful bursae over the metal implants.

2. Malunion, that is, undercorrection, overcorrection, malrotation, or even retroversion, which is noticed in PAO only.
3. Breakage of the implant.
4. Delayed union and nonunion.
5. Penetration of the implant into the hip joint.
6. Loss of the original fixation.
7. Changes in the leg length.
8. Weakness of the abductors with subsequent limp.
9. Difficulty in subsequent total hip replacement (THR).
10. Nerve injury, especially the lateral cutaneous nerve, which is commonly involved in PAO.
11. Intra-operative fracture of the femoral neck or the acetabulum.
12. Clinical failure despite a well-performed osteotomy, in the form of hip stiffness or persistent residual pain.

Of all these listed complications, the most commonly seen is trochanteric bursitis, and routine removal of the implants usually avoids this problem. An adequate radiographic workup and skillful preoperative tracing or computer templating for many osteotomies. Rigid internal fixation is critically important for stability by osteosynthesis. A preoperative Trendelenberg limp can be improved after osteotomy or possibly by greater trochanter advancement, which improves the abductor mechanics. Osteotomy can make subsequent THR surgery more difficult on both the pelvic and femoral sides. In some cases, a revision osteotomy of the femur may be necessary prior to proceeding with a THR. Simultaneous implant removal and THR surgery results in slightly increased operative time and possibly an increased infection rate for the THR. One of the more dreaded complications is AVN. Myositis ossificans can appear after an otherwise uncomplicated osteotomy, more commonly on the pelvic side. It is usually an incidental finding but can cause symptomatic stiffness.

REFERENCES

1. Ganz R et al. A new periacetabular osteotomy for the treatment of hip dysplasias. Technique and preliminary results. *Clin Orthop Relat Res* 1988; 232: 26–36.

2. Judet J, Judet R. The use of an artificial femoral head for arthroplasty of the hip joint. *J Bone Joint Surg Br* 1950; 32-B: 166–73.

3. Siguier T, Siguier M, Brumpt B. Mini-incision anterior approach does not increase dislocation rate: A study of 1037 total hip replacements. *Clin Orthop Relat Res* 2004; 426: 164–73.

4. Matta JM, Shahrdar C, Ferguson T. Single-incision anterior approach for total hip arthroplasty on an orthopaedic table. *Clin Orthop Relat Res* 2005; 441: 115–24.

5. Haddad FS, Garbuz DS, Duncan CP. Osteotomies around the hip: Radiographic planning and postoperative evaluation. *Instr Course Lect* 2001; 50: 253–61.

6. Weber MA, Egermann M, Thierjung H, Kloth JK. Modern radiological postoperative diagnostics of the hip joint in children and adults. *Rofo* 2015; 187(7): 525–42.

PART 1

Pediatric Hip Preservation Techniques

6

Salter's osteotomy and Dega osteotomy

MOHAMED M. H. EL-SAYED

SALTER'S INNOMINATE OSTEOTOMY

Prerequisites

- Capacity to bring the femoral head to the level of the acetabulum. Originally, Salter recommended preoperative traction.
- Contractures of the adductors and the iliopsoas muscles must be released.
- Concentric reduction of the femoral head in the true acetabulum must be performed.
- Appropriate congruity of the acetabulum and femoral head. Joint should have a rounded circumference.
- No fixed deformity. Good motion of the hip joint is necessary, especially flexion, abduction, and internal rotation.
- Patient must be over 18 months of age.
- A flexible symphysis pubis is required.

Indications

- To correct acetabular maldirection from developmental dysplasia of hip (DDH) in children over 18 months of age
- To correct acetabular dysplasia
- To cover the anterolaterally exposed femoral head
- To stabilize a concentrically reduced hip in a functional position of weight bearing
- For dislocation after the age of 2 years when closed reduction is contraindicated (a concentric reduction is a prerequisite)
- Residual subluxation following previous treatment failure in patients from 18 months to approximately 6 years of age (a concentric reduction is a prerequisite)
- Residual dislocation following previous treatment failure in patients from 18 months to approximately 6 years of age (a concentric reduction is a prerequisite)

Contraindications

- Patient older than 6 years with dislocation (relative contraindication)
- Incapacity to carry the femoral head to the acetabulum
- Incapacity to reduce the femoral head into the true acetabulum
- Joint incongruity
- Range of motion significantly limited

Technique

Salter's innominate osteotomy is based on redirection of the acetabulum as a unit by hinging and rotation through the symphysis pubis, which is mobile in children. It is performed by making a transverse linear cut above the acetabulum at the level of the greater sciatic notch and the inferior iliac spine.[1]

The whole acetabulum with the distal fragment of the innominate bone is tilted downward and laterally by rotating it while maintaining contact at the posterior osteotomy site. The new position of the distal fragment is maintained by a triangular bone graft taken from the proximal portion of the ilium and inserted in the open wedge osteotomy site. Internal fixation is provided by two threaded Kirschner wires.[1]

During this rotation, the acetabulum is redirected so that it is extended and adducted relative to its preoperative position. Through the rotation and redirection of the acetabulum, the femoral head is covered adequately with the hip in a normal weight-bearing position.[1]

THE OPERATIVE TECHNIQUE

The patient is taken to the operating room and placed supine with a roll (or radiolucent sandbag) under the back.[1-3] General anesthesia is obtained. The skin is prepared with the patient in the side-lying position, so that the abdomen, lower part of the chest and affected half of the pelvis can be draped to the midline anteriorly and posteriorly; the entire lower limb is also prepared and draped to allow free motion of the hip during the operation. Appropriate catheters are used.

The skin incision used is an oblique "bikini" incision, as the bikini incision results in excellent exposure and cosmoses. The anterior inferior iliac spine is palpated and marked. The incision begins about two-thirds of the distance from the greater trochanter to the iliac crest, crosses the inferior spine and extends 1 or 2 cm beyond the inferior spine.

The incision is then retracted over the iliac crest and the dissection is carried down to the apophysis of the crest. The anterior superior iliac spine is identified. The lateral femoral cutaneous nerve is visualized as it travels just medial to the tensor-Sartorius interval and just distal to the inferior iliac spine; it is always protected and marked with a vessel loop extending by an angle roughly equivalent to the angle of the osteotomy opening.

The tensor-Sartorius interval is bluntly dissected beginning distally and working proximally. The interval is widened with blunt dissection, and the rectus femoris is identified, as it inserts into the anterior inferior iliac spine.

Just inferior to the iliac apophysis, a sharp incision is made (using a scalpel or cautery), and the apophysis is reflected in a medial direction (with the aid of periosteal elevators), giving exposure to the iliac crest. The outer pelvic musculature abductors are stripped subperiosteally, and on the inside of the pelvis, the iliacus musculature is stripped subperiosteally all the way posteriorly to the sciatic notch. Care must be taken to keep the periosteum intact, as it protects the iliac muscles and prevents bleeding and injury to the superior gluteal vessels (laterally) and injury of the sciatic nerve. Bleeding points on the iliac wings are controlled using bone wax. A dry wound makes subsequent steps in the procedure easier. Further subperiostal dissection clears the Sartorius medially and the tensor laterally, exposing the rectus femoris as it arises from the anterior inferior spine.

The Sartorius muscle could usually be reflected medially with the cartilaginous iliac apophysis. If it is difficult to do so, or if more distal exposure is desired, the Sartorius is detached from the anterior superior iliac spine, its free margin is marked with whip sutures for later re-attachment, and the muscle is medially and distally reflected.

The interval is widened, the iliac apophysis incised and reflected, and the rectus femoris and the underlying capsule exposed. The rectus femoris is elevated from the hip capsule, the straight head (from the anterior inferior iliac spine), and the reflected head (from the superior margin of the acetabulum) are identified, tagged, sectioned, and reflected distally. The hip capsule is exposed laterally, first with a periosteal elevator to clear muscle attachments from the capsule.

Next, the medial portion of the capsule is exposed, again using the periosteal elevator to dissect between the capsule and the iliopsoas tendon. Flexion of the hip relaxes the iliopsoas and provides good medial exposure.

The capsule beneath the iliopsoas is exposed, and a strong medial retraction with army-navy retractors is necessary to access the acetabulum.

The iliopsoas tendon is sectioned (the psoas tendon is isolated from within the iliacus muscle at the pelvic rim and sectioned at one or two levels). The divided edges of the tendinous portion are retracted and the muscle fibers separated, releasing contractures of the iliopsoas without disturbing the continuity of the muscle. A percutaneous adductor longus tenotomy is usually performed at this point (if it has not been done before).[4]

Once the medial exposure is adequate, the capsule is opened with a knife. A hemostat is inserted under the capsule, and the capsule is opened over it and parallel to the acetabular margin, leaving about a 5-mm margin of the capsule. The incision is carried out from the lateral to medial direction and should extend medially all the way to the transverse acetabular ligament and laterally to above the greater trochanter. Another capsular incision is then done extending along the femoral neck and forming a T-shaped incision.

The ligamentum teres is cut free from its base in the acetabulum with curved sharp scissors, and bleeding is controlled with electrocautery. Pulvinar tissue present within the acetabulum is now moved with a curette and rongeur until a clear acetabulum is developed. The transverse acetabular ligament is then incised to increase the acetabular volume.

The labrum of the acetabulum is then inspected. When the labrum is found infolded with trials of head reduction, that indicates that the medial obstacles to reduction (capsule, iliopsoas, transverse ligament) have been inadequately released. After adequate through release medially, the head should be reducible beneath the labrum, which will elevate the labrum out of the acetabulum. Excision of the labrum is never attempted.

The medial and lateral walls of the iliac bone are then exposed subperiosteally to the sciatic notch posteriorly. Two medium-sized Hohman elevator retractors, one from the lateral side and the other from the medial side, are placed subperiosteally in the sciatic notch. This step is crucial; besides keeping neurovascular structures out of harm's way, the Hohman retractors maintain continuity of the proximal and distal innominate segments at the sciatic notch.

A right-angle forceps is then passed subperiosteally from the medial side of the ilium and guided through the sciatic notch to the outer side with the index finger of the surgeon's opposite hand. An umbilical tape is then passed using the right-angle

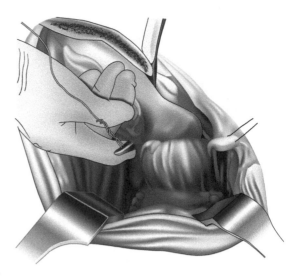

Figure 6.1 Passage of Gigli saw. (From Lovell WW, Winters RB. In: *Dysplasia of Hip*, edited by Lovell WW, Winters RB. Philadelphia: JB Lippincott; 2013.)

force through the sciatic notch from the lateral side and then grasped and pulled (subperiosteally) from the medial side. The Gigli saw is then tied to the medial end of this umbilical tape and easily passed through the sciatic notch. This will protect the important structures within the sciatic notch from direct injury from the passage of the Gigli saw (Figure 6.1).[5]

The tissues are retracted medially and laterally from the ilium. The operation table is then lowered. The osteotomy line extends from the sciatic notch to the anterior inferior iliac spine, perpendicular to the sides of the ilium. It is vital to begin the osteotomy well inferiorly in the sciatic notch; the tendency is to start too high.

The handles of the Gigli saw are kept widely separated and at continuous tension in order to keep the saw from binding in the soft cancellous bone. The osteotomy emerges anteriorly immediately above the anterior inferior iliac spine. The use of an osteotome is avoided, as that may subject the superior glutal vessels and the sciatic nerve to iatrogenic damage (Figure 6.2).

The Hohman retractors are kept constantly at the sciatic notch by an assistant to prevent posterior or medial displacement of the distal segment and loss of bony continuity posteriorly. A full thickness graft (triangular shaped) from the anterior part of the iliac crest is then taken using an

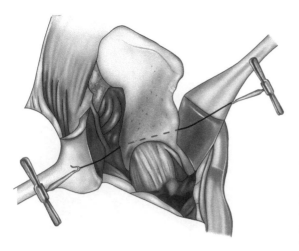

Figure 6.2 Direction of osteotomy. (From Lovell WW, Winters RB. In: *Dysplasia of Hip*, edited by Lovell WW, Winters RB. Philadelphia: JB Lippincott; 2013.)

oscillating saw (a double-action bone cutter is also used) (Figure 6.3).

The proximal fragment of the innominate bone is held steady with a large towel clip forceps, and the distal fragment is grasped with a second stout towel

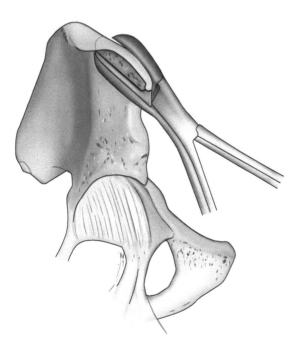

Figure 6.3 Harvesting triangular iliac graft. (From Lovell WW, Winters RB. In: *Dysplasia of Hip*, edited by Lovell WW, Winters RB. Philadelphia: JB Lippincott; 2013.)

forceps. Next, a curved elevator is inserted into the sciatic notch, levering the proximal fragment anteriorly. The affected hip is placed in 90° of flexion, maximal abduction, and 90° of lateral rotation (figure-of-four position); a second assistant applies distal and lateral traction on the thigh. With the second towel clip placed well posteriorly on the distal fragment, the surgeon rotates the distal fragment downward, outward, and forward, thus opening the osteotomy site anteriorly. The site must be kept closed posteriorly. Leaving the osteotomy site open posteriorly displaces the hip joint distally without adequate rotation and redirection of the acetabulum at the symphysis pubis; furthermore, it will lengthen the lower limb unnecessarily (Figure 6.4).

Opening the osteotomy site with a laminectomy spreader or a self-retaining retractor is also a common technical fault. This would only move the distal fragment downward but without rotation at the symphysis.

The bone graft fragment is then inserted into the osteotomy site, traction on the inferior fragment is released, and thus the graft is firmly locked between the two segments of the iliac bone. The distal fragment of the innominate bone should be kept slightly anterior to the proximal fragment (Figure 6.5).

Two stout, threaded no. 1.8 Kirschner wire (KW) are then drilled through the remaining superior part of the ilium, through the graft, and into the inferior fragment posterior to the acetabulum. Care is taken not to penetrate the hip joint, as this would cause chondrolysis. Inadequate penetration of the wires into the distal fragment results in loss of alignment of the osteotomy. The femoral head is then reduced into the acetabulum and stability is re-evaluated (Figure 6.6).

Radiographs are obtained to check the adequacy of correction of the acetabular maldirection. Reduction at this moment should be stable with the hip either in adduction or in slight external rotation.

Another modification of the Salter osteotomy was described by Kalamachi,[6] where displacing the distal fragment into the posterior botch of the proximal fragment was done, thereby avoiding increased pressure from the femoral head (Figure 6.7).

A Sutherland double innominate osteotomy[7] is usually indicated in DDH and following a Salter osteotomy in the age group between 5 and 15 years. This is a second pubic osteotomy, which is medial to the obturator foramen in the interval between the pubic symphysis and the pubic tubercle, and

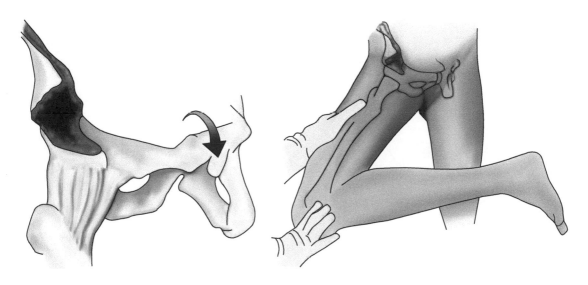

Figure 6.4 Figure-of-four and opening of osteotomy site. (From Lovell WW, Winters RB. In: *Dysplasia of Hip*, edited by Lovell WW, Winters RB. Philadelphia: JB Lippincott; 2013.)

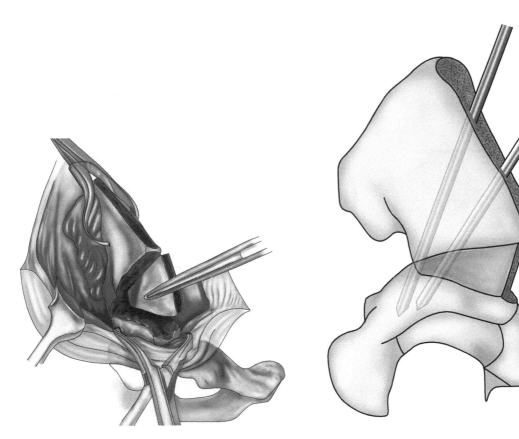

Figure 6.5 Graft insertion. (From Lovell WW, Winters RB. In: *Dysplasia of Hip*, edited by Lovell WW, Winters RB. Philadelphia: JB Lippincott; 2013.)

Figure 6.6 K wire insertion. (From Lovell WW, Winters RB. In: *Dysplasia of Hip*, edited by Lovell WW, Winters RB. Philadelphia: JB Lippincott; 2013.)

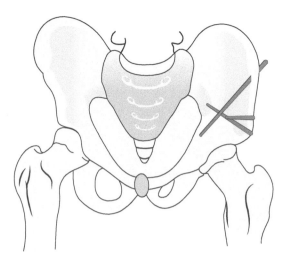

Figure 6.7 Kalamchi modification of Salter osteotomy.

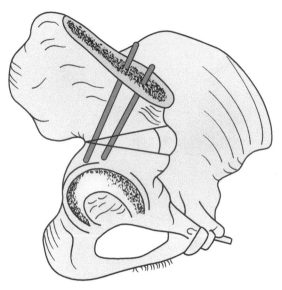

Figure 6.9 Double innominate osteotomy as described by Sutherland, where it uses a supra-pubic supplementary incision to osteotomize the pubis just lateral to the symphysis pubis to remove a small wedge, which allows some joint medialization when the freed pelvic fragment is rotated santerolaterally with towel clips and pinned under direct vision followed by routine flexion of the innominate osteotomy, which is immobilized by a Spica cast for 4–6 weeks postoperatively.

1. The addition of the pubic osteotomy increases the amount of acetabular rotation and thus coverage of the femoral head.
2. The femoral head could be then shifted medially, thus reducing the length of the femoral lever arm.

DEGA OSTEOTOMY

Surgical technique

The patient is positioned supine with the involved hip tilted up approximately 30–40° by a bump placed at the midlumbar level.[8-15] An extended anterolateral incision is made starting 1 cm inferior and posterior to the anterior superior iliac spine and extending distally over the proximal part of the femur, centered over the greater trochanter (Figure 6.10).

The interval between the tensor fasciae latae. muscle posteriorly and the Sartorius muscle anteriorly is developed, and the Sartorius is released from its origin on the anterior superior iliac spine.

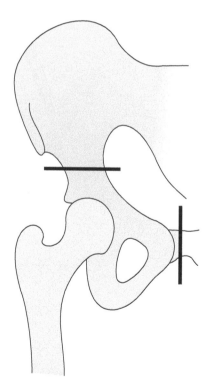

Figure 6.8 Sutherland innominate osteotomy.

consists of a wedge of bone about 7–13 mm in diameter that is just lateral to the symphysis pubis and parallel to it (Figures 6.8 and 6.9). It displaces the acetabular fragment distally and anteriorly. Its main advantages are twofold:

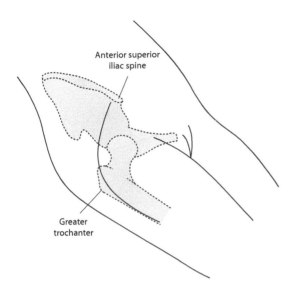

Figure 6.10 The anterolateral incision is made starting 1 cm inferior and posterior to the anterior superior iliac spine and extending distally over the proximal part of the femur, centered over the greater trochanter.

The abductor muscles are sharply reflected off of the lateral wall of the ilium just distal to the iliac apophysis. The apophysis itself is not split. The abductor muscles and the periosteum are completely separated from the ilium and the hip capsule back to the sciatic notch, which is fully exposed, and an adult-sized blunt Hohmann retractor is then inserted into the notch.

Neither the muscles nor the periosteum are dissected off of the inner wall of the ilium. The reflected head of the rectus femoris muscle is separated from the hip capsule and is incised. The tendon of the straight head of the rectus femoris muscle is detached from the anterior inferior iliac spine only when necessary for proper visualization of the capsule. The tendinous portion of the iliopsoas muscle is isolated from the capsule and is transected either over the anteromedial aspect of the capsule just distal to the pelvic brim or more distally, near its insertion. Open reduction of the hip and/or concomitant femoral osteotomy with shortening and rotation to correct excessive anteversion are performed at this time if required.

The vastus lateralis fascia and muscle are split, exposing the proximal part of the femur. If valgus correction was planned preoperatively, we use a 90° AO (Association of Osteosynthesis, AO Foundation, Switzerland) infant blade-plate for

fixation and reduce the true neck-shaft angle to 110–120°.

If shortening and rotation without valgus correction are planned, then a straight one-third tubular AO plate is used. Two small Kirschner wires are inserted into the femur, one above the osteotomy plane and the other below the level of the desired shortening, to aid in determining the amount of anteversion correction.

The femur is osteotomized in the subtrochanteric or intertrochanteric region, and the fragments are allowed to overlap as the femoral head is reduced deeply into the acetabulum. A femoral shortening equivalent to the amount of overlap is then performed. Preliminary fixation of the straight plate or 90° blade-plate is achieved with a bone clamp. The hip is flexed to 90°, and the clamp is loosened so that enough external rotation of the distal fragment is added to make internal and external rotation of the hip symmetrical.

Observation of the guide wires at this point reveals an estimated anteversion correction ranging from 10–40°. At this point, the femoral head will rest deeply in the still steep acetabulum and have a diminished tendency to dislocate with the lower limb in neutral position.

Next, the Dega osteotomy is performed to decrease acetabular dysplasia and enhance containment of the femoral head. The orientation of the osteotomy is first marked on the lateral cortex of the ilium (Figure 6.11).

The direction of the osteotomy is curvilinear when viewed from the lateral cortex, starting just above the anterior inferior iliac spine, curving gently cephalad and posteriorly to reach a point superior to the midpoint of the acetabulum, then continuing posteriorly to end approximately 1–1.5 cm in front of the sciatic notch.

The most cephalad extent of the osteotomy is in the middle of the acetabulum, at a point on the ilium determined by the steepness of the acetabulum. Very steep acetabular inclinations require a correspondingly higher midpoint. A guide wire is inserted under fluoroscopic control at the most cephalad point of the curvilinear marking line, directed caudally and medially to ensure that the osteotomy will exit at the appropriate level just above the horizontal limb of the triradiate cartilage.

A straight 0.25- or 0.5-in (0.64- or 1.3-cm) osteotome is used to perform the bone cut, which extends obliquely medially and inferiorly,

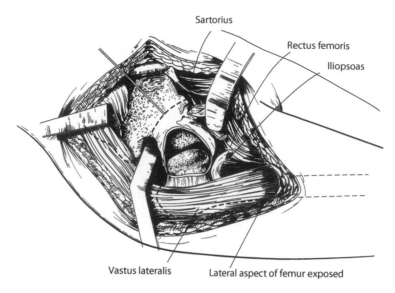

Figure 6.11 The Dega incomplete transiliac osteotomy line is marked on the lateral cortex of the ilium, and a guide wire is inserted under fluoroscopic control to exit just above the horizontal limb of the triradiate cartilage.

paralleling the guide wire to exit through the inner cortex just above the iliopubic and ilioischial limbs of the triradiate cartilage (Figure 6.12a), leaving the posterior one-third of the inner cortex intact (Figure 6.12b).

If predominantly anterior coverage is desired, the medial (inner) cortex is cut over the anterior and middle portion, leaving only the posterior sciatic notch hinge intact. If more lateral coverage is desired, more of the medial cortex is left intact, resulting in

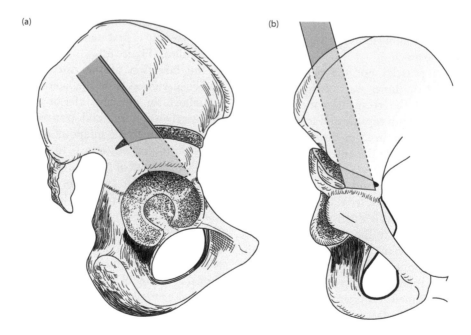

Figure 6.12 (a) The osteotome penetrating the inner cortex, viewed from the lateral aspect of the ilium. (b) View from the inner side of the pelvis, showing an intact posteromedial cortical hinge. The length of the intact cortex depends on the amount of anterior or lateral coverage desired.

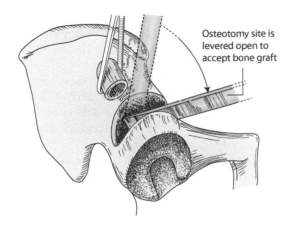

Osteotomy site is levered open to accept bone graft

Figure 6.13 The osteotomy site is levered open with either an osteotome or a small laminar spreader.

a posteromedial hinge based on the posteromedial inner cortex and the entire sciatic notch. In most cases, approximately one-quarter to one-third of the inner pelvic cortex is left intact posteriorly. With experience, the osteotomy cut might be performed safely without fluoroscopic guidance, as per Dega's original description; however, we prefer to use fluoroscopy.

A 0.5-in (1.27-cm) osteotome is then used to gently lever open the osteotomy site either anteriorly or laterally in a controlled manner (Figure 6.13).

A small laminar spreader is also useful for this maneuver. Quite often, while the osteotomy site is being opened, the osteotomy cut on the outer cortex of the ilium propagates toward the sciatic notch as a greenstick fracture.

However, since the posterior portion of the inner cortex is still intact, the outer cortical greenstick fracture does not weaken the recoil and stability at the osteotomy site. The osteotomy site is kept open by inserting two correctly sized bone grafts (Figure 6.14a and b).

The grafts are fashioned from a bicortical segment of iliac crest bone or, alternatively, if femoral shortening had been performed, the segment of the femur that was removed is used as a graft. In cases in which there is a substantial gap at the osteotomy site, an autogenous femoral or iliac crest graft may not be sufficient.

Under these circumstances, the height of the graft can be increased by using freeze-dried fibular allograft cut into trapezoidal sections. The correct graft height is determined by simply noting the opening of the osteotomy gap created by the laminar spreader or the levering osteotome. In congenital dysplasia, acetabular deficiency is most pronounced anteriorly, mandating placement of the larger graft more anteriorly. A smaller graft is then wedged more posteriorly, just in front of the intact sciatic notch. Care is taken to ensure that both grafts are of an appropriate height and that the amount of correction of the dysplastic acetabulum provides enough coverage of the femoral head.

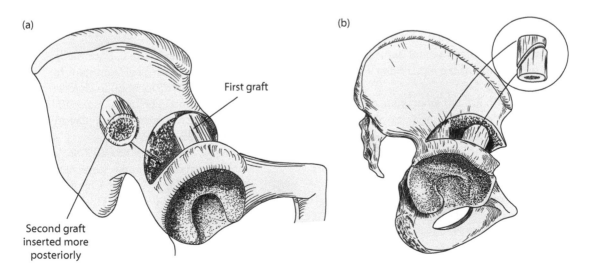

(a)

First graft

Second graft inserted more posteriorly

(b)

Figure 6.14 (a) Two grafts that are large enough to keep the osteotomy site open at the premeasured height are inserted. (b) A larger graft is inserted anteriorly. The posterior graft should be smaller in order not to loosen the anterior graft.

Once the grafts have been inserted, they are stable because of the inherent recoil at the osteotomy site produced by the intact sciatic notch. Metallic internal fixation is not necessary.

The more posterior the extent of the outer cortical cut, and the greater the amount of the inner cortex left intact, the more lateral the tilt of the acetabulum. A more cephalad starting point and a steeper osteotomy angle allow for more lateral coverage. A more extensive cut through the inner cortex allows for more anterior coverage of the hip. Finally, the closer the osteotomy is to the acetabulum, the thinner and more pliable the acetabular fragment will be, theoretically allowing for more reshaping and less redirection to occur. These three-dimensional changes in the osteotomy are admittedly difficult to quantify, as is the true anatomical nature of a dysplastic hip. Once the osteotomy is performed, satisfactory femoral head coverage can be appreciated and the hip should be stable during flexion and rotation.

After closure, a one and one-half Spica cast is applied with the hip in neutral extension, approximately 20° of internal rotation, and 20–30° of abduction. The cast is worn for 8 to 12 weeks depending on the healing of the osteotomy site. After the cast is removed, progressive walking and range of motion are begun, but no formal physical therapy is prescribed.

REFERENCES

1. Salter RB. Innominate osteotomy in the treatment of congenital dislocation and subluxation of the hip. *J Bone Joint Surg* 1961; 43B: 518.
2. Salter RB. Role of innominate osteotomy in the treatment of congenital dislocation and subluxation of the hip in the older child. *J Bone Joint Surg Am* 1966; 48(7): 1413–39.
3. Salter RB, Dubos JP. The first fifteen years' personal experience with innominate osteotomy in the treatment of congenital dislocation and subluxation of the hip. *Clin Orthop* 1974; 98: 72–103.
4. Bassett GS, Engsberg JR, McAlister WH, Gordon JE, Schonenecker PL. Fate of the psoas muscle after open reduction for developmental dislocation of the hip. *J Pediatr Orthop* 1999; 19: 425–32.
5. Lovell WW, Winters RB. Developmental. In: *Dysplasia of Hip*, edited by Lovell WW, Winters RB. Philadelphia: JB Lippincott; 2013.
6. Kalamachi A. Modified Salter osteotomy. *J Bone Joint Surg Am* 1982; 64(2): 183–7.
7. Sutherland DH, Greenfield R. Double innominate osteotomy. *J Bone Joint Surg Am* 1977; 59(8): 1082–91.
8. Ward WT, Grudziak JS. Dega osteotomy for the treatment of congenital dysplasia of the hip. *J Bone Joint Surg* 2011; 83(A): 845–54.
9. Dega W. Selection of surgical methods in the treatment of congenital dislocation of the hip in children. *Chir Narzadow Ruchu Ortop Pol* 1969; 34: 357–66.
10. Grudziak JS, Labaziewicz L, Kruczynski J, Nowakowski A, Wierusz-Kozlowska M, Schwartz R. Combined one-staged open reduction, femoral osteotomy, and Dega pelvic osteotomy for developmental dysplasia of the hip. *J Pediatr Orthop* 1993; 13: 680.
11. Labaziewicz L, Piskorski Z. Early results of treatment of congenital hip dislocation by means of a one-stage operation consisting in open reduction, transiliac osteotomy and detorsion-devalgization osteotomy with femur shortening. *Chir Narzadow Ruchu Ortop Pol* 1974; 39: 615–20.
12. Pucher A, Piskorski Z. Early results of surgical treatment for congenital dislocation of the hip by the Degi method in young children. *Chir Narzadow Ruchu Ortop Pol* 1992; 57: 199–203.
13. Pucher A, Labaziewicz L, Kaczmarczyk J. Early results of surgical treatment for congenital hip dislocation in children using Degi's method in children under 18 months of age. *Chir Narzadow Ruchu Ortop Pol* 1994; 59: 135–42.
14. Senger A, Pucher A, Piskorski Z. Isolated transiliac osteotomy in the surgical treatment of congenital hip dysplasia. *Chir Narzadow Ruchu Ortop Pol* 1988; 53: 175–81.
15. Senger A, Wlodarczyk R, Kesa P, Grudziak J. Results of the surgical treatment of residual dysplasia of the hip joint with or without subluxation by transiliac osteotomy and corrective osteotomy of the proximal end of the femur. *Chir Narzadow Ruchu Ortop Pol* 1988; 53: 182–9.

7

Pemberton osteotomy

MEHMET BÜLENT BALIOĞLU

INTRODUCTION

Treatment for developmental dysplasia of the hip (DDH) varies according to the age of the patient. For children under 3 months, the preferred treatment is Pavlik bandaging and/or dynamic hip orthosis; for children of 3–18 months (with/without arthrography), closed and open reductions (ORs) are most common; and for children 18 months and older, pelvic osteotomies are used.[1–9] Pemberton described an acetabuloplasty, now called the Pemberton pericapsular osteotomy (PPO), where an iliac osteotomy ended at the posterior limb of the triradiate cartilage and the anterolateral rim of the acetabulum was hinged downward and laterally.[3] PPO performed with OR may be adequate for DDH patients over 18 months, but femoral shortening (FS) osteotomy is often performed alongside pelvic osteotomy for patients aged 3 years plus.[10,11] At this age, soft tissue and muscle have developed to the point where femoral head reduction of the acetabulum is not possible. FS, which permits the muscles surrounding the hip to perform like a lengthened muscle and thereby reduces the force required to achieve concentric reduction, helps to ensure reduced pressure on the femoral head, which may otherwise result in avascular femoral head necrosis (AVN).[12] The use of FS has been shown to decrease such complications as redislocation and AVN.[13,14] The patient age is often an unclear indication for surgery.[10]

Owing to the risks involved in surgical treatments, such as AVN, joint stiffness, shortening of extremities, and ongoing complications like subluxation and dysplasia due to insufficient covering of the femoral head, PPO, rather than OR, has become the most commonly used treatment, as it provides better coverage for the acetabular roof of the femoral head in patients over 2 years of age. On the other hand, FS is also often necessary in older patients. There has, however, been a debate about at what age FS may be necessary. Sankar et al. used the term *older* to refer to children over 3 years of age.[10] Klisic and Jancovic[15] reported good results in a patient series over 5 years of age, whereas Galpin et al.[12] uniformly performed FS over the age of 2 years. Wenger et al. even advocated FS in certain children younger than 2 years of age,[13] while evaluation of clinical and radiological results should be used, such as acetabular index (AI),[16] center-edge (CE) angle (Wiberg), Severin classification,[17] Tönnis grading,[5] Kalamchi–MacEwen,[18] and McKay's[19] criteria.

SURGICAL TECHNIQUE

Indication

In dysplastic hips between the age of 18 months and 6 years, 10–15° correction of acetabular index is required. Small femoral head, large acetabulum.

Procedure

- Pericapsular osteotomy of the ilium.
- Osteotomy is made through the full thickness of the bone from just superior to the antero-inferior iliac spine anteriorly to the triradiate cartilage posteriorly.
- The triradiate cartilage acts as a hinge on which the acetabular roof is rotated anteriorly and laterally.

Advantages

1. Osteotomy is incomplete and therefore more stable.
2. Internal fixation is not required.
3. A greater degree of correction can be achieved with less rotation of the acetabulum.

During the operation, a tricortical trapezoidal iliac graft is placed in the osteotomy space (Figure 7.1). K wire or fixation materials are not used in patients who receive only PPO. For FS patients, a Harris–Müller plate (three or four holes) is applied for stabilization. Patients undergo an adductor tenotomy immediately prior to the PPO, and an iliopsoas tenotomy is performed during the course of the operation. Patients

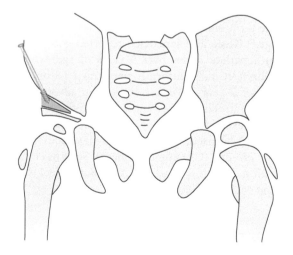

Figure 7.1 The osteotomy is made through the full thickness of the bone from just superior to the anteroinferior iliac spine anteriorly to the triradiate cartilage posteriorly, with the triradiate cartilage acting as a hinge on which the acetabular roof is rotated anteriorly and laterally.

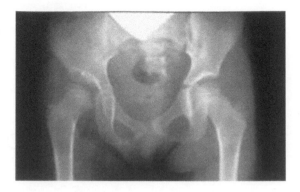

Figure 7.2 Symptomatic residual acetabular dysplasia in an 8-year-old girl after treatment of congenital dislocation of right hip.

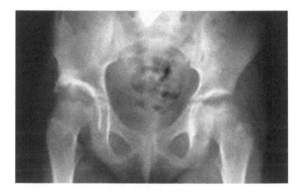

Figure 7.3 After Pemberton acetabuloplasty.

receive OR, during which a ligamentum teres and pulvinar excision are made and the transverse ligament released. OR patients have hip capsule plications applied (Figures 7.2 and 7.3).

Increased femoral anteversion often occurs in DDH patients. To avoid this complication, the FS patients in the study are received derotation. An anterolateral oblique incision was made for PPO and OR, and for FS patients, a separate lateral incision was made to the proximal femur. Patients received a single surgery. Following the operation, a hip spica cast was applied for 1.5 months, and following the removal of the cast, a Dennis–Brown bar was prescribed for 1 month. At 2.5 months postoperative, the patient should start mobilization with physiotherapy and partial weight bearing of the lower extremities. Follow-up is done for the 1st, 6th, 12th, and 24th months postoperatively, with an ongoing annual checkup of the hip.

The grade of displacement is calculated according to Tönnis[5] grading, and AI[16] is determined preoperatively and postoperatively, and CE post-operatively. Clinical evaluations are made according to the modified McKay's[19] criteria, which include assessments of pain, range of motion of the affected and contralateral hips, instability, limp, and Trendelenburg sign; radiological assessments are made according to Severin's[17] classification, which is a system that helps surgeons rate the long-term outcomes of an operation against future possible osteoarthritis, and femoral head AVN measurements are taken with criteria proposed by Kalamchi and MacEwen.[18]

DISCUSSION

The aim of any DDH treatment is to provide sufficient coverage of the acetabular roof, which must be provided in order to prevent displaced hips from developing and to allow for a concentrated reduction of the hip joint. Both incomplete (Pemberton, Dega) and complete (Salter) iliac osteotomies can be used successfully in DDH patients.[3,4,6-9] However, incomplete osteotomies are advantageous since they do not require an internal fixation.

One of the most important factors in DDH surgery is matching the correct surgical method to the right age group. Since the AI of DDH patients is normally high, PPO is a preferred choice to reduce the AI angle and allow for better coverage of the acetabular roof. The effect of PPO on AI is expected to be different according to age group. Periacetabuler osteotomy/PPO aims to reduce AI and provide coverage for the femoral head, while PPO + FS helps to reduce the femoral head, protect against vascularization, and prevent AVN in patients aged 3 years and older. The recommended age period for the performance of a Pemberton osteotomy is 1.5–14 years.[3] However, there has been some debate about the fixing of recommended ages for procedures since, according to Sankar et al., patient age is also an unclear indication for surgery.[10] Developmental dysplasia of the hip patients who receive acetabular osteotomies or PPO with FS may develop AVN of the femoral head.

It is known that PPO provides a notable correction in AI and allows for the rotation of the acetabulum.[20,21] For DDH patients with a clear defect in the anterior and superolateral walls of the acetabulum, PPO is the preferred choice. The rotation center is located near the hip joint, and PPO allows

for good coverage.[3,22,23] Although Tachjian[22] demonstrated that there is a decrease in the volume of the acetabulum, Solomczykowski et al.[24] showed that PPO increases the volume.

REFERENCES

1. Akel I, Tumer Y. Residual acetabular dysplasia-natural history and indication for surgery. *Turkiye Klinikleri J Orthop Traumatol Spec Top* 2010; 3: 10–3.
2. Bursali A, Tonbul M. How are outcomes affected by combining the Pemberton and Salter osteotomies? *Clin Orthop Relat Res* 2008; 466: 837–46.
3. Pemberton PA. Pericapsular osteotomy of the ilium for treatment of congenital subluxation and dislocation of the hip. *J Bone Joint Surg Am* 1965; 47: 65–86.
4. Salter RB, Dubos JP. The first fifteen year's personal experience with innominate osteotomy in the treatment of congenital dislocation and subluxation of the hip. *Clin Orthop Relat Res* 1974; 466(98): 72–103.
5. Tönnis D. An evaluation of conservative and operative methods in the treatment of congenital hip dislocation. *Clin Orthop Relat Res* 1976; 466(119): 76–88.
6. Tukenmez M, Perc S, Tezeren G, Cingoz MA. The outcomes of Salter innominate osteotomy in the treatment of developmental dysplasia of the hip. *Turkiye Klinikleri J Med Sci* 2006; 26: 390–5.
7. Utterback JD, MacEwen GD. Comparison of pelvic osteotomies for the surgical correction of the congenital hip. *Clin Orthop Relat Res* 1974; 466(98): 104–10.
8. Bhuyan BK. Outcome of one-stage treatment of developmental dysplasia of hip in older children. *Indian J Orthop* 2012; 46: 548–55.
9. El-Sayed M, Ahmed T, Fathy S, Zyton H. The effect of Dega acetabuloplasty and Salter innominate osteotomy on acetabular remodeling monitored by the acetabular index in walking DDH patients between 2 and 6 years of age: Short- to middle-term follow-up. *J Child Orthop* 2012; 6: 471–7.
10. Sankar WN, Tang EY, Moseley CF. Predictors of the need for femoral shortening osteotomy during open treatment

of developmental dislocation of the hip. *J Pediatr Orthop* 2009; 29: 868–71.

11. Vitale MG, Skaggs DL. Developmental dysplasia of the hip from six months to four years of age. *J Am Acad Orthop Surg* 2001; 9: 401–11.

12. Galpin RD, Roach JW, Wenger DR, Herring JA, Birch JG. One-stage treatment of congenital dislocation of the hip in older children, including femoral shortening. *J Bone Joint Surg Am* 1989; 71: 734–41.

13. Wenger DR, Lee CS, Kolman B. Derotational femoral shortening for developmental dislocation of the hip: Special indications and results in the child younger than 2 years. *J Pediatr Orthop* 1995; 15: 768–79.

14. Schoenecker PL, Strecker WB. Congenital dislocation of the hip in children. Comparison of the effects of femoral shortening and of skeletal traction in treatment. *J Bone Joint Surg Am* 1984; 66: 21–7.

15. Klisic P, Jankovic L. Combined procedure of open reduction and shortening of the femur in treatment of congenital dislocation of the hips in older children. *Clin Orthop Relat Res* 1976; 466(119): 60–9.

16. Berkeley ME, Dickson JH, Cain TE, Donovan MM. Surgical therapy for congenital dislocation of the hip in patients who are twelve to thirty-six months old. *J Bone Joint Surg Am* 1984; 66: 412–20.

17. Severin E. Congenital dislocation of the hip; development of the joint after closed reduction. *J Bone Joint Surg Am* 1950; 32-A: 507–18.

18. Kalamchi A, MacEwen GD. Avascular necrosis following treatment of congenital dislocation of the hip. *J Bone Joint Surg Am* 1980; 62: 876–88.

19. Classic. Translation: Hilgenreiner on congenital hip dislocation. *J Pediatr Orthop* 1986; 6: 202–14.

20. Balioğlu MB, Öner A, Aykut ÜS, Kaygusuz MA. Mid-term results of Pemberton pericapsular osteotomy. *Indian J Orthop* 2015; 49(4): 418–24.

21. Omeroglu H, Biçimoglu A, Agus H, Tümer Y. Measurement of center-edge angle in developmental dysplasia of the hip: A comparison of two methods in patients under 20 years of age. *Skeletal Radiol* 2002; 31: 25–9.

22. Coleman SS. The incomplete pericapsular (Pemberton) and innominate (Salter) osteotomies; a complete analysis. *Clin Orthop Relat Res* 1974; 466(98): 116–23.

23. Herring JA, editor. Developmental dysæplasia of the hip. In: *Tachdjian's Pediatric Orthopedics*. 3rd ed., Vol. 1. Philadelphia: W.B. Saunders; 2002. pp. 513–654.

24. Solomczykowski M, Mackenzie WG, Stern G, Keeler KA, Glutting J. Acetabular volume. *J Pediatr Orthop* 1998; 18: 657–61.

8

Triple innominate osteotomy (Steel)

K. MOHAN IYER

References   48

Steel's redirectional pelvic osteotomy (1973) divides the ischial ramus, superior pubic ramus, and ilium above the acetabulum and allows the acetabulum to be rotated anterolaterally. There are few reports of the results of triple innominate osteotomy for acetabular dysplasia after poliomyelitis. Steel (1977) initially documented 18 such cases in a total of 175 osteotomies.[1]

Steel's triple innominate osteotomy was originally created for correcting dysplastic acetabulum in adolescents and young adults. A modification was devised with two anterior incisions and ramus cuts as close to the acetabulum as possible to improve the mobility of the fragment to get better coverage of the hip. This modified technique gave better mobility of the rotated fragment in correcting acetabular dysplasia with a short learning curve and, most importantly, provided greater coverage and medialization of the femoral head for better long-term results.[2]

It is a total redirectional reconstruction, obtained by osteotomies through the ilium, ischium, and pubis that achieves coverage of a dislocated or subluxated femoral head where other iliac osteotomies are ineffective or incomplete. The majority of patients had a satisfactory result, while it was infective in patients with cerebral palsy, myelodysplasia, and peroneal muscular atrophy and associated with uncontrolled muscle contractures or progressive disease[3] Femoral head resection with valgus subtrochanteric osteotomy in nonambulatory patients with painful, chronically

dislocated hips due to spastic paralysis benefited them due to pain relief, ease of perineal care, and ability to sit up. Certain other complications, such as proximal migration of the remaining femur, recurrence of adduction deformity, hip stiffness, and excessive heterotopic bone formation, which were seen in other procedures used for this condition, were not evident.[4]

The triple pelvic osteotomy is the most effective surgical management of both Legg–Calvé–Perthes (LCP) disease due to secondary insufficient coverage of the femoral head and dysplasia of the hip.

A. *Triple pelvic osteotomy in the treatment of Legg–Calvé–Perthes disease*: In LCP disease, triple pelvic osteotomy is used mostly in older children where hip containment is not easy to achieve using the Salter pelvic osteotomy. It is also used because at the end of the disease course, all that remains is a large, insufficiently covered femoral head that will later require surgical coverage, and it is also used for those who reject varisation osteotomies because of the functional problems manifested by postoperative shortened leg and waddling gait. The added shortening of the femur in the Salter pelvic osteotomy in older children with more severe subluxations enables us to achieve the required containment more easily and obtain good anatomical and functional treatment results.[5] Initially, following femoral osteotomy, immobilization in children was used, which in the later course of treatment necessitated prolonged rehabilitation. With time, immobilization during the postoperative period was stopped, which enabled early rehabilitation. However, weight bearing was only allowed after the femoral osteotomy healed, which usually took longer than the bone consolidation of the pelvic side. By using triple pelvic osteotomy, statistically significantly better coverage of the femoral head is achieved. The main advantages of triple pelvic osteotomy are in the achievement of excellent containment, quick bone healing, and reliable bone fixation, which postoperatively allows patients to avoid immobilization and undergo early rehabilitation with early full limb weight bearing. Hence, triple pelvic osteotomy is the method of choice in the treatment of severe LCP disease in all patients in whom treatment cannot be achieved using Salter osteotomy due to the patient's age, regardless of the disease stage, initial containment, and degree of damage.[6]

B. The triple pelvic osteotomy has been shown to be reliable for acetabular dysplasia in the adolescent and young adult, alone or in association with proximal femoral osteotomy and/or great trochanter distal advancement.[7]

Certain complications of the triple osteotomy are as follows:

1. Deep wound infection, which can be treated by early wound debridement and parenterally applied antibiotics.
2. Peroneal palsy, treated with corticosteroids, B vitamins, and physical therapy.
3. Pseudoarthrosis of the pubis and pseudoarthrosis of both pubis and ischium. Clinically, all pseudoarthroses are asymptomatic.

The triple osteotomy has proved very reliable and effective in the management of acetabular dysplasia and hip joint incongruence in adolescents (in cases where good results could not be accomplished using the Salter pelvic osteotomy and when the Chiari osteotomy does not lead to a good long-term result).

Triple innominate osteotomy is indicated in adolescents and skeletally mature adults with residual dysplasia and subluxation in whom remodeling of the acetabulum is no longer anticipated (Figure 8.1).

Indications:

1. Developmental dysplasia of hip (DDH) in an older child
2. Needs good range of movements

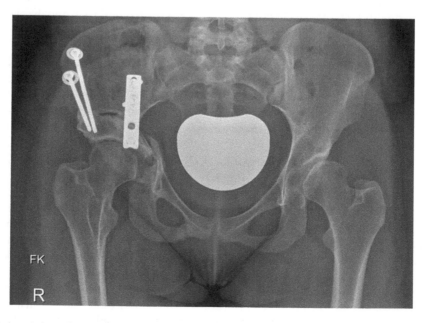

Figure 8.1 Right triple pelvis osteotomy with a dysplastic left hip. (Courtesy of Rajesh Botchu, MSK Radiologist, Birmingham, UK.)

3. Secure bone graft with Arbeitsgemeinschaft für Osteosynthesefragen—which in English is Association for Osteosythesis (AO) screw fixation

The contraindications are:

1. Limited range of movements
2. Significant joint space narrowing with degenerative arthritis
3. Incongruous reduction

Its main advantages are that it has better coverage of the femoral head by the articular cartilage and better hip joint stability and hence no need for a spica cast (Figure 8.2).

Its main disadvantages are that it is technically more difficult, as it does not change the size of the acetabulum, and it distorts the hip such that natural childbirth is not possible (Figure 8.3).

It is best done by a two-incision approach, and the ischium, superior pubic ramus, and ilium, which is superior to the acetabulum, are repositioned and stabilized by a bone graft. This method of osteotomy is safe and has a relatively shallow learning curve compared with other triple pelvic osteotomy procedures.

A triple pelvic osteotomy as described by Tönnis through the ilium, pubis, and ischium was performed, followed by an intrapelvic and

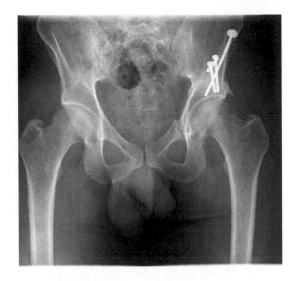

Figure 8.2 Left triple pelvis osteotomy. (Courtesy of Rajesh Botchu, MSK Radiologist, Birmingham, UK.)

anterior and posterior dissection of the hip. In order to assess pelvic anatomy in relation to surgical approach and osteotomy sites, 12 cadaver hips were studied,[8] and the findings are as follows:

1. At the ischium, the pudendal and inferior gluteal neurovascular bundles are most at risk medially and proximally, respectively.

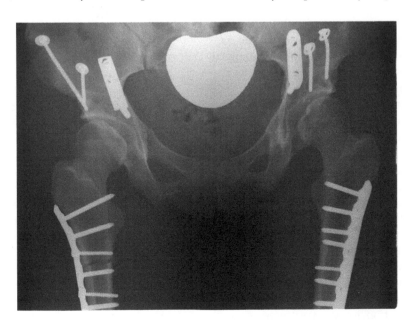

Figure 8.3 Bilateral triple pelvis osteotomy done. (Courtesy of Rajesh Botchu, MSK Radiologist, Birmingham, UK.)

2. Much less in danger is the sciatic nerve, as it runs 1–3 cm lateral to the osteotomy site.
3. At the pubis osteotomy the femoral vein lies close on the bone and is prone to damage. The artery lies further off the bone.
4. The ilium osteotomy starts just proximal to the anterior inferior iliac spine and exits posteriorly at the sciatic notch. Here, the sciatic nerve and the superior gluteal neurovascular bundle may be damaged.

In summary, the conclusions were as follows: the practical surgical implications of these three osteotomies are discussed, especially with respect to the requirement of meticulous subperiosteal dissection and accurate placement of retractors.

The Tönnis triple pelvic osteotomy (TPAO) is one of the popular surgical osteotomies described and still used since 1978. The Tönnis triple osteotomy technique differs from other periacetabular osteotomies, mainly with the additional ischial osteotomy. The osteotomies of ischium, pubis, and ilium are close enough to the hip joint to allow satisfactory rotation of the acetabulum.[16] There are many papers about the TPAO surgery reporting improved femoral head coverage, decreased acetabular inclination, and also an improvement in hip pain and function scores.[9]

The technique in brief is as follows:

1. A long ischial cut connects the obturator foramen with the sciatic notch so that the cut finishes proximal to the sacrospinous ligament, thus preventing it from tethering from the acetabular fragment during correction.
2. The long cut provides good contact after displacement to prevent a pseudoarthrosis.
3. The iliac cut is slightly curved, while the pubic cut is the same as in the Steel procedure (Figure 8.4).
4. The fixation is with screws and attaching a cerclage wire from the screw in the pubis to the pin in the ilium.

In another article, the aim of the study was to compare the midterm clinical and radiological outcomes of the Salter osteotomy (SO) and Tönnis lateral acetabuloplasty (TLA) with concomitant open reduction for the treatment of developmental dysplasia of the hip. Both osteotomy techniques showed similar satisfactory outcomes

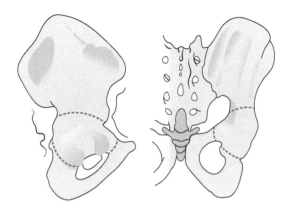

Figure 8.4 Tönnis osteotomy lines. (Redrawn from Tönnis D et al. *J Pediatr Orthop* 1981; 1: 243.)

for the treatment of DDH in patients older than 18 months of age.[10]

A minimally invasive Tönnis osteotomy has also been described in literature,[11] where the authors described in detail a modified single-incision approach to perform the Tönnis triple pelvic osteotomy by a minimally invasive approach, and they concluded a minimally invasive Tönnis osteotomy is a viable option based on the results. This technique is recommended for those who are conversant with traditional pelvicosteotomies.[11]

REFERENCES

1. Steel HH. Triple osteotomy of the innominate bone. *J Bone Joint Surg [Am]* 1973; 55-A: 343–50.
2. Li YC, Wu KW, Huang SC, Wang TM, Kuo KN. Modified triple innominate osteotomy for acetabular dysplasia: For better femoral head medialization and coverage. *J Pediatr Orthop B* 2012; 21(3): 193–9.
3. Steel HH. Triple osteotomy of the innominate bone. A procedure to accomplish coverage of the dislocated or subluxated femoral head in the older patient. *Clin Orthop Relat Res* 1977; (122): 116–27.
4. McHale KA, Bagg M, Nason SS. Treatment of the chronically dislocated hip in adolescents with cerebral palsy with femoral head resection and subtrochanteric valgus osteotomy. *J Pediatr Orthop* 1990; 10(4): 504–9.

5. Vukašinović Z, Slavković S, Miličković S, Siqeca A. Combined Salter innominate osteotomy with femoral shortening versus other methods of treatment for Legg–Calvé–Perthes disease. *J Pediatr Orthop B* 2000; 9: 28–33.

6. Vukasinovic Z, Spasovski D, Vucetic C, Cobeljic G, Zivkovic Z, Matanovic D. Triple pelvic osteotomy in the treatment of Legg–Calvé–Perthes disease. *Int Orthop* 2009; 33(5): 1377–83.

7. Vukasinovic Z, Pelillo F, Spasovski D, Seslija I, Zivkovic Z, Matanovic D. Triple pelvic osteotomy for the treatment of residual hip dysplasia. Analysis of complications. *Hip Int* 2009; 19(4): 315–22.

8. de Kleuver M, Kooijman MAP, Kauer JMG, Kooijman M, Alferink C. Anatomic basis of Tönnis' triple pelvic osteotomy for acetabular dysplasia. *Surg Radiol Anat* 1998; 20(2): 79–82.

9. Tonnis D, Behrens K, Tscharani F. A modified technique of the triple pelvic osteotomy: early results. *J Pediatr Orthop* 1981; 1: 241–9.

10. Bayhan IA, Beng K, Yildirim T, Akpinar E, Ozcan C, Yagmurlu F. Comparison of Salter osteotomy and Tönnis lateral acetabuloplasty with simultaneous open reduction for the treatment of developmental dysplasia of the hip: Midterm results. *Journal of Pediatric Orthopaedics B* 2016; 25(6): 493–8.

11. Balakumar B, Racy M, Madan S. A technical annotation and review of short term results. *J Orthop* 2018; 15(1): 253–8.

9

Bernese periacetabular osteotomy

DIANZHONG LUO AND HONG ZHANG

The Bernese periacetabular osteotomy (PAO) was originally introduced in 1988 by Ganz et al. for the treatment of adult hip dysplasia.[1] Nowadays, the surgical technique of PAO is widely accepted and applied for early osteoarthritis stages of young adults and adolescents with hip dysplasia.[2-4]

INDICATIONS

Indications of PAO for hip dysplasia include:[1,4]

1. The patient has started to feel hip pain or discomfort.
2. The range of motion of the hip joint is normal or nearly normal.
3. The age of patients is between the closure of the triradiate cartilage of the acetabulum and around 50 years.
4. Only mild hip dysplasia and subluxation with good joint congruency and Tönnis hip osteoarthritis grade I-II should be considered to receive PAO.

SURGICAL PROCEDURES

The patient is positioned supine on a radio translucent operation table under general anesthesia. The surgeon should wear radiation protection clothing because part of the surgery is performed under the monitoring of a C-arm. The following steps are designed after the four bone cuts of PAO: the ischial cut, the pubic cut, the iliac cut, and the posterior column cut (Figure 9.1a–e).

A modified Smith-Peterson approach is applied for exposure. Taking the anterior superior iliac spine (ASIS) as the center, the incision is about 12–15 cm long. Open the superficial fascia to expose the iliac crest and fascia over the tensor fasciae latae muscle. From ASIS, aponeurosis of the external oblique muscle of abdomen is severed proximally along the lateral edge of the iliac crest. The ASIS is osteotomized (Figure 9.1a) and reflected medially with the attachment of the sartorius and inguinal ligament. The periosteum of the inner surface of the ilium is stripped from the lower end of the sacroiliac joint to the bottom of the pubic ramus.

The fascia over the tensor fasciae latae muscle is incised along the muscle fiber 1 cm lateral to the interval between sartorius and tensor. Blunt separation of the sartorius and tensor is done under the fascia. The hip was positioned into about 40° flexion. The sartorius and medial part of the fascia over the tensor fasciae latae muscle as well as the lateral femoral cutaneous nerve in the fasciae are reflected medially. Meanwhile, the tensor fasciae latae muscle is reflected laterally. This dissection is extended into the deep layer to expose the tendon of the rectus femoris. Medial to the rectus, the hypertrophic

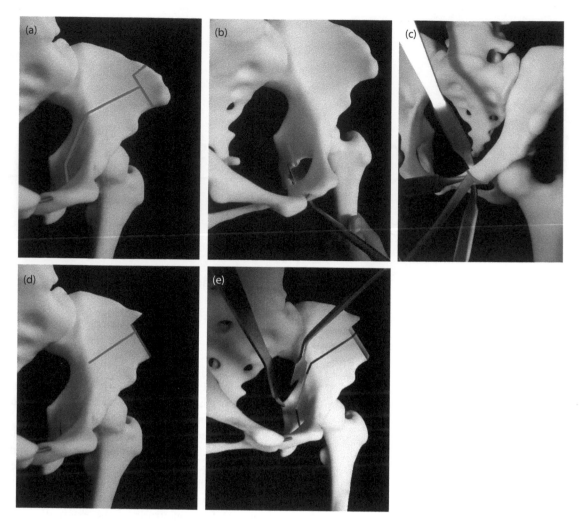

Figure 9.1 Schematic bone cutting lines of periacetabular osteotomy. (a) Cutting lines of PAO. (b) The ischial two-thirds cut is performed from anterior to posterior via the interval space between the hip joint capsule and iliopsoas muscle. (c) The pubic complete cut located at 0.5–1.0 cm medial to the iliopectineal eminence. (d) The iliac cut is about 3.0–4.0 cm proximal to the joint of the acetabular. (e) The posterior column cut is about 0.5–1.0 cm anterior to the sciatic notch.

iliocapsularis muscle lies on the anterior articular capsule. The iliocapsularis muscle is dissected from the capsule and reflected medially.

Using a pair of Metzenbaum scissors, dissect the soft tissue between the hip joint capsule and iliopsoas muscle to reach the ischial ramus. A curved double-pointed 15 mm osteotome is used for ischium osteotomy. Under the monitoring of 30° oblique fluoroscopy view, the ischial osteotomy is performed at the infracotyloid groove to the direction of the ischial spine (Figure 9.1b). The depth of the ischial osteotomy is approximately one-half the ischial width, about 10–15 mm in depth. The tips of

the osteotome must not be out of the bone during the lateral cortex cut to minimize the risk of sciatic nerve injury. When finished with the ischial osteotomy, the hip is flexed and adducted to expose the pubic ramus. Peeling away the periosteum of the pubic ramus, two blunt Homan tractors are placed at the superior and inferior aspects of the pubic ramus subperiosteally. The pubic osteotomy is made just medial to the iliopectineal eminence (Figure 9.1c). Mobility between the two fragments of the ramus is confirmed to ensure that the osteotomy is completed.

A blunt Homan tractor is placed along the lateral side of the iliac wing to protect the gluteus medius muscle. The medial surface of the quadrilateral bone is stripped subperiosteally. A reverse Homan tractor is placed on the ischial spine. The ischial spine is an important landmark and guidepost. Osteotomy anterior to the ischial spine can ensure that the posterior column of the hemipelvis is intact. A notch is made by wide curved osteotome on the arcuate line in the pelvis, about 1 cm lower than the sacroiliac joint, 3–4 mm superior to the top of the hip joint (Figure 9.1e). The iliac cut is made by oscillating saw from ASIS to the notch (Figure 9.1d).

With the hip adducted, the posterior acetabular cut is along the medial cortex of the quadrilateral surface cortex to the ischial cut. A Schanz screw is placed into the acetabular fragment in the anterior inferior iliac spine (AIIS). The Schanz screw is levered to open the osteotomy gap slightly. With the help of the Schanz screw, the lateral cortex of the pelvis is divided. The acetabular fragment is completely mobilized.

KEY POINTS IN PERIACETABULAR OSTEOTOMY

The sequence is the osteotomy of the ischium, the osteotomy of the pubic ramus, the osteotomy superior to the acetabulum, and the osteotomy posterior to the acetabulum. The osteotomy line superior to the acetabulum extends into the ischial cut. After the acetabular fragment is freely mobilized, reposition of the acetabulum to optimize the surgical correction is the core and essence of the surgery (Figure 9.2a–d).

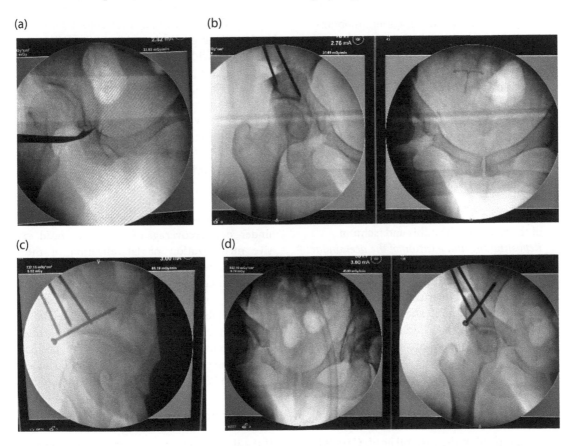

Figure 9.2 Assessment during the operation. (a) The ischial osteotomy is performed at the infracotyloid groove to the direction of ischial spine, under the monitoring of 30° oblique fluoroscopy view. (b) Temporary fix with Kirschner wires after repositioning the acetabular fragment, symmetry of bilateral foramina, and adequate repositioning of the acetabular fragment by fluoroscopy. (c) Under the monitoring of 65° oblique fluoroscopy view, assess integrity of the posterior column and accurate position of the nails. (d) Satisfaction of position of the acetabular and nails under standard fluoroscopy, with symmetry of bilateral foramina postoperation (AP view).

1. *Ischial osteotomy*: On the infracotyloid groove, approximately two-thirds of the ischium is cut from anterior to posterior. Both the medial and lateral cortex must be broken. The other one-third of the ischium is maintained to keep the continuity of the pelvic ring. This cut should be done under the C-arm to ensure the osteotomy site is precise (Figure 9.2a).

2. *Osteotomy of pubic ramus*: The core technique of osteotomy of the pubic ramus is the management of the periosteum. The osteotomy site is on the iliopectineal eminence. The angle between the pubic ramus and osteotomy line is about 20°. It is very easy to injure the obturator nerve and its concomitant vessels if the osteotome cuts through the ramus and goes too deep.

3. *Mobilization of the acetabular fragment*: One key point of acetabular fragment mobilization is that the iliac cut may be made 3–4 cm superior to the top of the acetabulum to ensure adequate supra-acetabular bone stock for reduction and to prevent the fracture of the weight-bearing part of the acetabulum. The second key point is that the posterior osteotomy must not break the posterior column and medial wall of the acetabulum (Figure 9.2c). The third key point is that the acetabulum fragment should be completely separate from the pelvis. If not, forceful correction of immobilized acetabulum may cause a stress fracture of the ramus of the pubis and ischium.

4. *Repositioning and fixation of the acetabular fragment*: After the acetabular fragment is freely movable, taking the posterior superior angle as the fulcrum, the acetabulum is repositioned with internal rotation, extension, and medial translation (Figure 9.2b). The following parameters are assessed in order: (1) Tönnis Acetabular Inclination (AI) angle 0°–10°. (2) Lateral Central Edge (LCE) angle 25°–40°. (3) Distance between medial femoral head to iliopubic line 0–10 mm. (4) anterior acetabular rim located on the superior medial on one-third of the femoral head. Care is taken to maintain the acetabular version in order to avoid limited range of motion or secondary impingement. (5) Anterior Central Edge (ACE) angle 30 ± 10°. (6) Shenton's line improved and its continuity resorted. Be cautious of the occurrence of under- and overcorrection.

Three 4.5 mm long cortical bone screws are used to fix the fragment. One of them is inserted from the AIIS to the sacroiliac joint. The other two are inserted from the iliac crest to the top of the reduced acetabulum. Hip flexion, extension, and rotation are tested to ensure the range of motion and stabilization of the acetabulum. Fluoroscopy is used to confirm if the screws are out of the articular gap (Figure 9.2d). One 3.5 mm cortical bone screw is used to fix the ASIS. Due to a smaller field of fluoroscopy, an intraoperative antero-posterior (AP) view pelvic radiograph will provide more comprehensive information (Figure 9.2d). If the optimal deformity correction is not achieved, recorrection is performed immediately.

PREVENTION OF COMPLICATIONS

The incidence of complications of PAO is relatively higher during the learning curve.[5] The occurrence of incidents may be as high as 78%. The most common complications include unsuccessful correction, intra-articular osteotomy, fracture of posterior column of the hemipelvis, fracture of ischium, delayed union of osteotomy sites, necrosis of acetabulum, and nerve injury.[6]

Unsuccessful correction of acetabulum

Unsuccessful correction of acetabulum includes[5] under- or overcoverage of the femoral head, excessive medialization or lateralization of the hip rotation center, insufficient or excessive anterior acetabular coverage, etc. The key method to avoiding these complications is the routine assessment of the acetabular position before the acetabulum is fixed. In the operation, the acetabulum is allowed to be repositioned to optimize the correction. Accurate acetabulum position is essential for a good result in a PAO; hence, greater focus is needed.

Intra-articular osteotomy

If the iliac osteotomy or posterior acetabular osteotomy is too close to the articular surface of the hip joint, the strong force generated from the correction of the acetabulum may lead to acetabular fracture.[5,6] Prevention methods include the following. First, the iliac osteotomy line should be at least 3–4 cm higher than the top of the articular surface. Second, when the quadrilateral surface is cut, the ischial spine and other bony landmarks should be fully exposed. If necessary, fluoroscopy should be used to ensure more than 1 cm posterior acetabular wall remains. If the fracture has happened on the weight-bearing area, it should be treated immediately following the conventional treatment of acetabular fracture. Treating the fracture on the medial wall of the acetabulum is not necessary, as it is not weight bearing. However, loose bodies should be taken seriously in that condition. When we perform osteotomy on ischium, pubis, and ilium, maintaining fluoroscopy monitoring in different directions may help us avoid intra-articular osteotomy. After the osteotomy is accomplished, the mobility of the fragment should be confirmed to avoid fracture caused by the force of manipulating the correction.

Nerve and blood vessel damage

In PAO, important vessels and nerves are not necessarily exposed; therefore, direct damage is rare. It is estimated that the average blood loss during the surgery is 600–800 mL.[6–8] In some difficult cases, the blood loss may be more than 1500–2000 mL. General anesthesia, low blood pressure, autologous blood transfusion, and tranexamic acid should be applied to reduce the volume of blood loss.[8,11] When the pubic ramus is exposed, the femoral nerve and femoral vein may be injured due to stretching. When performing an ischial or iliac osteotomy, the sciatic nerve is prone to be injured if the osteotome goes too deep. When fixing the acetabular fragment, the sciatic nerve is likely to be damaged if the screw goes into the greater sciatic notch.[9,10]

Delayed union of osteotomy sites

After repositioning of the acetabular fragment, gaps appear around the osteotomy lines. Large gaps (>10 mm) are prone to nonunion. Therefore, continuity of the bone should be maintained. Large gaps should be filled with bone graft.

Necrosis of acetabulum

To avoid ischemic necrosis of the acetabulum, iliac osteotomy should be performed on the site 4 cm superior to the top of the acetabulum. In addition, soft tissue on the lateral surface of the ilium should be maintained. To avoid damage to the inferior branch of the superior gluteal artery, at least 10 mm of bony surface above the acetabular should be covered by soft tissue.

Deep vein thrombosis

Deep vein thrombosis (DVT) is rare in younger patients undergoing PAO.[12] The prophylaxis of DVT is not advised routinely. We prefer early mobilization and a foot pump to prevent DVT.

PROGNOSTIC FACTORS

For patients who have complex deformities, additional surgery will give them a better outcome than only performing PAO. For instance, surgical dislocation and intra-articular surgery can be used in a deformed or avulsed acetabular labrum.[13,14] Osteochondroplasty and femoral head reduction can be used in deformity of the femoral head. Intertrochanteric or femoral neck osteotomy can be used in the correction of coxa vara and coxa valga. Derotation osteotomy can be used in the abnormal femoral neck ante version.[15–18] The other category of factors is surgery-related factors. Most of them concern acetabulum repositioning, such as under- or overcorrection of the acetabulum, abnormal acetabular version, and lateralized hip center.[19] These factors can be resolved by the routinization and refinement of the PAO procedure.

AFTERCARE

In PAO, the posterior column of hemipelvis is preserved. An intact pelvis ring makes early function training possible. (1) Ankle pumps and quad sets begin on the surgery day and during exercise in bed to avoid deep venous thrombosis. (2) With the help of the others, patients should sit by the bed with legs drooping. This is good for the adaption of the cardiovascular and venous systems on lower extremities. Twice every day is suggested, once in the morning and once in the afternoon. (3) Two or 3 days after the surgery, ambulation with crutches is allowed. Weight bearing is forbidden for the involved limb for 6 weeks. (4) Six weeks postoperatively, partial burden with crutches and lateral leg raises are added to train muscle strength around the hip. (5) From 10–12 weeks after surgery, according to the bony healing condition, which is verified roentgenographically, walking without crutches is allowed. Gait training starts at the same time.

OUTCOMES

It has been widely reported that the PAO surgery has very a satisfactory clinical outcome.[2,20,21] With adequate indications, precise techniques, and individual rehabilitation protocols, most patients with hip dysplasia can be benefit from PAO combined with other hip preservation procedures (Figure 9.3).

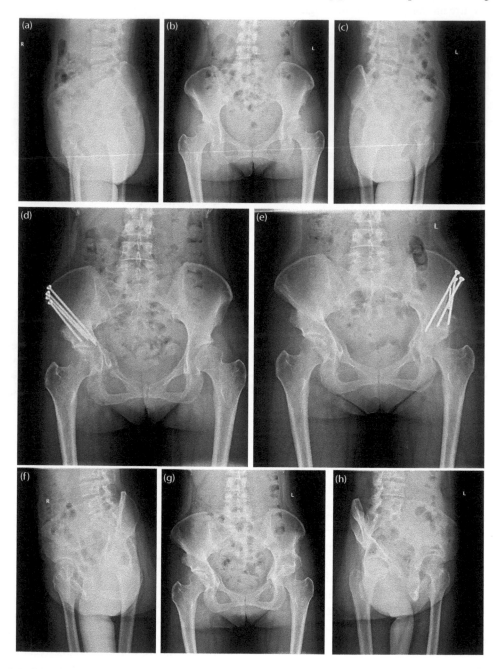

Figure 9.3 Female, 35 years old, bilateral hip pain for 1 year. (a) Right-side false oblique view pre-op, 2010.09; (b) standard AP pelvic view pre-op, 2010.09; (c) left-side false oblique view pre-op, 2010.09; (d) pelvic AP view after right side post-op, 2010.09; (e) pelvic AP view after post-op left side, 2011.08; (f) right-side false oblique view 7 years post-op, 2017.08; (g) standard AP pelvic view 6–7 years post-op, 2017.08; (h) left-side false oblique view 6 years post-op, 2017.08, no pain with normal range of motion and gaits.

REFERENCES

1. Ganz R et al. A new periacetabular osteotomy for the treatment of hip dysplasias. Technique and preliminary results. *Clin Orthop Relat Res* 1988; 232(7): 26–36.
2. Steppacher SD et al. Mean 20-year followup of Bernese periacetabular osteotomy. *Clin Orthop Relat Res* 2008; 466(7): 1633–44.
3. Clohisy JC et al. Patient-reported outcomes of periacetabular osteotomy from the prospective ANCHOR cohort study. *J Bone Joint Surg Am* 2017; 99(1): 33–41.
4. Yasunaga Y, Yamasaki T, Ochi M. Patient selection criteria for periacetabular osteotomy or rotational acetabular osteotomy. *Clin Orthop Relat Res* 2012; 470(12): 3342–54.
5. Hussell JG, Rodriguez JA, Ganz R. Technical complications of the Bernese periacetabular osteotomy. *Clin Orthop Relat Res* 1999; 363(6): 81–92.
6. Zaltz I et al. Complications associated with the periacetabular osteotomy: A prospective multicenter study. *J Bone Joint Surg Am* 2014; 96(23): 1967–74.
7. Lee CB et al. Predictors of blood loss and haematocrit after periacetabular osteotomy. *Hip Int* 2013; 23(Suppl 9): S8–13.
8. Wingerter SA et al. Does tranexamic acid reduce blood loss and transfusion requirements associated with the periacetabular osteotomy? *Clin Orthop Relat Res* 2015; 473(8): 2639–43.
9. Sierra RJ et al. Prevention of nerve injury after periacetabular osteotomy. *Clin Orthop Relat Res* 2012; 470(8): 2209–19.
10. Kalhor M et al. Reducing the risk of nerve injury during Bernese periacetabular osteotomy: A cadaveric study. *Bone Joint J* 2015; 97-B(5): 636–41.
11. Novais EN et al. Surgical treatment of adolescent acetabular dysplasia with a periacetabular osteotomy: Does obesity increase the risk of complications? *J Pediatr Orthop* 2015; 35(6): 561–4.
12. Polkowski GG et al. Screening for deep vein thrombosis after periacetabular osteotomy in adult patients: Is it necessary? *Clin Orthop Relat Res* 2014; 472(8): 2500–5.
13. Ganz R et al. Surgical dislocation of the adult hip a technique with full access to the femoral head and acetabulum without the risk of avascular necrosis. *J Bone Joint Surg Br* 2001; 83(8): 1119–24.
14. Fujii M et al. Effect of intra-articular lesions on the outcome of periacetabular osteotomy in patients with symptomatic hip dysplasia. *J Bone Joint Surg Br* 2011; 93-B: 1449–56.
15. Michael L, Reinhold G. Relative neck lengthening and intracapital osteotomy for severe Perthes and Perthes-like deformities. *Bull NYU Hosp Jt Dis* 2011; 69(Suppl. 1): S62–7.
16. Kamath AF et al. Subtrochanteric osteotomy for femoral mal torsion through a surgical dislocation approach. *J Hip Preserv Surg* 2015; 2(1): 65–79.
17. Clohisy JC et al. Periacetabular osteotomy for the treatment of acetabular dysplasia associated with major aspherical femoral head deformities. *J Bone Joint Surg Am* 2007; 89(7): 1417–23.
18. Ganz R, Horowitz K, Leunig M. Algorithm for femoral and periacetabular osteotomies in complex hip deformities. *Clin Orthop Relat Res* 2010; 468(12): 3168–80.
19. Clohisy JC et al. Medial translation of the hip joint center associated with the Bernese periacetabular osteotomy. *Iowa Orthop J* 2004; 24: 43–8.
20. Lerch TD et al. One-third of hips after periacetabular osteotomy survive 30 years with good clinical results, no progression of arthritis, or conversion to THA. *Clin Orthop Relat Res* 2017; 475: 1154–68.
21. Wells J et al. Survivorship of the Bernese periacetabular osteotomy: What factors are associated with long-term failure? *Clin Orthop Relat Res* 2016; 475(2): 1–10.

10

The Staheli shelf procedure

SWAPNIL M. KENY

INTRODUCTION

The Staheli shelf, as a procedure, is often spoken about in the same breath as periacetabular osteotomies around the hip. Unlike periacetabular osteotomies, which are redirectional procedures, the Staheli shelf procedure is purely an acetabular augmentation procedure. It is neither an osteotomy nor an arthroplasty, which it is commonly misunderstood to be.

Augmentation, by definition, is a process of making or becoming greater in size or amount. A shelf procedure by design is also a process of augmenting either a shallow acetabulum or increasing the coverage of a misshapen femoral head.

HISTORY OF SHELF PROCEDURES

Shelf procedures are the oldest acetabular procedures described in history (Figures 10.1 through 10.6).[1-5]

The use of this procedure steadily declined as more and more periacetabular osteotomies were described.[6-9]

There have been numerous descriptions of the various shelf procedures. Some placed the grafts intracapsularly, while others placed them outside the capsule. Because of the variability in methods of graft placement, problems abounded in early shelf procedures. A graft placed too high would be resorbed due to lack of loading, and one placed too low would impinge on the acetabulum.

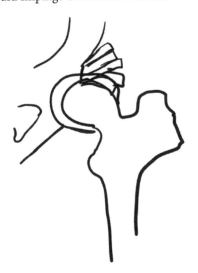

Figure 10.1 Iliac flap augmentation. (Konig F. *Verhandle Deutch Gesellsch Chir* 1891;20:75–80; Albee FH. *New York Med J* 1915;102:433–5; Jones E. *Journal of Orthopaedic Surgery* 1920;2:183; Dickson FD. *J Bone Joint Surg* 1924;6:262–77; Gill B. *Surg Clin North Am* 1926;6:147–53; Lowman CL. *JBJS* 1931;13(3):511–14; Wainwright D. *J Bone Joint Surg [Br]* 1976;58-B:159–63.)

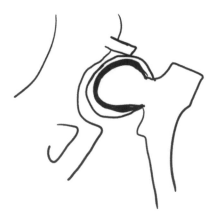

Figure 10.2 Peg augmentation. (Hey Groves EW. *Br J Surg* 1927;14:486–517; Ghomrmley RK. *JBJS* 1931;13:784–98; Compere EL. *Am J Surg* 1939;43:404–13; Flinchum D. *South Med J* 1979;72:1512–5; Love et al. *JBJS* August 1980;62B(3).

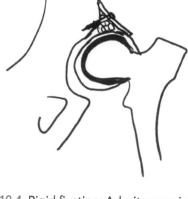

Figure 10.4 Rigid fixation: Arbeitsgemeinschaft für Osteosynthesefragen, or Association for Osteosynthesis in English (AO) screw. (Wagner H. Osteotomies for congenital hip dislocation. In: *The Hip: Proceedings of the Fourth Open Scientific Meeting of the Hip Society.* St Louis: Mosby, 1976:45–66.

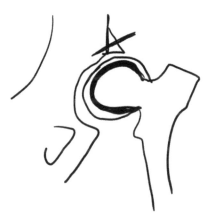

Figure 10.3 Rigid fixation: Steinmann pin. (Wilson JC. *Clin Orthop Rel Res* 1974;98:137–45.)

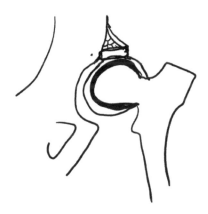

Figure 10.5 Butress. (Saito S, Takaoka K, Ono K. *J Bone Joint Surg [Br]* 1986;68-B:55–60.)

It was in these settings in the late 1960s that slotted acetabular augmentation (SAA) procedures were described. SAA was designed to provide a congruous extension to the acetabulum to augment the acetabular edge to improve coverage of the femoral head.

INDICATIONS

The Staheli procedure allows lateral, anterior, or posterior acetabular coverage. The indications are aspherical (Perthes) or eccentric incongruence (cerebral palsy, myelodysplasia, and congenital dysplasia). This extra-articular procedure is simple, effective, and harmless of morbidity.

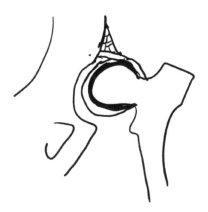

Figure 10.6 Intracapsular shelf. (Heyman CH. *J Bone Joint Surg (Am)* 1963;45:I-113–6.)

The Staheli procedure is also useful to augment redirectional periacetabular osteotomies or to manage persistent slippage due to head flattening after a proximal femoral varus osteotomy.

TECHNIQUE

Planning

The width of the augmentation is determined from an anteroposterior pelvic radiograph. The existing center edge angle and the desired width to be covered are measured.

In developmental hip dysplasia, the goal is to achieve an angle of 35°–40°. In cerebral palsy and other neuromuscular disorders, an additional 10° is added to compensate for the muscle imbalance.

In children less than 10 years, the augmentation should be wider and thicker for future appositional growth. In children less than 5 years, an additional 10° is recommended, and in children between 5 and 10 years, an additional 5° is recommended (Figure 10.7).

Arthrography

Plain x-rays depict only the ossified portion of the proximal femoral epiphysis. The largely cartilaginous portion of the femoral head remains obscured on plain x-rays. There is a definitive role of arthrography in the planning of a shelf acetabuloplasty.

Arthrography helps differentiate between spherical vs aspherical congruity, containment vs noncontainment, and coverage vs an uncovered femoral head (Figure 10.8).

Execution

The hip is opened by a standard Smith-Peterson approach. The reflected head of the rectus femoris is split, and the ends are held together by sutures.

Step 1

Making a supra-acetabular slot: A supra-acetabular slot is made about 1–1.5 cm in depth just proximal to the attachment of the hip joint capsule. A few superficial fibers of the capsule may be teased off the pelvis to gain better assess to the supra-acetabular region. The extent of the slot is determined by the extent of the desired coverage (Figure 10.9).

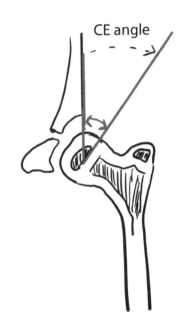

Figure 10.7 Planning the shelf by measuring the desired CE angle.

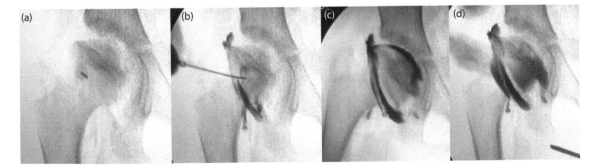

Figure 10.8 **(a–d)** Arthrographic findings of coxa magna and an uncovered femoral head in a patient of Legg–Calvé–Perthes disease where a shelf procedure was planned.

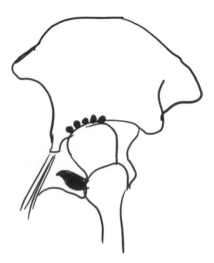

Figure 10.9 The supra-acetabular slot.

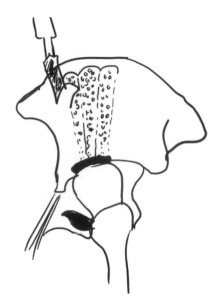

Figure 10.11 Harvesting bone grafts.

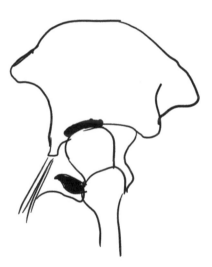

Figure 10.10 Extending the supra-acetabular slot.

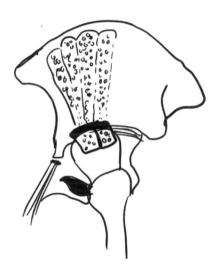

Figure 10.12 Inserting the cortical grafts in the slot.

Step 2

Extending the slot by connecting the holes: The holes of the slot are connected with the help of a bone chisel. At times, a Kerrison ronguer and a cone curette are also used to make this slot uniform (Figure 10.10).

Step 3

Harvesting strips of cortical bone from the iliac crest: Vertical strips of bone are harvested from the iliac crest with the help of a sharp osteotome (Figure 10.11).

Step 4

Placing the cortical bone grafts in the slot: The harvested strips of cortical bone graft are placed in the slot and adjusted to fit the depth of the slot in two layers to achieve a press fit (Figure 10.12).

Step 5

Securing the grafts: The grafts are secured to the shelf by suturing the cut ends of the reflected head of the rectus femoris over them (Figure 10.13).

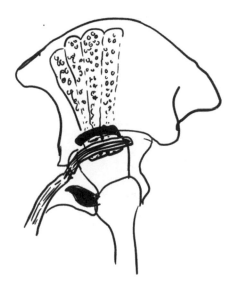

Figure 10.13 Securing the cortical bone grafts.

Step 6

Placing cancellous grafts: Harvested pure cancellous bone grafts are placed over the layers of secure cortical bone grafts beneath the abductor muscles (Figure 10.14).

Step 7:

The author recommends and has now switched over to a modification of the Staheli shelf procedure wherein a contoured reconstruction plate is secured to the iliac wing with unicortical screws and used to additionally secure the graft (Figures 10.15 through 10.17).

CLINICAL IMPLICATIONS

1. *Developmental hip dysplasia:* SAA is advisable as a procedure when periacetabular

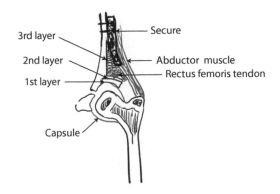

Figure 10.15 The secure shelf.

osteotomies are deemed ineffective[10] or when the severity of dysplasia is such that no other procedure can help resolve it completely. Bilateral residual acetabular dysplasia is another indication for the use of SAA, as it is a comparatively less morbid procedure than more complex osteotomies. A dysplasia with a Centre Edge Angle (CEA) angle of less than 20° is an appropriate indication for SAA.[11] However, in mature individuals, there is no clarity on the absolute indications in asymptomatic individuals.

2. *Cerebral palsy:* SAAs are effective in treating walking children with low grades of spasticity in cerebral palsy. The shelf should be planned in such a way that the CEA is greater than or equal to 50°[12] with the aim to overcorrect acetabular dysplasia. It is often performed in conjunction with a bilateral, femoral varus osteotomy.

3. *Myelodysplasias:* The results of SAAs have been reported to be excellent in adults.[13-15] This procedure is probably best suited for individuals in their second or third decade of life.

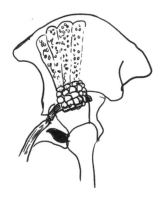

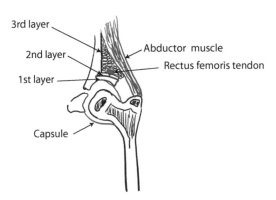

Figure 10.14 The layered shelf.

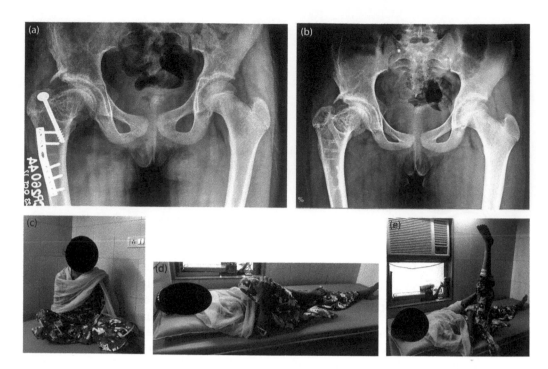

Figure 10.16 **(a–e)** Long-term results of a classic Staheli shelf procedure done for aspherical incongruity in a case of Perthes disease.

THE SLOTTED ACETABULAR AUGMENTATION AS AN ACCESSORY PROCEDURE

The Pemberton osteotomy in combination with slotted acetabular augmentation

This combination is indicated in children with neuromuscular disorders who have severe subluxation or dislocation.[12] The Pemberton procedure reduces the radius of curvature of the acetabulum, and the SAA provides an additional lateral augmentation buttress. This improves the acetabular configuration, provides a stable hip, and moves the hyaline cartilage of the hip into an weight-bearing area.

The Chiari procedure and slotted acetabular augmentation

A combination of the Chiari osteotomy and SAA[16,17] is indicated when the hip is lateralized and the CEA is <10°. A lateralized hip is in a compromised position due to increased head loading and impaired abductor function. Excessive medialization unloads the hip but also impairs function. To achieve adequate coverage, the Chiari procedure alone would require excessive medialization, thereby compromising abductor function.

Innominate osteotomies and slotted acetabular augmentation

Combined innominate osteotomies and SAA are indicated in children in the second decade. The Salter osteotomy alone increases the CEA by about 10°. When greater degrees of coverage are required, a technically easier procedure, i.e., a Salter with SAA, may be preferred to the technically demanding triple innominate osteotomy.[12]

Femoral osteotomy and slotted acetabular augmentation

The combination of augmentation and femoral osteotomy is common, simple, and effective. The surgery may be done in cases of residual uncovered head after a femoral osteotomy or for late lateral subluxation after femoral varus osteotomy.

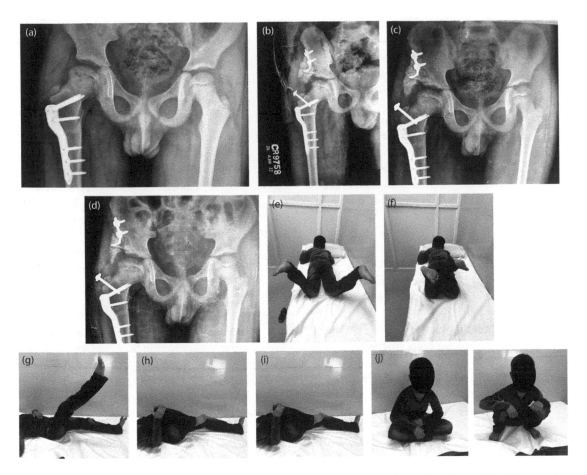

Figure 10.17 (a–j) Long-term results of the secure Staheli shelf procedure done for residual femoral head dysplasia secondary to coxa magna.

LONG-TERM RESULTS

Diab et al.[18] did a 30-year analysis and histopathological follow-up of three patients who had undergone the surgery in adolescence and in whom the block was excised for secondary hip osteoarthritis. They found that the lining of the block was essentially that of type 1 collagen, which is found in bone and capsular structures, and not type 2 collagen, which is found in the cartilage. They concluded that the shelf does not undergo cartilage metaplasia and that the head articulates with the shelf via a capsular interposition.

Pompe and Antolib[19] studied the results of shelf acetabuloplasty in adults with developmental hip dysplasia. The mean age of their patients was 38.4 years and the mean follow-up was 4 years.

They found the procedure reliable and safe and found that there were added advantages of pain relief, adequate acetabular roof coverage, and reduced peak stress on the weight-bearing area of the acetabulum.

Yoshii et al.[20] did acetabular augmentation with a glass ceramic block fixed to the acetabular edge with screws. They noted that the advantages of their surgical procedure were: (1) correct and solid fixation of the implant, (2) a shorter surgical procedure, (3) less blood loss since an autogenous graft is not used, (4) customized sizing of glass-ceramic block for coverage, (5) improved stability of the joint, (6) rapid clinical recovery with no need for cast or a brace, and (7) major improvement in pain and Harris hip scores. However, their series had only three patients with a 4-year follow-up.

REFERENCES

1. Albee FH. The bone graft wedge: Its use in the treatment of relapsing acquired and congenital dislocation of the hip. *NY Med J* 1915; 102: 433–5.
2. Dickson FD. Operative treatment of old congenital dislocations of the hip. *J Bone Joint Surg* 1924; 6: 262–71.
3. Gill AB. Discussion on paper of Dickson FD: The operative treatment of old congenital dislocation of the hip. *J Bone Joint Surg* 1924; 6: 271–7.
4. Gill AB. Operation for old or irreducible congenital dislocation of the hip. *J Bone Joint Surg* 1928; 10: 696–711.
5. Hey Groves EW. Some contributions to the reconstructive surgery of the hip. *Br J Surg* 1926; 14: 486–517.
6. Chiari K. Beckenosteotomie als pfannen-dachplastik. *Wein Med Wochenschr* 1953; 103: 707–10.
7. Colonna PC. Capsular arthroplasty for congenital dislocation of the hip: Indications and technique. Some long-term results. *J Bone Joint Surg (Am)* 1965; 47: 437–49.
8. Pemberton PA. Pericapsular osteotomy of the ilium for treatment of congenital sub-luxation and dislocation of the hip. *J Bone Joint Surg [Am]* 1978; 60: 575–85.
9. Salter RB. Innominate osteotomy in the treatment of congenital dislocation and subluxation of the hip. *J Bone Joint Surg [Br]* 1961; 43: 518–39.
10. Coleman SS. *Congenital Dysplasia and Dislocation of the Hip.* Saint Louis: C.V. Mosby, 1978.
11. Winery G. Reduction and the shelf operation for hip dysplasia in overage dislocations. *Acts Orthop Scand* 1951; 21: 32–9.
12. Staheli L, Chew D. Slotted acetabular augmentation in childhood and adolescence. *J Pediatr Orthop* 1992; 12: 569–80.
13. Courtois B, Le Saout J, Lefevre C, Kerboul B, Robin L, Miroux D, Lagdani R. The shelf operations for painful acetabular dysplasia in adults. A continuous series of 230 cases. *Int Orthopaedics* 1987; 11: 5–11.
14. Flinchum D. Shelf reconstruction for hip dysplasia. *South Med J* 1979; 72: 1512–5.
15. Van dear Ham WJ, Van dear Heyden AM. Long-term results of the shelf operation in 56 patients with early coxarthrosis. *Acta Orthop Scand* 1986; 57: 386.
16. Bailey TE Jr, Hall JE. Chiari medial displace-ment osteotomy. *J Pediatric Orthop* 1985; 5: 635–41.
17. Fernandez DL, Isler B, Muller ME. Chiari's osteotomy. A note on technique. *Clin Orthop* 1984; 185: 53–8.
18. Diab M, Clark JM, Weis MA, Eyre DR. Acetabular augmentation at 6–30 year follow up. *J Bone Joint Surg [Br]* 2005; 87-B: 32–5.
19. Pompe B, Antolib V. Slotted acetabular augmentation for the treatment of residual hip dysplasia in adults: Early results of 12 patients. *Arch Orthop Trauma Surg* 2007; 127: 719–23.
20. Yoshii S, Oka M, Yamamuro T, Ikeda K, Murakam H. Acetabular augmentation using a glass-ceramic block. *Acta Orthop Scand* 2000; 71(6): 580–4.
21. Konig F. Osteoplastische behandlung der kongenitalen heuftgelensluxation mit dem-onstration eines pareparates. *Verhandle Deutch Gesellsch Chir* 1891; 20: 75–80.
22. Albee FH. The bone graft wedge: its uses in the treatment of relapsing acquired, and congenital dislocation of the hip. *New York Med J* 1915; 102: 433–5.
23. Jones E. The operative treatment of irreduc-ible paralytic dislocation of the hip joint. *Journal of Orthopaedic Surgery* 1920; 2: 183.
24. Dickson FD. The operative treatment of old congenital dislocation of the hip. *J Bone Joint Surg* 1924; 6: 262–77.
25. Gill B. Operation for old congenital disloca-tion of the hip. *Surg Clin North Am* 1926; 6: 147–53.
26. Lowman CL. The double-leaf shelf opera-tion for congenital dislocation of the hip. *JBJS* 1931; 13(3): 511–14.
27. Wainwright D. The shelf operation for hip dysplasia in adolescence. *J Bone Joint Surg [Br]* 1976; 58-B: 159–63.
28. Hey Groves EW. Some contributions to the reconstructive surgery of the hip. *Br J Surg* 1927; 14: 486–517.
29. Ghomrmley RK. Use of anterior superior spine and crest of ilium in surgery of hip joint. *JBJS* 1931; 13: 784–98.

30. Compere EL. The shelf operation for congenital dislocation of the hip. *Am J Surg* 1939; 43: 404–13.
31. Flinchum D. Shelf reconstruction for hip dysplasia. *South Med J* 1979; 72: 1512–5.
32. Love et al. *JBJS* August 1980; 62B(3).
33. Wilson JC. Surgical treatment of the dysplasia acetabulum in adolescents. *Clin Orthop Rel Res* 1974; 98: 137–45.
34. Wagner H. Osteotomies for congenital hip dislocation. In: *The Hip: Proceedings of the Fourth Open Scientific Meeting of the Hip Society*. St Louis: Mosby, 1976: 45–66.
35. Saito S, Takaoka K, Ono K. Tectoplasty for painful dislocation or subluxation of the hip: Long-term evaluation of a new acetabuloplasty. *J Bone Joint Surg [Br]* 1986; 68-B: 55–60.
36. Heyman CH. Long term results following a bone shelf operation for congenital and some other dislocations of the hip in children. *J Bone Joint Surg (Am)* 1963; 45: I-113-6.

11

Chiari osteotomy

K. MOHAN IYER

References 74

The Chiari osteotomy is a procedure designed by Karl Chiari in the 1950s. In general, young patients with fixed subluxations and/or femoral head deformities are well suited for this procedure. It is mainly a salvage procedure for treatment of pain in an incongruous hip. It is a capsular interposition arthroplasty and an extra-articular acetabular augmentation using a slightly inclined (distal–lateral to proximal–medial) supra-acetabular iliac osteotomy. Chiari's original methods included relatively minimal exposure through an anterolateral approach. He made a slightly upsloping, inferiorly concave osteotomy just above the joint capsule. He rarely used internal fixation, and patients were immobilized in a hip spica cast. Although the Chiari procedure is one of the easier pelvic osteotomies with an easier learning curve, its results are very dependent on precise surgical technique.

It mainly increases the coverage of the hip joint by medializing the hip center, where there is fibrocartilaginous transformation of the superior capsule. When he initially presented 200 procedures, it had about two-thirds good to excellent outcomes, while one-third were improved in the result. Similar results were also reported by others.[1] The main aspect of pain relief was predictable, while the Trendelenburg gait still persisted when trochanteric advancement was considered to alleviate the Trendelenburg gait.

The Chiari procedure mainly results in the accomplishment of two goals:

1. The displaced superior fragment forms a lateral shelf over the pathologically lateralized and uncovered femoral head, while the proximal fragment can be manipulated anteriorly as well as laterally. Through the process of metaplastic transformation, this new buttress and the interposed capsule produce a fibrocartilaginous articular surface, which broadens the surface area available for weight bearing and also prevents progression of the subluxation.
2. The medialization of the hip joint, usually around 1.5 cm, which decreases the resulting joint reaction forces. The inferior fragment is hinged on the symphysis pubis, and displacement actually slightly increases the already abnormal inclination of the acetabulum.

It is primarily a greater load-bearing osteotomy. The indications are as follows:

1. Unique: It is the only pelvic osteotomy that is indicated primarily when the hip is incongruous and when femoral head coverage cannot be achieved by other methods of reconstruction.
2. It is recommended when the femoral head is irregular or cannot be centered in the acetabulum by abduction and internal rotation of the hip.

3. It can also be performed in the presence of severe instability.
4. It is also used in the prevention or treatment of pain, rather than primary improvement in hip function, as the principal objective of this procedure.

It is an oblique osteotomy in a proximal and medial direction, beginning at the lateral margin of the dysplastic acetabulum at an angle of 10°. The optimal location to begin the osteotomy is within 1 cm or less of the capsular insertion on the lateral margin of the dysplastic acetabulum. An osteotomy that is too distal may enter the joint or place increased pressure on the femoral head when the hip is displaced medially. An osteotomy that is too proximal may fail to provide adequate load bearing for the femoral head.

Technique:

1. The osteotomy is made precisely between the insertion of the capsule and the reflected head of the rectus femoris.
2. It ends distal to the Anterior Inferior Iliac Spine (AIIS) anteriorly and in the sciatic notch posteriorly (Figure 11.1).
3. With a straight, narrow osteotome, start osteotomy on lateral table with plane direction. The distal fragment is now displaced medially by forcing the limb into abduction hinging at the symphysis pubis.

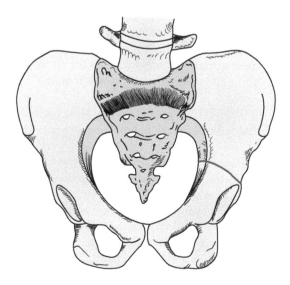

Figure 11.1 Line of osteotomy.

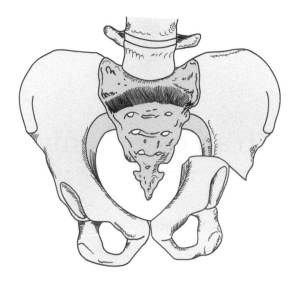

Figure 11.2 Medial displacement of the proximal fragment.

4. It is displaced enough medially so that the proximal fragment completely covers the femoral head, i.e., about half of the thickness of the bone (Figure 11.2).
5. If necessary, the fragments may be transfixed by screws driven obliquely directed 10° superiorly toward the inner table.

Disadvantages:

1. The insertions of the hip abductor muscles are displaced medially and proximally as the hip is displaced along the slope of the osteotomy.
2. It reduces the strength of the hip abductor muscles and decreases their mechanical advantage.

Technical considerations:

1. Risk of posterior displacement of the distal osteotomy fragment.
2. Greater risk when the osteotomy is more horizontal.
3. The osteotomy that is curved from anterior to posterior will help resist posterior displacement of the acetabulum.
4. A dome-shaped osteotomy also provides more anterior and posterior support to the hip capsule and femoral head.
5. It is recommended that 80% of the femoral head should be covered following displacement.

Most patients who are candidates for a Chiari osteotomy have a limp and a Trendelenburg gait preoperatively. Usually only the antalgic portion of a limp will be improved by the procedure. In general, advise patients that their Trendelenburg lurch may not improve and can worsen postoperatively because the traditional surgical approach involves stripping of the tensor and much of the abductor musculature from the lateral iliac wall. Some authors have reported an improvement in the Trendelenburg lurch in a majority of patients, attributing the improvement to the medialized hip center and to advancement of the greater trochanter in some patients.

There are certain contraindications to the Chiari osteotomy, as follows:

1. Marked joint stiffness.
2. A relative contraindication is physiologic age over 45 years because of the poorer results in this age group.
3. Totally uncovered hip.
4. Severe proximal migration prohibiting access to the appropriate iliac slope for the osteotomy, resulting in insufficient breadth of the iliac wing and dangerous proximity to the sciatic notch.

When there is significant coxa vara or incongruity (femoral head flattening), a valgus-extension and inter trochanteric osteotomy (ITO) can be combined with the Chiari procedure, which moves the broader surface of the head into the weight-bearing zone, where superior–lateral eccentric loading of the head would otherwise occur. This decision to perform a valgus-extension osteotomy is guided by preoperative adduction and abduction radiographs.

The Chiari medial displacement osteotomy is a procedure that uses cancellous bone of the ilium to contain the femoral head and bear weight. The Chiari osteotomy can produce good or excellent results in adolescent or young adult patients who have specific indications, including painful dysplasia or uncoverage of the femoral head, in which incongruity or poor acetabular development make other reconstructive procedures inappropriate.[2]

It is an acetabular osteotomy salvage procedure that is indicated in patients without a concentrically reducible hip; modified shelf osteotomy above acetabulum with or without medial displacement of

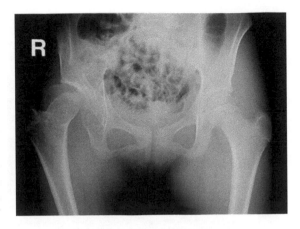

Figure 11.3 Anteroposterior radiograph of the patient at the age of 13, showing residual acetabular dysplasia with a center-edge angle of 9° and 59% femoral head coverage. (Reproduced with the kind permission of Dr. Khalid A. Bakarman, Department of Orthopedics, College of Medicine and King Khalid University Hospital, King Saud University, Riyadh, Kingdom of Saudi Arabia.)

acetabulum. The distal fragment is displaced medially and upward as the osteotomy hinges on the symphysis pubis when the hip capsule is interposed between the newly formed acetabular roof and femoral head, when medialization will decrease the lever arm and hence reduce joint loading, thereby altering the biomechanics of the hip joint to result in an elimination of the Trendelenburg gait. The level of pelvic osteotomy is crucial (Figure 11.3).

It should be less than 5 mm from the joint space and directed with a cephalic inclination of 10° toward the sacroiliac joint. A high-level osteotomy will create an undesired step (Figure 11.4) between the femoral head and the new acetabulum.

A modified technique (Figure 11.5) used the distal transfer of the lateral part of the iliac bone without the need to dismantle the Chiari osteotomy (Figure 11.6) and resulted in good outcome.[3] The Chiari osteotomy is a supra-acetabular medial displacement pelvic osteotomy, which was developed by Chiari in the 1950s, mainly to cover the femoral head completely by enlarging the inadequate acetabular roof as seen in primary hip dysplasia, where there is a discrepancy between acetabular and femoral head size, as seen in early Perthes disease. The Chiari osteotomy provided an improvement in femoral head coverage and hip congruency, as indicated by radiographs that showed progressive spherical remodeling of the femoral head and

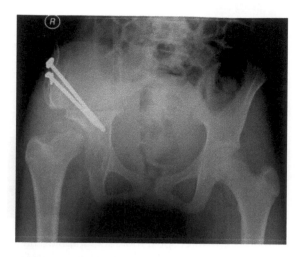

Figure 11.4 Anteroposterior radiograph immediately after Chiari osteotomy showing a high-level osteotomy (14 mm). (Reproduced with the kind permission of Dr. Khalid A. Bakarman, Department of Orthopedics, College of Medicine and King Khalid University Hospital, King Saud University, Riyadh, Kingdom of Saudi Arabia.)

improvement of the concentricity.[4] The main aim in the treatment of Legg–Calvé–Perthes disease is to prevent femoral head deformation by containing the head within the acetabulum. Currently, surgical containment methods are the mainstay of treatment, and pelvic osteotomies have been shown to be successful, including triple pelvic osteotomy (TPO), Salter osteotomy, Chiari osteotomy, and shelf procedure. Total hip arthroplasty after a successful Chiari osteotomy leads to medium-term results similar to those of other dysplastic hips. A Chiari osteotomy may delay the need for total hip arthroplasty and may facilitate acetabular reconstruction, but does not seem to compromise the medium-term clinical or radiographic outcome.[5] Early developmental dysplasia of hip (DDH) is considered a good indication for Chiari pelvic osteotomy because of the good results at 10 years or more. Even with advanced DDH, a flat femoral head predicts a good surgical outcome, but patients with a spherical femoral head may experience early progression to osteoarthritis.[6]

In this procedure, there is a capsule that is interposed between the newly formed acetabular roof and the femoral head, and it is mainly indicated in congenital subluxation in children 4–6 years or older, including adults. It is also indicated in dysplastic hips with osteoarthritis, coxa magna after Perthes disease, or vascular necrosis after treatment of congenital dysplasia. In addition, it is indicated for paralytic dislocation due to muscular weakness or spasticity routine preoperative antibiotic and thromboembolic prophylaxis are given before the procedure, The patient is placed supine on a radiolucent table, with the leg slightly abducted and externally rotated. A 10-cm-long anterolateral ilioinguinal incision beginning at the iliac crest and extending medially or a Smith-Peterson approach may be preferred for more exposure, in larger patients, or for combined pelvic and femoral osteotomies through one incision.

The hip is approached by a Smith-Peterson approach anterolaterally between the capsule and the reflected head of the rectus femoris, ending

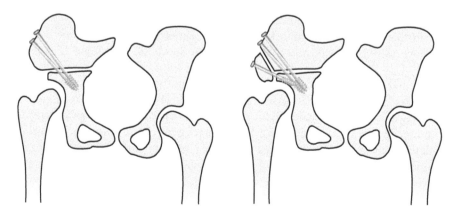

Figure 11.5 Distal transfer of the proximal outer iliac bone table to solve the problem of the step that was created by a high-level cut during Chiari osteotomy. (Reproduced with the kind permission of Dr. Khalid A. Bakarman, Department of Orthopedics, College of Medicine and King Khalid University Hospital, King Saud University, Riyadh, Kingdom of Saudi Arabia.)

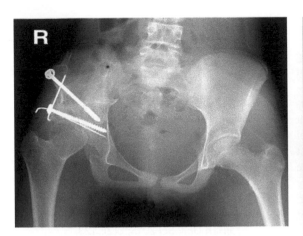

Figure 11.6 Postoperative standing antero-posterior radiograph showing center-edge angle of 40° and 100% femoral head coverage. (Reproduced with the kind permission of Dr. Khalid A. Bakarman, Department of Orthopedics, College of Medicine and King Khalid University Hospital, King Saud University, Riyadh, Kingdom of Saudi Arabia.)

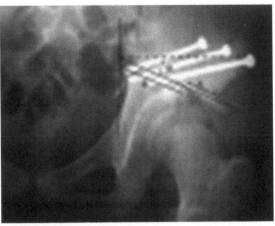

Figure 11.7 Radiographic parameters of Chiari osteotomy. Angle of Chiari (α), the angle between the line parallel to the reference line (intertear drop line), and the osteotomy line. (Reproduced with the kind permission of Mohsen Karami and the *Journal of Children's Orthopaedics*.)

distal to the anterior inferior iliac spine anteriorly and in the sciatic notch posteriorly. With a straight, narrow osteotome, the osteotomy is started on the lateral table with a plane directed 20° superiorly toward the inner table. The distal fragment is then displaced medially by forcing the limb into abduction hinging at the symphysis pubis. It is displaced enough medially so that the proximal fragment completely covers the femoral head (about half the thickness of bone), and if need be, the fragments may be transfixed with a screw driven obliquely (Figure 11.7).

The interval between the sartorius and tensor fascia lata muscles is developed with retraction of the tensor laterally and preserving the lateral femoral cutaneous nerve medially. Expose the iliac wing by subperiosteal dissection medially and laterally, and release the tensor, sartorius, and direct head of the rectus femoris from their origins off the ilium, which exposes the anterior and lateral hip joint capsule. Separate the tendon of the rectus femoris from the capsule and divide the reflected head, which serves as a marker for the level of the osteotomy. Dissect subperiostially from the capsule to the sciatic notch posteriorly and place a blunt retractor, such as a relatively radiolucent flexible metal ribbon and likewise place a retractor medially after careful dissection to the greater

sciatic notch. This is confirmed radiographically as the starting point and direction of the osteotomy with a pin drilled into the pelvis just superior to the capsule. A curved osteotome is used to complete the semicylindrical osteotomy, inclining 15° superiorly from inferolateral to superomedial. A Gigli saw can be used to cut the most posterior portion from the sciatic notch anteriorly about 1 cm, which reduces the danger of injuring the neurovascular structures in the sciatic notch from an osteotome or bone splinters or spikes. After carefully completing the osteotomy of the medial cortex, displace the osteotomy. Release any traction on the leg and abduct the hip. Displace the inferior fragment medially 1–1.5 cm but at times up to 2.5 cm as needed to provide 80–100% lateral coverage of the femoral head. Then, harvest a supplemental corticocancellous shelf graft from the iliac wing as needed and wedge this into the osteotomy or otherwise secure the graft. Use internal fixation from the iliac wing across the osteotomy to eliminate the need for a spica cast in adults. In cases where more than 75% displacement of the osteotomy is required, consider placement of a bone graft medially to assist with healing and confirm this by x-ray. Close the wound in layers with a suction drain. Repair all muscles, suturing the tendons back to bone through drill holes where the initial release was from bone, and also avoid injury to the lateral femoral cutaneous nerve.

Postoperatively, start partial weight bearing after 6 weeks, followed by graduated full weight bearing after 3 months.

Pain relief is significant in 80–90% of patients since pain relief is the primary aim in adults. Gait improvement is less dramatic than pain relief because a positive Trendelenburg limp may persist in some and normalize in others. Osteotomy of the greater trochanter with advancement shows more significant improvement in the Trendelenburg test. Although abduction may improve, overall range of motion does not. If the capsule is opened at the time of surgery, either for inspection or resection of a labral tear, secure repair is essential, as an intact capsule is a prerequisite for a successful Chiari result. Gadolinium-enhanced MRI is now the preferred method for evaluating the labrum.

In adults, the results are best and most durable in patients who are younger and have no signs of arthritis at the time of surgery. There are 80% good results for patients younger than 45 years of age at operation (age range 30–44 years) and only 50% good results for patients older than 44 years of age.

The conversion of a Chiari to a total hip replacement (THR) is difficult, and revision of the acetabulum with the presence of scars, bone defects, and anatomic distortions should be anticipated strictly.

REFERENCES

1. Hogh J, MacNicol MF. The Chiari pelvic osteotomy: A long-term review of clinical and radiographic results. *J Bone Joint Surg Br* 1987; 69: 365–73.
2. Karami M, Fitoussi F, Ilharreborde B, Penneçot G-F, Mazda K, Bensahel H. The results of Chiari pelvic osteotomy in adolescents with a brief literature review. *J Child Orthop* 2008; 2(1): 63–8.
3. Bakarman KA. New technique to overcome surgical pitfall during Chiari osteotomy. *J Taibah Univ Sci* 2013; 8(2): 123–5.
4. Reddy RR, Morin C. Chiari osteotomy in Legg–Calvé–Perthes disease. *J Pediatr Orthop B* 2005; 14(1): 1–9, Hip.
5. Hashemi-Nejad A, Haddad FS, Tong KM, Muirhead-Allwood SK, Catterall A. Does Chiari osteotomy compromise subsequent total hip arthroplasty? *J Arthroplasty* 2002; 17(6): 731–9.
6. Yanagimoto S, Hotta H, Izumida R, Sakamaki T. Long-term results of Chiari pelvic osteotomy in patients with developmental dysplasia of the hip: Indications for Chiari pelvic osteotomy according to disease stage and femoral head shape. *J Orthop Sci* 2005; 10(6): 557–63.

12

Pelvic support osteotomy: The Schanz method

MANDAR AGASHE

INTRODUCTION

The problem of an unstable or damaged hip that is unsuitable for arthrodesis or arthroplasty is still present, especially in developing countries.[1,2] In such a scenario, the pelvic support osteotomy is a useful salvage procedure in adolescents and young adults who are incapacitated due to pain, limp, or both.[3,4] The surgery not only reduces pain and instability but also improves hip biomechanics by providing anatomical support to the unstable hip joint.[4]

HISTORICAL PERSPECTIVE

This procedure was primarily designed for untreated congenital dislocation of the hip (CDH), especially before the era of complex reconstructive procedures for CDH like the Salter and Pemberton osteotomies.[5] The credit for coining the term "pelvic support osteotomy (PSO)" should be given to Lance, who used it in 1936 for the subtrochanteric osteotomies used for the treatment of CDH.[6] The various types of osteotomies in this group are named after the surgeons who first described them and are different in terms of the level of osteotomy and the principle by which they provide stability to the unstable hip. Interestingly, some of these osteotomies predate the description of Lance. Lorenz was in fact the first to describe a procedure of a sort in which the osteotomy was performed in the subtrochanteric region and the proximal fragment abutted against the acetabulum by its almost vertical and proximal displacement.[7] A few years later, Schanz developed and described his own osteotomy in which the osteotomy, though performed at a similar location as the Lorenz osteotomy, was not accompanied by a proximal migration of the shaft but only a valgus and extension component of the same.[8] Von Baeyer also described an osteotomy where the cut is at the level of the lesser trochanter and it is the lesser trochanter that abuts against the acetabulum and provides stability.[5]

Over the years, there were some problems associated with these pelvic support osteotomies, namely abduction contractures, loss of parallelism of the limbs, valgus knee thrust and knee pain, and inability to correct limb-length discrepancy (LLD), which is invariably present in unilateral cases.[2,9] It was Ilizarov in 1988 who solved this conundrum by adding a second distal osteotomy at the metadiaphyseal level that would cause varus, thus inducing parallelism to the limb and also enabling lengthening so as to correct the LLD. This method has become immensely popular, especially after Rozbruch and Paley published their article on reconstruction of postseptic sequelae with the Ilizarov hip reconstruction (IHR) method.[10] In the last few years, the IHR has become the treatment of choice and the indications for performing an isolated Schanz procedure have dwindled.

INDICATIONS

The indication for performing a Schanz pelvic osteotomy is any hip that is unstable or in severe varus, which is not amenable to more standard reconstructive procedures like total hip replacement (THR). It is especially useful in developing countries with lower socioeconomic strata who cannot afford the more expensive option of THR and would like a more mobile hip, unlike an arthrodesed hip.[11]

The indications for a pelvic support osteotomy (PSO) (Schanz type) are:

1. Untreated unilateral DDH (more than 12 years of age)[12]
2. Untreated bilateral DDH (more than 8–9 years of age)—relative indication[12]
3. Septic hip sequelae—Hunka type 4A/4B and 5[13-15]
4. After girdlestone arthroplasty
5. Chronic spastic hip dislocation in severely involved cerebral palsy with nonreconstructable hip with poor femoral head cartilage[3]

PRINCIPLE AND PREOPERATIVE PLANNING

The basic principle of a valgizing proximal femoral osteotomy is to create a proximal valgus that is enough to eliminate the adduction of the limb completely. This creates an adequate tightening of the abductors and is the most important factor for eliminating the abductor lurch.

It is important to note the difference between the two main osteotomies for pelvic support, namely the Lorenz and Schanz osteotomies, in order to correctly implement the principles used in both.

The Lorenz subtrochanteric osteotomy is a valgus osteotomy at the subtrochanteric level that has a medial as well as proximal displacement of the femoral shaft, so much so that the almost vertical disposition of the femoral shaft "supports" the pelvis from abutment. However, it has been noted that the severe prominence of the proximal fragment on the pelvis itself limits the range of motion and produces a very unsightly deformity that is difficult to correct or remodel.[5,7]

The Schanz osteotomy, on the other hand, works on a different principle. In this osteotomy, a valgus and extension component is present but without the proximal migration. The distal fragment is medialized in order to lock the valgus at a particular angle. The valgus increases the tension in the abductors and thus improves the Trendelenburg sign, and the extension reduces the excessive load on the false socket and reduces lumbar lordosis and thus prevents or decreases lumbar pain. Since there is no proximal migration of the distal fragment, there is a theoretical advantage of less abutment. However, it has been found in clinical studies that there is always some abutment that occurs when the limb is brought to neutral by adduction.[2,5,8]

This concept was further explained by Milch, who put forth an angle known as "postosteotomy angle" and its relation with the "pelvic inclination angle" (Figure 12.1).

He said that if the postosteotomy angle is more than the pelvic inclination angle, then impingement occurs on attempted adduction of the limb to neutral. Though the excessive valgus angle eliminates the Trendelenburg gait effectively, it has to be compensated for by tilting of the pelvis, valgus thrust on the knee, and eversion of the foot. This is even more difficult to compensate for in the case of bilateral hip affections.

PREOPERATIVE PLANNING

The preoperative planning is divided into two parts: clinical and radiological.

Clinical method

A. *Range of abduction-adduction*: This is the most important of all ranges. It is important to note

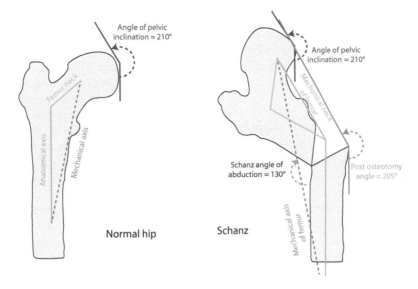

Figure 12.1 Schematic figure of the pelvic inclination angle in a normal hip and in a hip where a Schanz pelvic support osteotomy has been performed, as described by Milch.

the adduction that is possible with the pelvis immobile. This can be done in two ways: one by adducting the limb and flexing it over the contralateral limb so that the popliteal fossa of the operative limb rests on the knee of the contralateral limb. The other method is a measure of pure adduction that can be done by maximally abducting the contralateral limb, then adducting the affected side so as to know the maximal adduction without flexion interfering with the measurement.

There is some controversy regarding how much valgus is to be added to the proximal osteotomy. Initial articles suggested valgus equal to the amount of adduction possible. However, there have been instances of significant remodeling and loss of correction. This was solved by later authors, especially Paley and Nayagam, where they suggested adding an overcorrection of around 10–15° to the osteotomy to compensate for the remodeling.

B. *Quantum of flexion deformity*: The flexion deformity is caused by a severe contracture of the anterior structures, especially the psoas. Correction of just the valgus without correcting the flexion deformity leads to persistence of hyperlordosis. Hence, it is imperative to determine the amount of flexion deformity of the hip during planning. In some cases, along with the flexion deformity, the actual total

flexion arc is restricted, even to less than 90°. This preoperative arc of motion needs to be documented, as after surgery, the patient may have an inability to flex the hip completely for activities like squatting when the flexion deformity is corrected.

C. *Rotations*: The third plane of movement that needs to be checked is the rotational plane. The rotations of the hip need to be checked in full adduction and correlated with the foot progression angle. Hip rotations need to be checked at the time of fixation of the osteotomy, as external rotation of the distal fragment is a common problem that occurs and leads to a very unsightly foot progression angle.

Radiological planning

Radiological planning is based on the following x-rays: an x-ray of the pelvis with both hips; anteroposterior view with the pelvis squared; anteroposterior view of the pelvis with the ipsilateral hip maximally adducted; and a long leg standing view of both lower limbs with the pelvis squared, limb lengths equalized with a block of appropriate size under the short limb, and patella facing forward. The x-ray with the limb in maximum adduction is very important, as it shows the position of the proximal fragment after the osteotomy and also the level and position of the osteotomy at the point where it coincides with the ischial tuberosity. The long leg x-ray is important to know the exact limb-length discrepancy, any distal femoral or tibial deformities, and the magnitude of the pelvic obliquity.

SURGICAL PROCEDURE

The procedure is performed under appropriate anesthesia, usually epidural anesthesia with a catheter in place so as to provide good postoperative analgesia. The position is supine with a small radiolucent bump under the ipsilateral buttock. The image intensifier TV (C-arm) is positioned on the opposite side of the table, perpendicular to the body. The entire lower limb is painted and draped free in order to check the rotation of the entire limb.

The osteotomy fixation can be done in two ways, either with an external fixator or a plate. Here, the process of performing the osteotomy and fixation with an external fixator will be described in detail.

For the external fixator, either a universal external fixator (Association for Osteosynthesis [AO] or Aesculup type) or a limb reconstruction system (LRS)–monolateral frame can be used. Some clinicians have used the Ilizarov ring fixator system for the same.

The first Schanz pin is placed proximally at the level of the greater trochanter. The limb is kept in maximal adduction with the ipsilateral popliteal fossa on the contralateral patella so as to recreate the flexion deformity. This pin is placed at an angle of around 10–15° to the horizontal. This will give the angle of adduction plus some amount of overcorrection. The second pin is inserted in the mid-diaphysis of the femur in the distal fragment. This pin is inserted with the limb parallel to the opposite limb in neutral adduction-abduction and rotation, and its direction should be perpendicular to the shaft of the femur.

After these two pins, the osteotomy is performed at the point where the shaft intersects the ischial tuberosity with the limb in maximal adduction. A small 3–5 cm incision is made anterolaterally and the fascia is incised widely proximally and distally. The vastus lateralis is separated by blunt dissection and the bone exposed. The periosteum is incised in a small area and soft tissues are protected using small pointed Hohmann's spikes subperiosteally. Multiple drill holes are made with

copious irrigation and the osteotomy completed using a sharp 10-mm osteotome. Once the osteotomy is completed, the two Schanz pins are made parallel to each other and fixed using the monolateral frame or the connecting rod. This automatically imparts a sufficient valgus to the osteotomy. Also, the flexion deformity is corrected since the first pin is inserted with some flexion of the limb. Once these two pins are connected together, the angulation at the osteotomy is confirmed on the C-arm, as any further change would be difficult after this stage.

Once the osteotomy is fixed, further pins are inserted in the proximal and distal fragments. These pins will be parallel to the first two pins and connected to the monolateral frame. Usually, two pins are inserted in the proximal fragment and three pins in the distal fragment. All pins need to be bicortical for good hold. Also, care needs to be taken so as to prevent soft tissue clumping and skin tethering between the proximal and distal set of pins. The osteotomy site is irrigated with normal saline and closed in layers. All screws and nuts are tightened in the fixator frame, and sterile dressing is applied.

A similar procedure can be performed using a 3.5- or 4.5-mm dynamic compression plate (DCP) that is bent at a particular degree to accommodate the valgus required (Figure 12.2a–d).

For higher degrees of correction, this method is slightly more difficult due to the difficulty in bending a plate to such a degree as well as a chance of plate failure due to the same.

POSTOPERATIVE CARE

Usually no plaster or immobilization is required. Generally a long knee brace is given for pain relief and support. Knee and hip range of motion are started soon after surgery as soon as pain becomes tolerable. Pin tract care is taught to the patient and caregivers. As a general rule, weight bearing is deferred until sound osteotomy union at around 6–8 weeks. Fixator removal is done at around 3 months after good healing.

COMPLICATIONS AND DIFFICULTIES

The commonest complication or difficulty is getting adequate valgus in the osteotomy in order to completely tension the abductors. The key to this

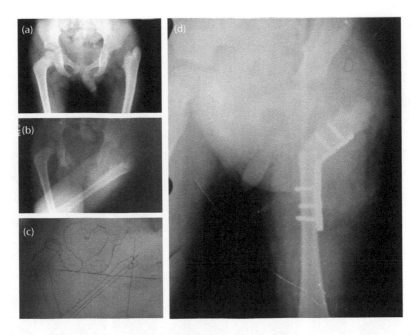

Figure 12.2 Series of figures showing a Schanz pelvic support osteotomy done using a bent 3.5-mm DCP. **(a)** Plain radiograph of the pelvis with both hips—anteroposterior view showing a Choi type 4 B septic hip sequelae of the left side. **(b)** Plain radiograph of the pelvis with both hips of the same patient with the operative hip in full adduction in order to know the available amount of adduction possible and the level of the osteotomy that coincides with the level of the ischial tuberosity. **(c)** Paper tracing of the same x-ray showing preoperative planning for the Schanz PSO. **(d)** Plain radiograph of the same child after the surgery showing excellent correction and fixation with a 3.5-mm DCP bent at around 50°.

step is to see to it that the periosteum is released well on the medial side of the osteotomy and the distal fragment is completely free and able to translate medially. The other reason for this loss of correction is performing this osteotomy too early in life. It has been seen that there is considerable remodeling of the proximal femoral osteotomy if it is performed before 11 years of age.

Pin tract infections: Pin tract infections are quite common in proximal femoral osteotomies fixed with external fixators. In the Schanz osteotomy, there is considerable mobilization of the proximal pin, with resultant clumping of the skin between the proximal and distal sets of pins. This results in skin stretching around the pin tracts, which is a precursor for pin tract infections. To prevent this occurrence, care should be taken to release the skin around the pin tracts and see to it that the skin does not get inverted into the pin tracts.

Delayed and nonunion: Delayed and nonunion is a complication seen very rarely, especially in younger patients. One of the causes of delayed union is unstable fixation, especially in patients with neurological disorders like cerebral palsy that have a high chance of pin loosening and pin walk-outs.

MODIFICATIONS OF THE TECHNIQUE

The major limitation of a Schanz proximal femoral osteotomy is the limitation of adduction of the hip with a severe valgus thrust on the knee.[2] This can be considerably disconcerting, especially in bilateral cases where the pelvis is unable to square with an abduction contracture of both hips. Also, limb-length discrepancy used to remain uncorrected with this technique. Ilizarov in 1988[10] and Rozbruch and Paley in 2005[2] solved this problem by adding a distal varizing osteotomy in the metadiaphyseal region of the femur where lengthening could also be performed (Figure 12.3a–c).

With the varus obtained in this osteotomy, adequate valgus could be given in the proximal osteotomy without fear of causing an abduction deformity and knee problems. Hence, in the last

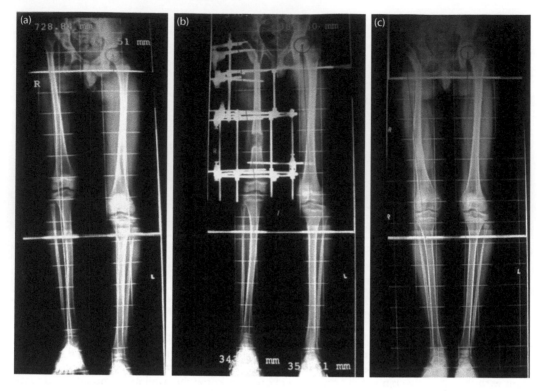

Figure 12.3 Series of figures showing a Schanz osteotomy coupled with a distal varizing osteotomy, as described by Ilizarov and Rozbruch for an untreated congenital hip dislocation in a 14-year-old boy. (a) Plain long leg film (scannogram) of both lower limbs—anteroposterior view of a 14-year-old with untreated right-sided congenital hip dislocation with a high riding femoral head with a 4.5 cm shortening. (b) Postoperative scannogram of the both lower limbs of the same patient showing a Ilizarov ring fixator being used for fixation of both the proximal and distal osteotomies. Lengthening is going on through the distal varizing osteotomy and good bone formation is seen. (c) Long leg scannogram of both lower limbs about 6 months after fixator removal, showing good healing of both osteotomies and good correction of limb-length discrepancy.

few years, the indications for performing an isolated Schanz osteotomy have decreased and the primary indications remain nonsalvageable hips in nonambulatory children with neurological conditions like cerebral palsy.

CONCLUSIONS

The Schanz low subtrochanteric valgus extension osteotomy is a worthwhile option in unstable nonsalvageable hips in which standard reconstructive options are not available. It provides adequate tension to the abductors and is helpful in decreasing the abductor lurch. The addition of a distal varizing osteotomy is a newer modification that also allows realignment of the mechanical axis and correction of limb-length discrepancy.

REFERENCES

1. Agashe M, Tong XB, Song SH, Park YE, Hong JH, Lee H, Song HR. Pelvic support osteotomy for unstable hips using hybrid external fixator: Case series and review of literature. J Orthop Sci 2012; 17(1): 9–17.
2. Rozbruch SR, Paley D, Bhave A, Herzenber JE. Ilizarov hip reconstruction for the late sequelae of infantile hip infection. J Bone Joint Surg Am 2005; 87: 1007–18.
3. Agashe M, Song SH, Tong XB, Hong JH, Song HR. Subtrochanteric valgus osteotomy with monolateral external fixator in hips for patients with severe cerebral palsy. Orthopedics 2013; 36(2): e139–46.

4. Pafilas D, Nayagam S. The pelvic support osteotomy: Indications and preoperative planning. *Strat Traum Limb Recon* 2008; 3: 83–92.

5. Milch H. The 'pelvic support' osteotomy. *J Bone Joint Surg Am* 1941; 23(3): 581–95.

6. Lance PM. *Osteotomies sous-trochanteri-enne dans le traitement des luxations con-genitales inveterees de la hanche*. Masson & Cie, Paris, 1936.

7. Lorenz A. Ueber die Behandlung der irreponiblen angeborenen Huftluxationen und der Schenkelhalspseudoarthrosen mittels Gabelung (Bifurkation des oberen Femurendes). *Wien Klin Wchnschr* 1919; XXXII: 997.

8. Schanz A. Zur Behandlung der veralteten angeborenen Huftverrenkung. *Munch Med Wchnschr* 1922; IXIX: 930.

9. Paley D. Hip joint considerations. In: *Principles of Deformity Correction*, edited by Paley D. Berlin: Springer; 2002. p. 647–94.

10. Ilizarov GA, Samchukov ML. Reconstruction of the femur by the Ilizarov method in the treatment of arthrosis deformans of the hip joint. *Ortop Travmatol Protez* 1988; 6: 10–3.

11. Sponseller PD, McBeath AA, Perpich M. Hip arthrodesis in young patients. A long-term follow-up study. *J Bone Joint Surg Am* 1984; 66(6): 853–9.

12. Kocaoglu M et al. The Ilizarov hip recon-struction osteotomy for hip dislocation: Outcome after 4–7 years in 14 young patients. *Acta Orthop Scand* 2002; 73(4): 432–8.

13. Hunka L et al. Classification and surgical management of the severe sequelae of sep-tic hips in children. *Clin Orthop Relat Res* 1982; 171: 30–6.

14. Choi IH et al. Surgical treatment of the severe sequelae of infantile septic arthritis of the hip. *Clin Orthop Relat Res* 2005; 434: 102–9.

15. El-Mowafi H. Outcome of pelvic support osteotomy with the Ilizarov method in the treatment of the unstable hip joint. *Acta Orthop Belg* 2005; 71(6): 686–91.

13

Lorenz osteotomy

K. MOHAN IYER

The main idea of the Lorenz osteotomy is to transform the upper end of the femur into a fork at the upper end of the shaft, or an inverted L, with the angle resting against the true acetabulum while the tip of its short limb is near the false acetabulum near the anterior inferior spine and the long limb is represented by the femoral shaft.

This was first shown at the meeting of the Dutch Orthopaedic Association in 1921 and has numerous advantages.

1. The commonest form of this procedure is a subtrochanteric osteotomy, where the lower fragment (the upper end of the shaft) is forced upward into the upper fragment as to lie at the bottom of the true acetabulum, which results in increasing the true shortening of the lower limb, thus bringing the two pieces of dense cortices into contact together and resulting in a delayed union.
2. This is followed by permanent fixation in an abducted limb by an intertrochanteric osteotomy done in the sagittal plane, which has the same drawbacks, while the upper fragment with the atrophied femoral head has to be very small.

Here, the upper end of the lower fragment is abducted and inserted into the acetabulum after making an intertrochanteric osteotomy, with the plane of the osteotomy from below and outward to above and inward (Figure 13.1).

Disadvantages:

1. Increased shortening
2. Less mobility with arthritic pain

By the Lorenz principle, wherein the osteotomy is done in the coronal (frontal) plane of the body, such that the upper end of the shaft is guided into the rue acetabulum, its raw posterior surface still continues to be in contact with the raw anterior surface of the upper fragment. This prevents it slipping backward, thus making hyperextension of the limb easy, and helps in early bony union. Once union has occurred, the abduction of the limb can be reduced with the limb comes with its pull on the head bringing the whole limb to a lower level, which is sometimes enough to compensate for the inevitable shortening of the osteotomy. This true

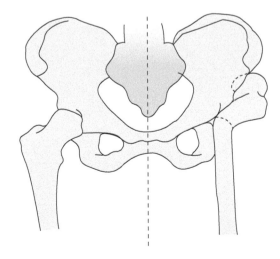

Figure 13.1 The limb abducted and extended so that the proximal end of the distal fragment is directed medially and anteriorly in the acetabulum.

shortening, which may be around 1/2 inch, may be abolished in young subjects by extra growth following improved function of the lower limb with extra weight bearing.

Following closure, a firm spica bandage is applied to force the greater trochanter area against the pelvis. The limb is fastened to a hip abduction frame in wide abduction, slight internal rotation, and full extension. Serial x-rays are taken every 3 weeks until sufficient callus is noticed that unites the bone ends. Usually 6 weeks is enough for the osteotomy to unite sufficiently with no need for manipulation. Graduated exercises are begun initially with parallel bars, with full weight bearing taking nearly 6 months in all. The results are evident in the stability offered, mobility, and muscle tone and redevelopment of the hip muscles gradually postoperatively.

14

Femoral valgus osteotomies

K. MOHAN IYER

CONGENITAL COXA VARA TREATMENT

Coxa vara in childhood may be clinically classified as developmental, congenital, dysplastic, or traumatic and may occur at the physis or in the trochanteric or subtrochanteric area. Always include a search for a family history of similar deformity, a history of trauma or infection, and evidence of associated skeletal abnormality. Radiographs will illustrate whether the deformity is unilateral or bilateral and whether it occurs at or below the physis. Surgical treatment of coxa vara in childhood is usually indicated when the disease is progressive, painful, unilateral, or associated with leg-length discrepancy.[1]

MEDICAL THERAPY

1. Spica cast immobilization and skeletal pin traction with bed rest, with generally unsatisfactory results.
2. Hence, it is generally accepted that no place remains for conservative nonoperative measures for individuals who require treatment of either symptomatic or progressive Congenital Coxa Vara (CCV).

SURGICAL THERAPY

The treatment of choice for CCV has followed the recommendations of early work by Amstutz, Freiberger, and Wilson in the use of either subtrochanteric or intertrochanteric osteotomies.

Of the intertrochanteric osteotomies, the Pauwels Y-shaped and Langenskiöld valgus-producing osteotomies have yielded good results; however, these osteotomies have a somewhat limited ability to correct the associated femoral neck retroversion.

On the contrary, the subtrochanteric valgus-producing osteotomies used by many authors have also provided good and lasting clinical results.

In summary, the actual type of osteotomy performed may be less important than ensuring that the goals of surgical correction, as outlined above, are achieved.

Many issues have been raised surrounding surgical intervention, including the following:

1. Amount of correction needed
2. Associated procedures at the time of surgery to aid in the osteotomy and decrease hip joint forces
3. Optimal age for operation

Postoperatively, good results have been achieved consistently when the Hilgenreiner-epiphyseal angle (HEA) has been corrected to less than 35–40°.

It is generally accepted that more important than the age at correction is the ability to correct the hip to meet the goals of surgery. Once the diagnosis is clear and progression is evident, few reasons remain to delay surgery beyond an age at which stable fixation can be achieved reliably, and long-term outcomes support the view that adequate realignment of the deformity is most important.

SURGICAL DETAILS

Complications

1. Premature closure of the proximal femoral physis has been consistently noted, occurring along with or shortly after healing of the inferomedial fragment of metaphyseal bone. Closure occurred at an average of 3 years after surgical correction. This, along with any residual shortening due to the osteotomy, requires follow-up with the aim of contralateral physeal arrest or ipsilateral lengthening at the appropriate time, should a clinically significant limb-length discrepancy exist near maturity.
2. Associated with premature closure of the proximal femoral physis is the often-encountered overgrowth of the greater trochanter. There was no overgrowth in cases where successful greater trochanteric apophysiodesis was achieved. All of these patents had a good clinical outcome.

Long-term monitoring: The patient should be seen every 2 weeks until early healing is present (~6–8 weeks after surgery). At that time, the spica cast is removed and physiotherapy is begun for mobilization and range-of-motion instruction. Close follow-up every 3–6 months is required to ensure that the deformity is resolving.

The Hilgenreiner-epiphyseal angle should be closed to 38–40° or less after surgery.[2]

Indications

The HEA is the angle subtended by the horizontal Hilgenreiner line through the triradiate cartilages and an oblique line through the proximal femoral capital physes (Figure 14.1).

A study of normal values of the HEA found that the angle in children younger than 7 years averages 20°, with a wide variation of 4–35°. The mean value for those aged 8 years to maturity is 23°.

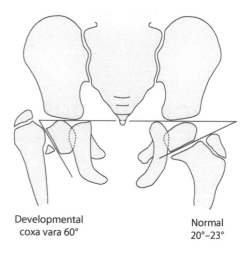

Hilgenreiner's epiphyseal angle

Developmental coxa vara 60°

Normal 20°–23°

Figure 14.1 The Hilgenreiner lines.

On the basis of this measurement, patients in whom surgery is indicated include the following:

1. A child with a clinical limp and an HEA of more than 60°
2. A child with a clinical limp and an HEA of 45–60° with documented progression of varus deformity

On the basis of the HEA, three relatively distinct groups have emerged, as follows:

1. In those with an HEA of less than 45°, the CCV is more commonly found to halt progression spontaneously and to heal without intervention.
2. In patients with an HEA of more than 60°, the CCV[3] follows a more traditional course of progressive deformity that can be aided only by surgical intervention.
3. An intermediate group, comprising patients with angle measurements of 45–60°, represents a so-called "gray zone"; these patients require observation for either healing or progression, the latter of which necessitates surgical intervention.

The main aims of surgical treatment are as follows:

A. Correction of the neck-shaft angle to a more physiologic angle and the HEA to less than 35–40°

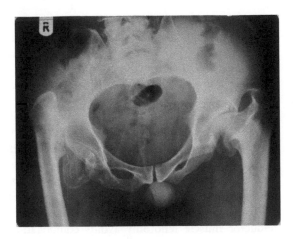

Figure 14.2 Congenital coxa vara. (Courtesy of Magdi E. Griess, Whitehaven, Cumbria, UK.)

B. Correction of femoral anteversion (or retroversion) to more normal values
C. Ossification and healing of the defective inferomedial femoral neck fragment
D. Reconstitution of the abductor mechanism through replacement of its normal length-tension relationship

Developmental coxa vara (also known as cervical or infantile coxa vara)[4]:

1. Represents coxa vara not present at birth but rather developing in early childhood.
2. Coxa vara is defined as any decrease in the femoral neck-shaft angle less than 120–135° (Figure 14.2).

Incidence

1. Relatively uncommon
2. Bilateral involvement is noted in 30%–50% of patients

Etiology-developmental abnormality, which causes faulty cartilage formation and maturation.

Clinical findings

1. Prominent and elevated greater trochanter
2. Positive Trendelenburg test
3. Limb-length inequality (usually less than 2.5 cm)
4. Decreased range of movements (ROM) with restrictions noted with abduction and internal rotation

Radiographic findings

1. Femoral-neck shaft angle below 90°
2. More vertical position of the epiphyseal plate with Hilgenreiner's-epiphyseal angle greater than 40° (normal is less than 25°)
3. Triangular metaphyseal fragment in inferior femoral neck surrounded by inverted Y (sine qua non)

Proper surgical treatment includes:

1. Adductor tenotomy, which allows for less forceful correction and improved stability.[5]
2. Proximal femoral shortening osteotomy if necessary to help relieve excessive femoral head pressure when the valgus angle is restored.
3. Stable internal fixation and hip spica cast if needed.
4. The aim of surgical treatment is to produce an overcorrection of the valgus angle to greater than 150–160°, as well as correction of the epiphyseal angle to less than 30°.

Complications

1. Recurrence of proximal femoral varus deformity.
2. Premature physeal closure—the incidence may be high.
3. Greater trochanteric overgrowth—associated with premature capital femoral physeal closure and commonly treated by greater trochanter transfer or epiphysiodesis.
4. Acetabular dysplasia—found to be greater in patients with premature physeal closure and in patients who have had an undercorrection of the neck-shaft angle less than 140°.
5. Other complications have included pseudarthrosis, avascular necrosis, leg-length discrepancy, and degenerative arthritis.

A simple valgus osteotomy is the treatment of choice in coxa vara. In children less than 8 years old, an epiphysiodesis of the greater trochanter is associated to prevent the high risk of recurrence, which depends on initial correction.

It is very useful when done in coxa vara and if the adduction x-ray film shows a concentric reduction.

This has also been reported in Logheswaren et al.[6] They emphasized that an ideal implant for fixation of osteotomy for this deformity of abnormal bone would be an intramedullary nail with proximal locking screw to the neck to maintain the correction of neck shaft angle (NSA), and a distal locking screw to provide stability.

One of the early methods of correcting coxa vara is the Wagner method that involves passing two Kirschner wires through the femoral neck and molding and fixing the external portion of the wires to the femoral shaft by cerclage wires. Fassier et al., in 2008,[7] showed a satisfactory outcome with this technique in 18 hips with osteogenesis imperfecta and three hips with fibrous dysplasia.

They advocate a retrograde entrance from the knee that allows protection of the whole femur from the intercondylar notch where the hook of the Rush rod sits firmly, through the shaft until proximal penetration in the piriformis fossa. Thus, they postulate that it is worth taking the risk of causing joint stiffness with the benefit of reducing the risk of recurrent fracture in osteogenesis imperfecta patients. Hence, they are of the opinion that our modified method can be an alternative when an appropriately sized interlocking nail is not available for correction of coxa vara or shepherd's crook deformity in abnormal bone.

A 15° medial bone wedge was removed from the intertrochanteric region, the osteotomy was closed, and stabilization was achieved with two Kirschner wires and a figure-8 cerclage (Figure 14.3).

The application of this fixation technique proved to be simple and effective, with few complications, and it is a good option for the fixation of proximal femoral varus osteotomy in children.[8]

There are multiple surgical techniques aimed to correct coxa vara/valga. A simpler technique is easier to perform, as it does not use other internal fixation materials besides the telescopic rod and avoids all complications that might arise from the tensions induced by the pelvic trochanteric muscles in coxa vara or by the adductor muscles in coxa valga. Diminishing the tension by using periosteal disinsertion of the pelvic trochanteric muscles and adductor muscle tenotomy avoids complications that might arise due to the tension produced by their contraction and retraction.[9]

A study was conducted to determine whether magnetic resonance arthrography can show differences in disorders of the labrum (tears, size, ganglion formation) expected in symptomatic patients with developmental dysplasia of the hip and anterior femoroacetabular impingement. Based on these data, the size of the labrum and the presence of soft tissue ganglia seem to be good predictors for the presence of developmental dysplasia, whereas the presence of tears did not differentiate between conditions. The capability of magnetic resonance arthrography to show these differences in labral disorders suggests this method is a helpful diagnostic tool that can aid in defining the most appropriate treatment strategy.[10]

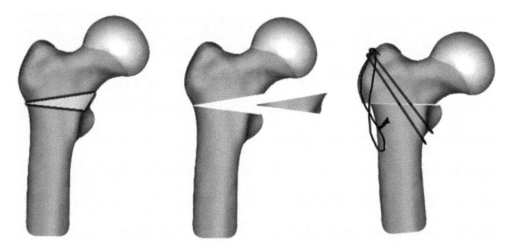

Figure 14.3 Tension band wiring for proximal femoral varus osteotomy. (Reproduced with kind permission of Maranho DA, Pagnano RG, Volpon JB. Tension band wiring for proximal femoral varus osteotomy fixation in children. *Medicine (Baltimore)* 2014; 93(7): e61.)

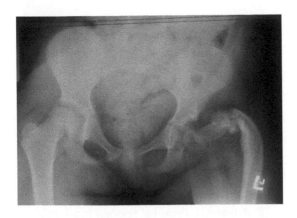

Figure 14.4 Proximal focal femoral deficiency (PFFD). (Courtesy of Magdi E. Griess, Whitehaven, Cumbria, UK.)

PROXIMAL FEMORAL FOCAL DEFICIENCY

It is a congenital defect of the proximal femur (Figure 14.4) and a spectrum of disease that includes (1) absent hip, (2) femoral neck pseudoarthrosis, (3) absent femur, and (4) shortened femur.

The main orthopedic manifestations include (1) fibular hemimelia (50%), (2) anterior cruciate ligament (ACL) deficiency, (3) coxa vara, and (4) knee contractures.

The clinical features include physical examination that shows severe shortening of one or both legs, along with a short bulky thigh that is flexed, abducted, and externally rotated.

Treatment:

A. *Nonoperative*:
  1. Observation, which is often done in children with bilateral deficiency, or
  2. An extension prosthesis, which is a less attractive option due to the large proximal segment of prosthesis, and assists the patient when attempting to pull self up to stand.
B. *Operative*:
  1. Ambulation without prosthesis to include limb lengthening with or without contralateral epiphysiodesis, with its main indication being a stable hip and functional foot, while the main contraindications are untreated coxa vara, proximal femoral neck pseudoarthrosis, or acetabular dysplasia.
  2. *Ambulation with a prosthesis*:
     a. Knee arthrodesis with foot ablation—indicated if ipsilateral foot is proximal to the level of contralateral knee and when the prosthetic knee will not be below the level of the contralateral knee at maturity.
     b. Femoral-pelvic fusion—indicated when the femoral head is absent (Aiken classifications C & D).[11,12]

        (C = Dysplasia of the acetabulum can be noted. There is no ossification of the head of the femur on that side, and the shaft of the femur rides proximal and posterior to the ilium. D = No ossification of the femoral heads has occurred and no acetabula are present. The femora are very short and are flexed, abducted, and externally rotated. No proximal tufts of ossification are evident on the femora.)
     c. Van Ness rotationplasty[13]—indicated when the ipsilateral foot is at the level of the contralateral knee along with an absent femoral head (Aiken classifications C & D as above).
     d. Amputation—indicated when the femoral length <50% of the opposite side.

REFERENCES

1. Beals RK. Coxa vara in childhood: Evaluation and management. *J Am Acad Orthop Surg* 1998; 6(2): 93–9.
2. Chotigavanichaya C, Leeprakobboon D, Eamsobhana P, Kaewpornsawan K. Results of surgical treatment of coxa vara in children: Valgus osteotomy with angle blade plate fixation. *J Med Assoc Thai* 2014; 97(Suppl. 9): S78–82.
3. Amstutz HC. Developmental (infantile) coxa vara—A distinct entity. *Clin Orthop* 1970; 72: 242.
4. Weighill FJ. The treatment of developmental coxa vara by abduction subtrochanteric and intertrochanteric femoral osteotomy with special reference to the role of adductor tenotomy. *Clin Orthop Relat Res* 1976; 116: 116–24.

5. Weinstein JN, Kuo DN, Millar EA. Congenital coxa vara: A retrospective review. *J Pediatr Orthop* 1984; 4: 70.

6. Logheswaren S et al. A modified technique of fixation for proximal femoral valgus osteotomy in abnormal bone: A report of two cases. *Malays Orthop J* 2017; 11(2).

7. Fassier F, Sardar Z, Aarabi M, Odent T, Haque T, Hamdy R. Results and complications of a surgical technique for correction of coxa vara in children with osteopenic bones results and complications of a surgical technique for correction of coxa vara in children with osteopenic bones. *J Pediatr Orthop* 2008; 28(8): 799–805.

8. Widmann RF, Hresko MT, Kasser JR, Millis MB. Wagner multiple K-wire osteosynthesis to correct coxa vara in the young child: Experience with a versatile "tailor-made" high angle blade plate equivalent. *J Pediatr Orthop B* 2001; 10(1): 43–50.

9. Callaghan JJ, Rosenberg AG, Rubash HE, editors. *Adult Hip*. 2nd ed., Philadelphia: Lippincott Williams & Wilkins; 2007, pp. 781–95.

10. Leunig M, Podeszwa D, Beck M, Werlen S, Ganz R. Magnetic resonance arthrography of labral disorders in hips with dysplasia and impingement. *Clin Orthop* 2004; 418: 74–80.

11. Aitken GT. Amputation as a treatment for certain lower extremity congenital abnormalities. *J Bone Joint Surg* 1959; 41A(7): 1267–85.

12. Aitken GT. Proximal femoral focal deficiency. In: *Limb Development and Deformity Problems of Evaluation and Rehabilitation*. Springfield, IL: Charles C Thomas; 1969.

13. Kostuik JP, Gillespie B, Hall JE, Hubbard S. Van Ness rotational osteotomy for treatment of proximal femoral focal deficiency and congenital short femur. *J Bone Joint Surg Am* 1975; 57: 1039.

15

Femoral varus osteotomy in children

K. MOHAN IYER

The main principles are that the lateral portion of the femoral head is intact, which is a prerequisite for the osteotomy, and that it can be combined with either a flexion or extension component.

Its main indications are as follows:

1. Hip joint instability before correction of the deformity, which corrects with internal rotation and abduction.
2. A pelvic osteotomy should be done when the center edge angle is less than 15°.
3. It is useful in some hip conditions such as developmental dysplasia of hip (DDH), slipped upper capital femoral epiphysis, Perthes disease, avascular necrosis, and nonunion or malunion of the femoral neck.

There are certain disadvantages with this procedure:

1. There is potential to shorten the limb.
2. Weakness of abductors.
3. Trendelenburg gait.
4. There is some difficulty in insertion of the femoral component in future arthroplasty.

There are two basic indications for this procedure:

1. The hips tend to gradually come out of their sockets due to spasticity of the hips. This is a painless process in the initial stages, but can become painful if there is a severe deformity of the whole hip joint. In children with severe cerebral palsy with an abnormal pull, the correction is not with growth and may require surgery (Figure 15.1a).

2. In children with severe femoral intorsion with their feet severely turned in. This variety may settle with the growth of the child with normal muscle power.

The basic surgery involves a subtrochanteric osteotomy of the femur, along with fixation by a plate and screws (Figure 15.1b) to hold the ends of the osteotomy together and hold the hip spica cast reinforced from chest to toes down on the operated side and halfway down on the other side. X-rays are done immediately and the cast is retained for 4–6 weeks postoperatively, with the bony union being monitored every 3 weeks.

The metalware can remain for 1 year altogether, after which it can be removed, or, if necessary, it can be removed earlier in case of bursitis or infection if it becomes painful. Alternatively, the metalware may be left inside indefinitely in the case of no problems arising from it.

Usually the operated-on leg is slightly shorter, which should not create any problems, but can be adjusted with measured heel raise.

A varus derotation osteotomy is best done in the early stages of Perthes disease, preferably under 7 years of age, where a lateral open-wedge osteotomy is done in children under 5 years of age and where the defect laterally rapidly fills up in children over 5 years of age (Figure 15.2).

In some cases, a salvage procedure is carried out after magnetic resonance imaging (MRI) or an arthrogram is done when surgery is mandatory in the form of a varus derotational osteotomy combined with an innominate osteotomy to follow

(a)

(b)

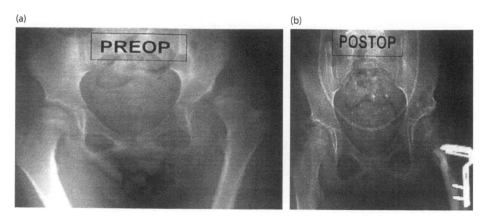

Figure 15.1 Subtrochanteric osteotomy of the femur, along with fixation by a plate and screws. (a) Preop and (b) postop. (Reproduced with the kind permission of Dr. John T Killain, MD, 2009, from the pamphlet OK. Orthopedics for Kids.)

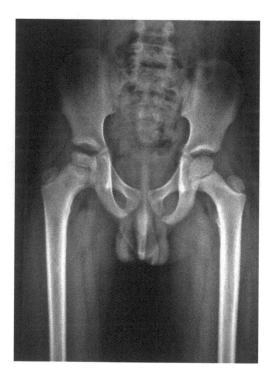

Figure 15.2 Perthes disease right hip. (Courtesy: K. Vinodh, Coimbatore, India.)

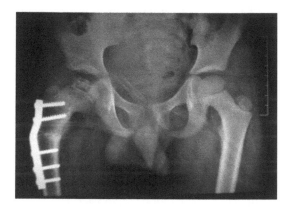

Figure 15.3 Perthes disease treated after varus derotational osteotomy, right hip. (Courtesy: K. Vinodh, Coimbatore, India.)

the principle of containment of the diseased femoral head in Perthes disease. Here the appropriate angled osteotomy is done and the wedge removed, and an osteotomy is made as proximal as possible just below the lag screw to ensure better healing and better correction of the deformity when the osteotomy is reduced and fixed with a plate and compressive screws (Figure 15.3).

Another alternative is a subtrochanteric derotation and varus osteotomy, which can be done with the aim of the surgery being to center the whole plastic epiphysis inside the joint cavity, keeping it well covered by the roof of the acetabulum and allowing the child to walk so that the redistributed intra-articular pressures will contribute to the molding of a normal joint. A small four-holed plate is then bent to the desired angle, and a subtrochanteric osteotomy is done, followed by derotation and angulation of the shaft. A double hip spica is given postoperatively and removed after 2 months, by which time the osteotomy will have united and the child is encouraged to walk, at first in a warm-water pool, then with walking aids, and finally without any support.

16

Three-dimensional trochanteric osteotomy for slipped capital femoral epiphysis based on flexion osteotomy

TAKUYA OTANI AND YASUHIKO KAWAGUCHI

TREATMENT FOR SLIPPED CAPITAL FEMORAL EPIPHYSIS

The treatment for slipped capital femoral epiphysis (SCFE) is complex and controversial, and a consensus regarding the optimal treatment has not been reached. In general, treatment is selected, or treatments are combined, from a list of options such as those in Table 16.1.

Previously, based on the notion that a poorly aligned epiphysis and deformed femoral head and neck can undergo remodeling over time, and thus are clinically not problematic, *in situ* fixation tended to be performed in moderate and even severe SCFE. Recently, however, residual deformities have been reported to cause femoroacetabular impingement (FAI) and frequently elicit damage to the cartilage and labrum, with resulting functional disorder;[1,2] thus, a more accurate improvement in epiphyseal alignment has been gaining interest.

TROCHANTERIC OSTEOTOMY FOR IMPROVED EPIPHYSEAL ALIGNMENT: CLASSICAL THREE-DIMENSIONAL OSTEOTOMY

The most effective method for improving epiphyseal alignment is realignment/osteotomy at the displaced and deformed portion, and the modified Dunn procedure has been increasingly reported in recent years.[3] However, since the displaced portion contains blood vessels that deliver nutrients to the epiphysis, surgical intervention of this portion carries the risk of femoral head necrosis in addition to various difficulties and problems in surgical technique.[4-6] In contrast, the method for safely improving epiphyseal alignment by performing an osteotomy at the trochanteric portion, apart from the vessels supplying the epiphysis, has long been used. Slipping of the epiphysis involves not just a pure medial or posterior displacement, but rather a

Table 16.1 Treatment options for SCFE

Prevention of further slipping
In situ static fixation (stable/unstable type)
In situ dynamic fixation (stable type)
Static fixation after gentle manual/open
  reduction (unstable type)
Improvement of epiphyseal alignment
Trochanteric osteotomy
Osteotomy at the base of femoral neck
Realignment/osteotomy at the slipping site
**Treatment of the femoroacetabular
  impingement**
Primary/secondary treatment
Open/arthroscopic treatment

combination of the two. Thus, a three-dimensional (3-D) osteotomy procedure is required for its correction, and classically used techniques have included the Imhäuser method[7] and the Southwick method.[8] These methods involve preoperative planning based on evaluation of the displacement using plain radiographic findings, and have been performed using classical surgical techniques. However, the techniques are rather complicated, and as a result of errors in radiography imaging, measurements, and osteotomy, issues such as the inability to accurately achieve the desired

correction have been reported. In particular, the affected lower extremity of most SCFE patients is externally rotated, leading to inaccurate evaluation by an anterior-posterior (AP) view, and posteriorly displaced elements tend to be falsely evaluated as medially displaced elements (Figure 16.1).

HOW WE DO IT: THREE-DIMENSIONAL TROCHANTERIC OSTEOTOMY BASED ON FLEXION OSTEOTOMY

In contrast to the classical 3-D osteotomy technique, some surgeons prefer to simplify the correction and perform mainly flexion osteotomy. Since the epiphyseal displacement in SCFE mainly involves posterior slippage in most cases, some studies have reported that simple flexion osteotomy leads to favorable outcomes for cases with 30–70° slip.[9,10] Furthermore, Kamegaya et al.[11] reported that while the main correction should be in flexion, obtaining a physiologic 20–30° varus angle of the physis in the postoperative radiographic AP view is also important. As such, they reported a surgical technique in which preoperative computed tomography (CT) is used to measure the direction of the epiphyseal displacement with reference to the lateral cortical surface of the femur, and some

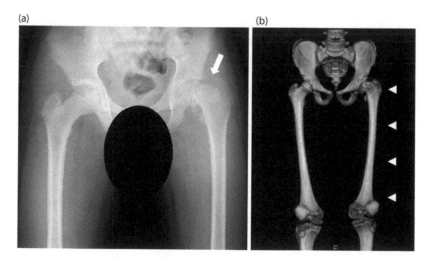

Figure 16.1 Case 1: 13-year-old male, stable-type SCFE (left hip; PTA = 64°). **(a)** Plain radiograph AP view; left femoral head and neck deformity due to stable-type SCFE is seen (arrow). Medial displacement of the epiphysis seems to be the primary element of the deformity on this view. **(b)** 3D-CT (pelvis~entire length of the femurs): It is clearly seen that the left femur is externally rotated significantly (arrow heads). It is also understood that the posterior displacement is a more significant element in epiphyseal slippage than is seen on the AP radiograph.

varus or valgus correction was added to the flexion osteotomy.

We perform an osteotomy based on the report by Kamegaya et al.[11] In other words, we mainly perform a flexion osteotomy to simplify the procedure and increase accuracy, but believe that ultimately 3-D osteotomy is required for SCFE. In addition, we have modified the method reported by Kamegaya et al.[11] as follows:

1. For the evaluation of SCFE and surgical planning, we always include the entire length of the femurs in the preoperative CT images.
2. We perform 3-D evaluation of the slippage with accurate coordinate settings having the femoral condyle as reference points. We then accurately evaluate how much varus or valgus should be added to the flexion osteotomy.
3. To prevent postoperative progression of slippage and to safely carry out rehabilitation, we perform a concomitant fixation of the epiphysis.
4. Because there are residual deformities in the displaced head–neck area following trochanteric osteotomy, we include treatment of the resulting FAI and consider the whole as one series of treatments.

Indications for surgery

As previously mentioned, the treatment for SCFE is not consistent and remains controversial. Of the treatment options in Table 16.1, various opinions exist in terms of the degree of slippage that would be an indication for epiphyseal alignment improvement surgery. For stable SCFE, we perform *in situ* dynamic single-screw fixation[12] for cases with a posterior tilt angle (PTA) ≤40°, and trochanteric osteotomy for cases with PTA >40°. For unstable SCFE, we consider a residual PTA >40° after initial treatment as an indication for the present osteotomy, but such cases are rare in clinical practice. We believe the reason to be that for unstable SCFE, we incise the hip joint through an anterolateral approach, and reduction and fixation is performed while confirming blood flow to the epiphysis with the epiphyseal drilling method,[13] and in most cases reduction to PTA ≤40° is possible while maintaining epiphyseal circulation. In contrast, we do not have an upper PTA limit for severe cases. This is because for one stable SCFE case with preoperative PTA of 94°, after we performed the present procedure with a correction angle of 50°, we secondarily performed FAI treatment by arthrotomy, with a good outcome (Figures 16.2 and 16.3).

Preoperative examinations and operative planning

PLAIN RADIOGRAPHY

We obtain AP and lateral views of both hip joints. The Lauenstein method is widely used for obtaining lateral views, and while this imaging technique is appropriate for observing the femoral diaphysis, the femoral head and neck are somewhat difficult to observe due to overlap. Therefore, imaging techniques such as the Dunn view or modified Dunlap lateral view, which allow for clear depiction of the femoral head to neck by decreasing abduction

(a)

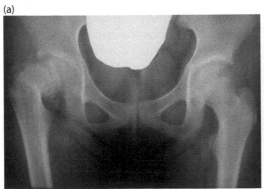

(b)

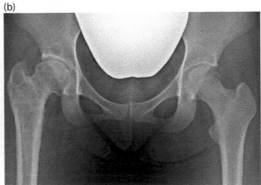

Figure 16.2 **Case 2:** 11-year-old female, stable-type SCFE (right hip; PTA = 94°). **(a)** Preoperative AP radiograph. **(b)** AP radiograph 10 years after the primary femoral flexion osteotomy.

(a)   (b)   (c)

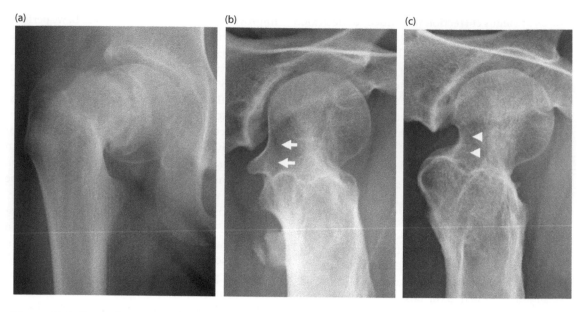

Figure 16.3 Secondary surgical treatment for FAI in Case 2. (a) Preoperative lateral radiograph of the right hip. (b) Lateral radiograph of the right hip after 50° flexion osteotomy; Significant residual FAI deformity is seen in anterior aspect of the femoral head to neck (arrows). (c) Lateral radiograph of the right hip after osteochondroplasty; open osteochondroplasty was performed (arrow heads) through the same skin incision as used in the primary osteotomy.

and elevating the femoral diaphysis, should be used. In unstable SCFE or in cases with significant pain, the cross-table lateral view, which allows for image acquisition even with the hip in extension, is useful.

COMPUTED TOMOGRAPHY IMAGING AND EXAMINATION

CT is necessary in the management of SCFE, which requires 3-D analysis. If only the region around hip joint is imaged by CT, accurate evaluation is difficult due to the effect of the external rotation deformity on the lower extremity (Figure 16.1b).

We therefore perform preoperative planning using the following imaging techniques and analysis. We believe all steps can be performed in most institutions by using widely used CT devices and image construction techniques.

- Images are obtained in 1–2 mm slices including the entire length of the bilateral femurs.
- Setting the coordinates in the image construction of the affected femur is important. We set the z-axis to be parallel to the proximal

femoral axis, then adjust the rotation so that the line connecting the posterior edges of the femoral medial and lateral condyles is parallel to the x-axis.
- Measurement of PTA by using CT.

In the correct sagittal plane of the femur, measure PTA from the proximal femoral axis slice and the epiphyseal slice (Figure 16.4).

- *Determination of the angle of flexion osteotomy*: The correction angle of flexion osteotomy is determined from the following three conditions: (1) measure preoperative PTA; (2) aim for a 10–20° postoperative PTA, but accept up to 40° of residual PTA; and (3) set the upper limit of the correction angle as 45–50°. Therefore, as previously mentioned, cases with severe slippage of up to around 90° are within the indication range of the present surgery.
- *Determination of varus or valgus angles:* We reset the z-axis in the image construction coordinates by posteriorly tilting by the determined flexion osteotomy angle (Figure 16.5a).

(a)

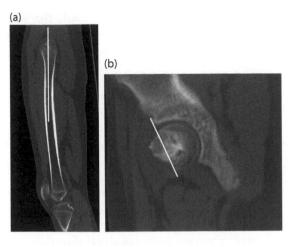

(b)

(a)

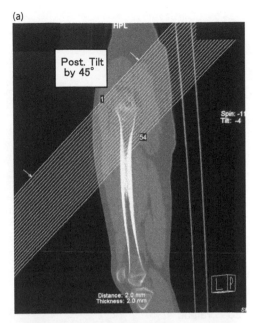

Figure 16.4 Correct sagittal plane of the left femur was constructed with CT in Case 1 (after the correct coordinates were set having the proximal femur and the femoral condyles as the reference points). PTA was measured from the proximal femoral axis slice (a) and the epiphyseal slice (b), and it was 64° in Case 1.

(b)

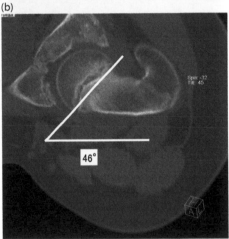

Once the coronal image of the femoral head is constructed in this condition, the frontal view after flexion osteotomy can be predicted. We measure the physeal inclination in a slice in which the epiphysis is clearly depicted (Figure 16.5b), and determine the varus or valgus correction angle so that the inclination becomes 20–30° varus postoperatively.

- *Comparison with the nonaffected side*: Image construction of the nonaffected femur using the same coordinate settings and creating a mirror image allows for accurate comparison with the normal side.

SURGERY PLANNING

We print an AP x-ray image of the affected proximal femur or a CT coronal image of the femur with the corrected coordinates as mentioned above, magnify it, and make a planning by tracing it on tracing paper. We set the osteotomy line so that it passes through the center of the lesser trochanter perpendicular to the bone axis, and apply the necessary varus or valgus. We apply the blade plate template and determine the plate type, length, and insertion level (Figure 16.6).

Figure 16.5 (a) CT analysis in Case 1: Reset of the z-axis in the image construction coordinates and construction of the coronal image of the femoral head in this condition. Flexion osteotomy angle was determined to be 45° in Case 1. Therefore, the z-axis in the image construction coordinates was reset to tilt it posteriorly by 45°. (b) CT analysis in Case 1: Reset of the z-axis in the image construction coordinates and construction of the coronal image of the femoral head in this condition. Once the coronal image of the femoral head is constructed in this condition, the frontal view after flexion osteotomy can be predicted. The inclination angle of the physis in this frontal view was 46° varus in Case 1. Therefore, the surgery was planned to have 20° valgus correction in addition to 45° flexion osteotomy.

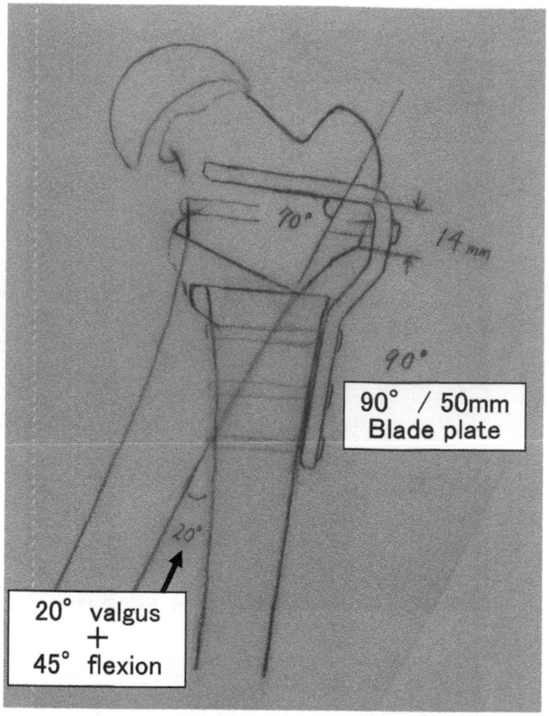

Figure 16.6 Surgery planning: The location, direction, and length of the blade plate to be inserted from the trochanter to the neck are planned.

Surgical technique

BODY POSITIONING AND EXPOSURE

Surgery is performed under general anesthesia with the patient in the lateral decubitus position. Intraoperative fluoroscopy is usually performed; thus, the device should be prepared preoperatively. Fluoroscopy is always performed such that the x-ray beams pass the patient in the anterior-to-posterior direction, and the frontal view is examined first. The lateral view is obtained with the femoral head and neck in the correct position for the lateral view, with the hip in 90° flexion and 45° abduction.

A lateral incision is made along the femoral axis, and the femoral fascia is incised longitudinally. The vastus lateralis muscle is longitudinally divided and the whole perimeter of the femur is exposed at the level of the lesser trochanter, during which the origin of the vastus lateralis muscle is released to adequately reduce its tension; these are later repaired. Proximally and medially to the lesser trochanter runs the medial circumflex

femoral artery, which gives off vessels that supply nutrients to the femoral head, so care must be taken not to damage this artery.

OSTEOTOMY AND OSTEOSYNTHESIS

The first and most important step is to accurately insert the blade of the blade plate from the trochanteric portion to the neck, as planned preoperatively. The insertion method of the blade chisel varies by system, but one that allows the use of a guidewire is convenient. The chisel should be inserted at 0° anteversion, and a Kirschner (K) wire is inserted into the trochanteric portion beforehand to serve as a guide for the 0° anteversion. For this step, the assistant observes from the distal direction with the knee in 90° flexion (Figure 16.7a).

Then, the guidewire is inserted accurately in the determined angle three-dimensionally; 0° anteversion and also at the determined angle from the subtrochanteric lateral cortex (determined from the varus or valgus angle and plate angle: Figure 16.7b) under AP fluoroscopy. After the guidewire is inserted, the location is checked with lateral view fluoroscopy. In performing flexion osteotomy at α°, the blade chisel is inserted so that the plate axis is tilted anteriorly by α° from the proximal femoral axis, and in systems with guidewires, the chisel can be rotated freely around the guide, thus allowing for more accuracy (Figure 16.7c).

Once the blade chisel is inserted accurately, the actual plate is hammered in, but since pediatric bone is soft, this must be done very carefully to avoid any change in the insertion angle. Before removing the blade chisel, a K-wire is inserted nearby, three-dimensionally parallel to the chisel, to use as a guide for plate placement (Figure 16.7d).

Once the plate has been inserted accurately, the next step is the femoral osteotomy, but the osteosynthesis condition after plate fixation is predicted and checked beforehand. Osteotomy is usually performed at the level of the center of the lesser trochanter, perpendicular to the bone axis, but if the blade insertion site and osteotomy level are far apart, it becomes difficult for the osteotomy surfaces to have appropriate contact with each other, so the osteotomy line is modified as necessary at this point. After osteotomy, the iliopsoas muscle is released from the lesser trochanter of the proximal bone piece, and the lesser trochanter is resected and preserved for bone graft. The plate is placed along the distal

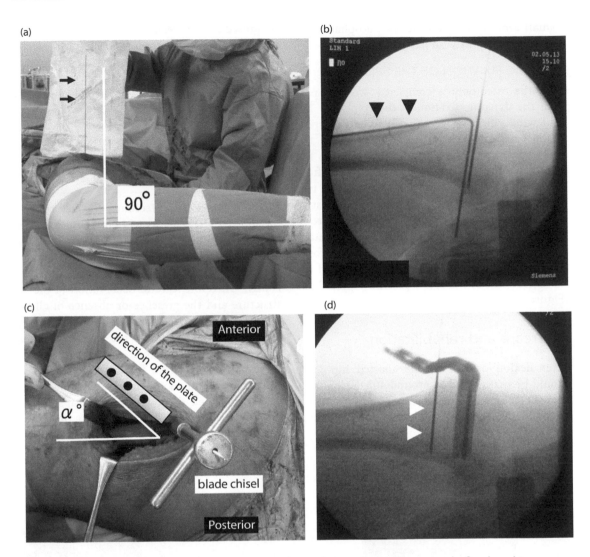

Figure 16.7 **(a)** A K-wire (black arrows) is inserted into the trochanteric portion beforehand to serve as a guide for the 0° anteversion. For this step, the assistant observes from the distal direction with the knee in 90° flexion to check the K-wire is perpendicular to the leg axis. **(b)** Then, the guidewire is inserted accurately in the determined angle three-dimensionally; 0° anteversion and also at the determined angle from the subtrochanteric lateral cortex (determined from the varus or valgus angle and plate angle; 70° in this case [black arrow heads]) under AP fluoroscopy. **(c)** In performing flexion osteotomy at α°, the blade chisel is inserted so that the plate axis is tilted anteriorly by α° from the proximal femoral axis. **(d)** Before removing the blade chisel, a K-wire (white arrow heads) is inserted nearby, three-dimensionally parallel to the chisel, to use as a guide for plate placement. The blade plate is then hammered in very carefully to avoid any change in the insertion angle.

bone piece, and once the rotation is set, is temporarily fixed with bone holding forceps. Under fluoroscopy, we confirm that the planned bone alignment has been achieved. We confirm the range of rotation of the hip joint and adjust rotation of the distal bone piece so that about 20° of internal rotation is possible. Care must be taken so that the distal bone piece is not fixed in external rotation. Next, the plate is fixed with screws. In order to avoid shortening of the femur, wedge osteotomy to obtain wide contact of the two bone pieces is not performed. We fill the space between the bone pieces with bone chips obtained from the proximal lesser trochanter, as well as with a small amount of β-tricalcium phosphate, and carefully cover this with periosteum.

DYNAMIC FIXATION OF THE EPIPHYSIS

Once the osteotomy is completed, we next perform the dynamic fixation of the epiphysis. The guidewire is inserted from the anterolateral aspect of the trochanter, passed carefully to avoid the upper surface of the blade, and inserted into the epiphysis. This step must be performed carefully while confirming the fluoroscopic image from two directions, and intra-articular perforation must be avoided. In order to prevent premature closure of the physis, we use short thread screws to contain all the threads inside the epiphysis, and perform the fixation using the dynamic method,[12] in which the lateral end of the screw protrudes by 1–2 cm (Figure 16.8).

Aftercare and rehabilitation

After flexion osteotomy, the affected hip joint should be maintained at around 40° flexion, and over the course of 1 week, extension of 0° should be gradually achieved. Transfer to a wheelchair is permitted after 1 week postoperatively. One-third weight bearing is permitted from postoperative week 6, and one-half weight bearing is permitted from postoperative week 8, after which weight bearing is further increased based on evaluation of the bone union.

Femoroacetabular impingement treatment with the internal fixation device removal

In the trochanteric osteotomy, the deformity of the slippage site remains without being corrected. While some remodeling can be expected during the postoperative course, the risk of a certain amount of residual deformity and resultant FAI is high. Therefore, careful observation of the 3-D structure and the presence or absence of clinical signs of FAI is important. Thus, bumpectomy or osteochondroplasty around the femoral head and neck portion is performed as necessary during the removal of internal fixation devices. For the surgery, we use the same incision used during the osteotomy, open the anterior joint capsule from the anterolateral approach (between the gluteus

(a)

(b)

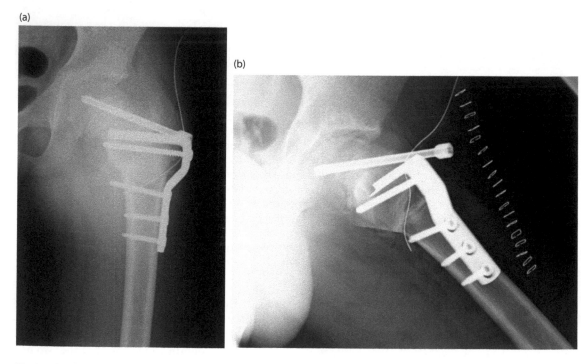

Figure 16.8 Postoperative radiographs (a: AP, b: lateral) in Case 1. A blade plate (90° and 50 mm blade) was used in this case. A short-thread/6.5-mm-diameter/cannulated screw was used for dynamic fixation of the epiphysis.

medius and tensor fasciae latae) with the hip joint in flexion and external rotation, and perform adequate osteochondroplasty using a high speed burr under direct visualization (Figure 16.3).

This postoperative observation of FAI and additional surgical treatment as needed are part of the whole treatment series, and before the primary osteotomy surgery, it is important to adequately inform the patient and family of the possibility of a secondary surgery at the time of removal of the internal fixation device.

CONCLUSION

SCFE has a complex pathology, with significant variation between cases. It is important to preoperatively perform detailed 3-D evaluation and meticulous surgery planning, and CT images must be obtained using the correct coordinates and including the entire length of the femurs. Key points during the surgery include correct insertion of the blade as planned using fluoroscopy, adjusting the blade position and osteotomy level while predicting the osteosynthesis state, and checking the rotation of the distal bone piece during fixation to avoid external rotation deformity of the hip. Postoperatively, continued 3-D evaluation for residual femoral head deformity and clinical evaluation for signs of FAI are performed, and secondary surgery is indicated as necessary at the time of internal fixation device removal. It is essential to understand that all the above steps are part of the whole treatment system and to plan the whole treatment accordingly.

REFERENCES

1. Leunig M et al. Slipped capital femoral epiphysis: early mechanical damage to the acetabular cartilage by a prominent femoral metaphysis. *Acta Orthop Scand* 2000; 71(4): 370–5.
2. Ilizaliturri VM Jr et al. Arthroscopic treatment of femoroacetabular impingement secondary to paediatric hip disorders. *J Bone Joint Surg Br* 2007; 89(8): 1025–30.
3. Ziebarth K et al. Capital realignment for moderate and severe SCFE using a modified Dunn procedure. *Clin Orthop Rel Res* 2009; 467: 704–16.
4. Sankar WN et al. The modified Dunn procedure for unstable slipped capital femoral epiphysis: A multicenter perspective. *J Bone Joint Surg Am* 2013; 95(7): 585–91.
5. Davis RL et al. Treatment of unstable versus stable slipped capital femoral epiphysis using the modified Dunn procedure. *J Pediatr Orthop* 2017 Mar 21. doi: 10.1097/BPO.0000000000000975, [Epub ahead of print].
6. Upasani VV et al. Iatrogenic hip instability is a devastating complication after the modified Dunn procedure for severe slipped capital femoral epiphysis. *Clin Orthop Relat Res* 2017; 475(4): 1229–35.
7. Imhäuser G. Spätergebnisse der sog. Imhäuser-Osteotomie bei der Epiphysenlösung. *Z Orthop* 1977; 115: 716–25.
8. Southwick WO. Osteotomy through the lesser trochanter for slipped capital femoral epiphysis. *JBJS-Am* 1967; 49: 807–35.
9. Ishii Y, Hoshi T. Intertrochanteric simple flexion osteotomy for slipped capital femoral epiphysis. *Hip Joint* 1993; 19: 62–6, in Japanese.
10. Takeuchi N et al. Treatment of slipped capital femoral epiphysis; anterior plating for trochanteric flexion osteotomy. *Hip Joint* 1993; 19: 57–61, in Japanese.
11. Kamegaya M et al. Preoperative assessment for intertrochanteric femoral osteotomies in severe chronic slipped capital femoral epiphysis using computed tomography. *J Pediatr Orthop Part B* 2005; 14: 71–8.
12. Kumm DA et al. Slipped capital femoral epiphysis: A prospective study of dynamic screw fixation. *Clin Orthop Rel Res* 2001; 384: 198–207.
13. Gill TJ et al. Intraoperative assessment of femoral head vascularity after femoral neck fracture. *J Orthop Trauma* 1998; 12(7): 474–8.

PART 2

Adult Hip Preservation Techniques

17

Challenges in subtrochanteric femur osteotomy management in adults in orthopedics

ZONG-KE ZHOU AND DUAN WANG

INTRODUCTION

In 1988, Sponseller and McBeath from Johns Hopkins Hospital used subtrochanteric osteotomy with intramedullary fixation for arthroplasty of the dysplastic hip.[1]

Until recently, total hip arthroplasty (THA) for the treatment of Crowe type IV–Hartofilakidis type III developmental dysplasia of the hip (DDH) was a technically demanding procedure due to triangular-shaped and hypoplastic acetabulum filled with fibrous tissue and fat; femoral deformities with straight and narrow medullary canal; soft tissue abnormalities, including hypertrophic capsule and shortened abductor muscle; and biomechanical alterations.[2–5] However, restoration of the anatomical hip rotation center can generally lead to a hip that is difficult to reduce due to soft tissue contracture and a limb that is excessively lengthened due to excessive soft tissue tension, abductor impairment, and nerve palsy. Moreover, leg lengthening of >3.5 cm may increase the risk of incidence of nerve injury.[6] Therefore, femoral shortening is a useful or sometimes necessary technique to facilitate reduction without stretching the sciatic nerve, equalize limb lengths, and overcome contractures.

Various subtrochanteric osteotomy techniques with different cutting shapes, such as transverse, oblique chevron, or Z-shaped, have been previously described with good clinical results. However, the risk of fracture and nonunion remains the major concern in the procedure. The transverse osteotomy has several advantages compared with other modified methods, including preservation of the proximal femoral metaphysis and simultaneous shortening and correction of rotational abnormalities, which may decrease the risk of torsional instability for the stem and provide more normal proximal femoral anatomy.[7]

Indications

- Crowe type III or IV DDH
- Combination of acetabular dysplasia and proximal femoral deformities
- Hip arthrosis
- Hip fusion
- Seriously insinuated acetabulum

Contraindications

- Active infection in hip
- Severe medical condition

- Severe osteoporosis (which may not allow stable internal fixation)
- Insufficient muscle strength of abductor
- Infection at the site of the surgical field

SURGICAL PROCEDURE

Preoperative planning

RADIOGRAPHY

Plain radiographs

A good-quality true anteroposterior (AP) and lateral radiograph of the hip is mandatory. An acetabular template was placed at the true anatomic hip center and a femoral template was placed for the femoral component. When the templating indicated that the maximum amount of lengthening was >3–4 cm, the length of the subtrochanteric shortening bone was planned to equalize the leg lengths and lengthen the limb by <3–4 cm.

Computed Tomography

Three-dimensional computed tomography (CT) scans were used on a routine basis to evaluate acetabular bone defects.

Intraoperative

STEP 1: POSITIONING AND APPROACH

All procedures were performed via a posterolateral approach with the patient in the lateral decubitus position.

- Place the patient in a lateral position.
- Begin the proximal limb of the incision at a point 6–8 cm anterior to the posterior superior iliac spine and just distal to the iliac crest, overlying the anterior border of the gluteus maximus muscle. Extend it distally to the anterior edge of the greater trochanter and farther distally along the line of the femur for 15–18 cm.

STEP 2: TOTAL HIP ARTHROPLASTY AND SUBTROCHANTERIC FEMUR OSTEOTOMY

- *Acetabular component implantation*: After total capsulotomy, we resected the femoral head and removed the osteophytes and fibrous scar tissue to recognize the true acetabulum before reaming. The acetabulum was gradually reamed with hemispherical reamers to reach the medial wall of the true acetabulum, with bleeding cancellous bone. The porous-coated acetabular component was inserted in the anatomic acetabular position with the use of the press-fit technique and fixed with dome screws in all hips. If the acetabular bone was deficient, bulk bone autografts with the resected femoral head were used to provide adequate coverage of acetabular cup.

- *Subtrochanteric Femur Osteotomy*: If the true acetabulum was not reachable due to the obstruction of the proximal part of the femur, a transverse femoral osteotomy approximately 1–2 cm distal to the lesser trochanter was performed. If there was a proximal femoral canal deformity, an osteotomy was conducted at the level of the deformity. Elevation or split of a short section of the vastus lateralis was performed to approach the subtrochanteric area. Next, the proximal femoral fragment was translated anteriorly to reach the true acetabulum after the performance of transverse osteotomy. The acetabulum was widened and deepened with use of hemispherical reamers at a designated angle of anteversion and abduction to obtain bleeding cancellous bone, which indicated an interference fit between the anterior and posterior columns (Figure 17.1a). For insufficient coverage or severe acetabular bone defects, augmentation of the acetabulum was conducted by a structural autograft or titanium alloy (Ti-alloy) mesh combined with bulk bone grafting from the resected femoral head. Femoral head structural bone autografts fixed with screws were used in 38 hips to improve coverage of the cup due to insufficient coverage, whereas Ti-alloy mesh and impaction bone grafting were used in 9 hips owing to severe acetabular bone defects according to the three-dimensional CT. Implantation of the acetabular cup was conducted using the press-fit technique (Figure 17.1b).

After the acetabular component was inserted, attention was then directed to the more distal femur. A second transverse subtrochanteric osteotomy was conducted to shorten the femur by the planned amount. If a proximal femoral canal deformity existed, correction of the rotational deformity of the proximal femur was conducted before axial reaming through subtrochanteric osteotomy. The straight axial intramedullary reaming

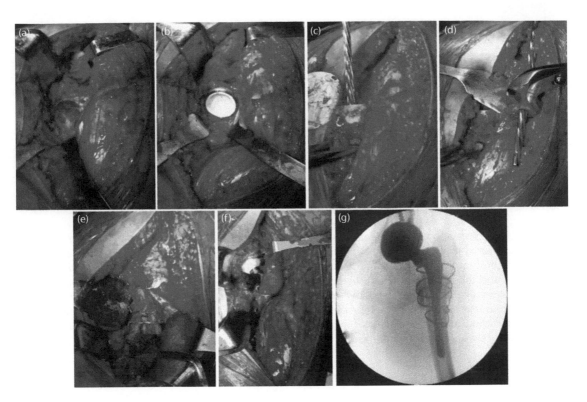

Figure 17.1 Intraoperative photographs of THA in a 31-year-old woman with Crowe type-IV DDH.
(a) Acetabulum was widened and deepened to obtain bleeding cancellous bone and femoral head autograft was applied. (b) The insertion of acetabular cup. (c) The straight axial intramedullary reaming process was conducted in the distal femur. (d) The proximal part of the femur was then prepared for the cementless implant. (e,f) The straight stem was then inserted into the femur across the osteotomy site, at which the gap was grafted with autogenous morselized bone and stabilized by cable fixation. (g) C-arm x-ray was used to ensure the position of the cup and stem.

process was conducted in the distal femur, and the proximal part of the femur was then prepared for the cementless implant (Figure 17.1c,d). Then, sequential rasping was performed until the appropriate femoral component size was achieved. The proximal and distal bone fragments were then aligned, and they were properly rotated on the trial component. If a trial reduction of the hip could not be achieved following the first cut of the osteotomy, an additional osteotomy was gradually performed in sequence with a transverse design to archive satisfactory hip reduction. After the proximal sleeve was implanted, the straight stem was then inserted into the femur across the osteotomy site when the rotational alignment of the two fragments was adjusted to allow approximately 15–20° of anteversion of the femoral component (Figure 17.1e). If necessary, prophylactic cable fixation can be used to prevent femoral fracture. After the insertion of femoral component, the gap at the osteotomy site was grafted with autogenous morselized bone and stabilized by cable fixation to enhance biologic healing in 46 cases (Figure 17.1f). After the insertion of femoral and acetabular components, C-arm x-ray was used in most patients to ensure the position of the cup and stem (Figure 17.1g).

Postoperative care

All patients were encouraged to conduct isometric exercises and active motion on a bed immediately after surgery. The patients walked with partial weight bearing under the protection of crutches for approximately 2 weeks. Then, gradually progressive full weight bearing was allowed at 4–6 weeks depending on the stability of the femoral stem and positively osseous healing at the osteotomy site.

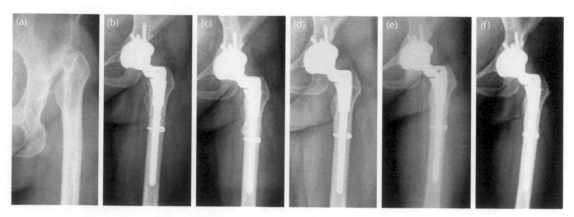

Figure 17.2 Radiographs of a 29-year-old woman with unilateral Crowe type-IV DDH. **(a)** Preoperative anteroposterior view. **(b)** Postoperative radiographic image at 4 months follow-up. Total hip arthroplasty was combined with simultaneous transverse osteotomy. Cerclage wires were placed at osteotomy site, and the acetabulum was reconstructed with screws. **(c)** Postoperative radiographic image at 1 year follow-up. **(d)** At 4 years follow-up, bone union was detected at the osteotomy site without radiolucent lines around the stem. **(e)** At 8 years follow-up, the femoral and acetabular components showed no radiographic signs of loosening. **(f)** Postoperative radiographic image at 11 years follow-up. The femoral and acetabular components were stable.

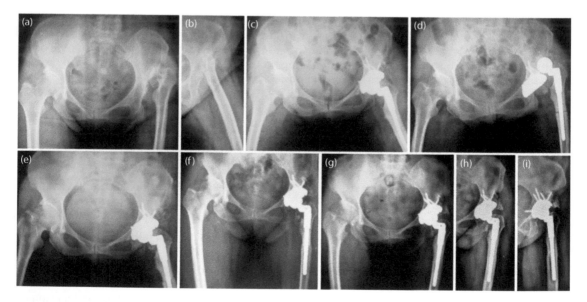

Figure 17.3 Radiographs of a 42-year-old woman with unilateral Crowe type-IV DDH. **(a, b)** Preoperative anteroposterior view. **(c)** Radiographic image at postoperative 1 day. Total hip arthroplasty was performed combined with transverse osteotomy in left hip. **(d,e)** Postoperative anteroposterior view showed dislocation at 1-week follow-up, which was treated successfully through closed relocation. **(f)** Radiographic image after 5 years follow-up showed that no radiolucent lines around the femoral and acetabular components were identified, but osteolysis around the stem at the distal tip and heterotopic ossification were identified. **(g–i)** At 11 years follow-up, the postoperative Harris hip score was 97, and the femoral stem was judged to be stable with bone ingrowth.

OUTCOMES

Our published studies have documented good long-term results in Crowe type IV–Hartofilakidis type III DDH. Our data demonstrate that the cementless, modular THA combined with transverse subtrochanteric shortening osteotomy was an effective and reliable technique with high rates of successful fixation of the implants and satisfactory clinical outcomes (Figure 17.2).[8] The modified Merle d'Aubigne and Postel hip score, hip dysfunction and osteoarthritis outcome score, and SF-12 significantly improved. However, there were three cases of postoperative dislocation (Figure 17.3), two cases of transient nerve palsy, one case of nonunion, and four cases of intraoperative fracture. Revision surgery was performed in two patients due to isolated loosening of the acetabular component and femoral stem, respectively.

Tips: Correspondent measures to prevent nonunion at the osteotomy site:

- The interface and canal diameters were congruent between proximal and distal segments, which may affect the union. Bone resection should be assisted by assistance with axial resistance at the knee to achieve a better anastomosis interface, and the two osteotomy interfaces should be cut smoother to keep the interfaces intact as much as possible.
- When preparing osteotomy sites and prophylactical cerclage wiring, we removed the circumferential periosteum and thereby damaged the osteoblastic activity of the periosteum. Therefore, the osteotomy site should be held with autologous cancellous bone and then stabilized with autogenous cortical bone plate affixed with cables or wires.
- Great care was taken to minimize damage to the periosteum circumferentially during preparation of osteotomy sites and prophylactic cerclage wiring to keep the osteoblastic activity of the periosteum.

Advantages of subtrochanteric femur osteotomy:

a. Restoration of the anatomical hip rotation center without extensive tissue release
b. Facilitate reduction without stretching the sciatic nerve
c. Overcome contractures
d. Early mobilization
e. Protect the metaphyseal structure
f. Does not damage the direction of the large rotor and abductor muscle, which can restore mechanical properties and avoid joint instability

Disadvantages of subtrochanteric femur osteotomy:

a. Subtrochanteric femur osteotomy may result in osteotomy site–related and other complications, including:
   - Delayed union or nonunion of the osteotomy site
   - Heterotopic ossification
   - Neurovascular injuries
   - Postoperative persistent pain of the osteotomy site
   - Hematoma
   - Femoral fracture
   - Hip dislocation
b. Prolonged surgical time and increased postoperative blood loss
c. Anemia

REFERENCES

1. Sponseller PD, McBeath AA. Subtrochanteric osteotomy with intramedullary fixation for arthroplasty of the dysplastic hip. A case report. *J Arthroplasty* 1988; 3(4): 351–4.
2. Ollivier M, Abdel MP, Krych AJ, Trousdale RT, Berry DJ. Long-term results of total hip arthroplasty with shortening subtrochanteric osteotomy in Crowe IV developmental dysplasia. *J Arthroplasty* 2016; 31(8): 1756–60.
3. Zhu J, Shen C, Chen X, Cui Y, Peng J, Cai G. Total hip arthroplasty with a non-modular conical stem and transverse subtrochanteric osteotomy in treatment of high dislocated hips. *J Arthroplasty* 2015; 30(4): 611–4.
4. Takao M, Ohzono K, Nishii T, Miki H, Nakamura N, Sugano N. Cementless modular total hip arthroplasty with subtrochanteric shortening osteotomy for hips with developmental dysplasia. *J Bone Joint Surg Am* 2011; 93(6): 548–55.

5. Charity JA et al. Treatment of Crowe IV high hip dysplasia with total hip replacement using the Exeter stem and shortening derotational subtrochanteric osteotomy. *J Bone Joint Surg Br* 2011; 93(1): 34–8.

6. Wang D, Li LL, Wang HY, Pei FX, Zhou ZK. Long-term results of cementless total hip arthroplasty with subtrochanteric shortening osteotomy in Crowe Type IV developmental dysplasia. *J Arthroplasty* 2016; 32(4): 1211–9.

7. Wang D et al. Subtrochanteric shortening osteotomy during cementless total hip arthroplasty in young patients with severe developmental dysplasia of the hip. *BMC Musculoskelet Disord* 2017; 18(1): 491.

8. Wang D, Li LL, Wang HY, Pei FX, Zhou ZK. Long-term results of cementless total hip arthroplasty with subtrochanteric shortening osteotomy in Crowe Type IV developmental dysplasia. *J Arthroplasty* 2017; 32(4): 1211–9.

18

Valgus osteotomy for femoral neck pseudoarthrosis

ASHOK S. GAVASKAR AND DAVID ROJAS

BACKGROUND

Femoral neck fractures in young patients have long been an enigma for treating surgeons. Nonunion rates as high as 43% have been reported in several series, which is considerably higher when compared to fractures in other regions of the skeletal system.[1,2] Several contributing factors, both mechanical and biological, have been implicated in the occurrence of femoral neck nonunion.[3,4] Mechanical factors, for example, poor fracture reduction and fixation leading to instability; comminution at the posterior and inferior cortices causing risk for failure of fixation; high fracture angle leading to shear forces at the fracture site; and small proximal segment in terms of volume and poor bone stock, can preclude secure and appropriate fixation.[3] Biological factors, for instance, injury to the retinacular arteries, which are the predominant blood supply to the femoral head in adults; capsular

tamponade compromising the blood supply to the femoral head; absence of the inner cambium layer of the periosteum; and lastly, the interference of the synovial fluid in consolidation of the fracture hematoma, have all been implicated.[5]

The proper management of femoral neck nonunion consists of a combination of biological and mechanical techniques to warrant a successful osteosynthesis treatment.[4] However, is biology more important than mechanical principles? Is it equally important, or vice versa? Conclusions remain controversial, and several treatment methods have been described in the peer-reviewed literature. Different bone grafting strategies (intrafocal cancellous grafting, free and vascularized cortical strut grafts, and muscle pedicle bone grafts) have been used, demonstrating variable results.[6–8] The combination of bone grafting and internal fixation techniques predominantly addressing the biological problem has not shown reliable results.[6]

Osteotomies, on the other hand, aim to generate an enhanced biomechanical environment for the proximal femur and/or femoral neck fracture's geometry, allowing fracture healing and union.[9] Two types of osteotomies have been described: (1) angular and (2) translational osteotomies. The classic medial translational osteotomy described by McMurray fell into disrepute due to concerns regarding gross distortion of the proximal femur anatomy and shortening.[10] The first description of an angular osteotomy is by Schantz, who described the subtrochanteric abduction angulation osteotomy. Angular osteotomies were believed to be more effective than translational osteotomies. The ideas were further expanded and refined by Friedrich Pauwels, who described the intertrochanteric valgization osteotomy.[11] The original osteotomy and its subsequent modifications by Mueller have stood the test of time and have provided consistently good results without the need for additional bone grafting practices.[12] This chapter describes different osteotomy techniques and the rationale for performing a valgus intertrochanteric osteotomy (VITO), highlighting the biomechanical advantages and limitations of VITO in treating a femoral neck nonunion.

PRINCIPLES AND RATIONALE OF VALGUS OSTEOTOMY IN FEMORAL NECK PSEUDOARTHROSIS

Compressive forces across the fracture tend to promote union, whereas shear forces impede union. Femoral neck nonunion is more commonly observed in vertical shear fracture patterns (Pauwels type III fractures).[9,13] During failure, the femoral head typically tends to drift and fail into varus, accentuating the degree of shearing, which ultimately leads to a nonunion. Shear forces do not favor fracture union; therefore, according to Pauwels, these biomechanical irregularities have to be addressed with proper osteosynthesis techniques.[14] The rationale for intertrochanteric valgus osteotomy for femoral neck nonunion is that valgization of the femoral head is capable of converting vertical shear forces into compressive forces at the nonunion site.[4] This can be achieved by transforming the vertical fracture plane into a more horizontal one. Consequently, the force along the line of

weight transmission will result in purely compressive forces, accelerating the process of union.[3,4,8,9]

The relevance of proximal femur biomechanics to understand the principles of valgus intertrochanteric osteotomy

To understand the fundamentals of VITO, it is important to recognize the normal loading patterns of the hip joint and how they can affect or influence outcomes in femoral neck nonunion when treated with VITO.[15]

Under normal loading circumstances, the hip joint is subjected to a compressive force "R," which is the result of all loads acting on the hip joint.[7,16] During normal gait, the hip joint is subjected to muscular forces "M" and the body weight "W." The direction of force R is a straight line representing the intersection of the muscle forces and the partial body weight acting during the single leg stance. The resultant force R, though, represents a sum of these two forces, and is primarily determined by the muscular forces acting on the hip joint (Figure 18.1).

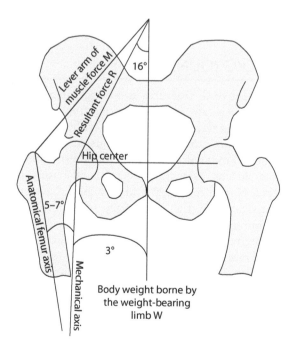

Figure 18.1 The different forces acting across the hip joint and their possible effects on healing of a femoral neck fracture.

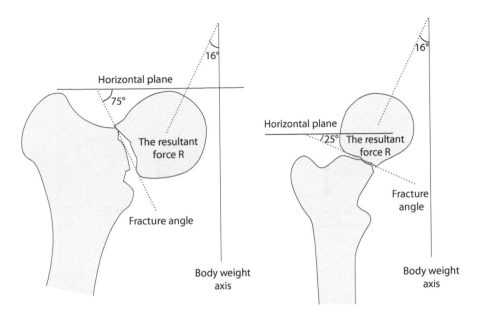

Figure 18.2 The effect of the fracture angle on the nature of forces at the fracture site after a femoral neck fracture. Low fracture angles (<30°) are subjected to predominantly compressive forces facilitating healing, while high fracture angles (>50°) are subjected to high shear forces that negatively influence fracture healing.

The muscle forces in turn depend on the abductor lever arm. To maintain equilibrium, the muscle forces must triple the body weight.[17]

The force R, however, is not entirely compressive because the line of action is not in line with the femoral neck axis, but slightly medial to it. This breaks down the resultant force R into two components: (1) a purely compressive force acting along the neck axis and (2) a shearing force acting perpendicular to it.[17] Therefore, femoral neck fractures are always exposed to some degree of bending and shearing forces (Figure 18.2), increasing with the verticality of the fracture line and resulting in a higher incidence of nonunion.[3,4,8,9,15]

The resultant force R acts on the center of rotation of the hip joint in an inclined direction, subtending an angle of 16° with the vertical (body axis).[13,17] A horizontal fracture plane will position the fracture perpendicular to the line of the resultant force R and hence will be subjected to predominantly compressive forces. This forms the biomechanical basis of VITO. Repositioning of the femoral neck will ensure stability. Once stable, the intervening fibrous tissue will be rapidly

mineralized and invaded by angiogenesis, allowing for endochondral ossification and successful osteosynthesis (Figure 18.3).

TYPES OF VALGUS INTERTROCHANTERIC OSTEOTOMY FOR FEMORAL NECK PSEUDOARTHROSIS

Pauwels described two types of osteotomies for femoral neck nonunion[11]: (1) a simple lateral closing wedge osteotomy, which moves the femoral head to valgus (Figure 18.4a). The amount and location of the wedge will depend on the degree of correction required and the angle of fixation device used. (2) A "Y" osteotomy, which he recommends for nonunion with a negative articulotrochanteric distance, indicating a serious disturbance in the head–shaft relationship with proximal migration of the trochanter and a femoral head that has fallen into gross varus (Figure 18.4b).[18] The "Y" osteotomy may also grossly distort the proximal femur anatomy and the mechanical axis, which can make a future arthroplasty much more difficult.

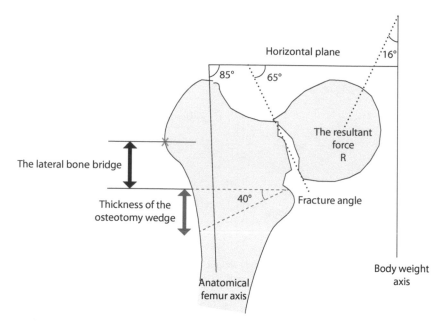

Figure 18.3 How a valgization osteotomy can reposition the nonunion more horizontally, subjecting the nonunion to more favorable compressive forces across the pseudoarthrosis.

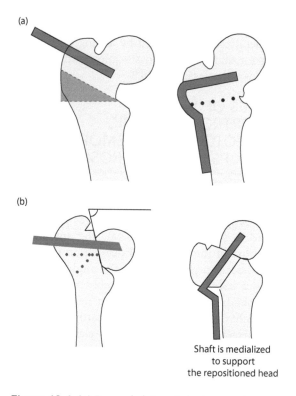

Figure 18.4 (a) Pauwels lateral closing wedge osteotomy. (b) Pauwels Y osteotomy used when there is gross varus with proximal migration of the shaft. This produces medial translation of the shaft fragment and laters the mechanical axis.

SURGICAL TECHNIQUE: VALGUS INTERTROCHANTERIC OSTEOTOMY

Indications

- Established femoral neck pseudoarthrosis[18]
- Delayed presentation with displaced fractures into varus
- Primary osteotomy for high Pauwels angle fractures (highly debatable, and there is not enough evidence to recommend a routine application of VITO for Pauwels type III fractures)

Prerequisite

A viable femoral head is an essential prerequisite for a good long-term outcome. However, the radiological presence of osteonecrosis without collapse of the femoral head is not a contraindication for VITO, and a successful osteosynthesis can still be achieved. The presence of avascular areas can lead to a quite rapid fragmentation and collapse of the femoral head, affecting long-term results of VITO, but this can still be attempted in young patients.[19]

Contraindications

- Advanced age[11,20]
- Gross osteopenia with poor bone stock
- Morbid obesity
- Smoking
- Poor bone stock in the femoral head (small volume) with severe neck resorption
- Advanced femoral head collapse

Preoperative planning

The aim of the surgery is to reposition the fracture perpendicular to the direction of the resultant force R.[21] The force R makes an angle of 16° with the sagittal body axis. The anatomical axis of the femoral shaft makes an angle of 8–10° with the sagittal body axis. So according to Mueller, placing the nonunion at an angle of 25° to a perpendicular dropped from the anatomical shaft axis will result in purely compressive forces at the nonunion.[22] The angle of correction (wedge) required will be calculated by subtracting 25° from the angle subtended by the fracture plane with the perpendicular dropped from the femoral shaft axis. The need for limb lengthening and rotational and sagittal plane correction should also be accounted for during preoperative planning based on clinical/physical examination results.[23] Careful preoperative planning is an absolute requisite for accurate correction of the deformities, limb length, and restoration of the proximal femur anatomy.

Always keep in mind the possible need for a future arthroplasty.[24,25]

Good quality anteroposterior (AP) and lateral x-rays are required for preoperative planning.[26] AP x-rays should be taken with the limb in internal rotation. Longitudinal traction while taking x-rays might help assess mobility of the pseudoarthrosis and provide information in regard to the extent of correction needed. Lateral x-rays help with the assessment of the sagittal plane deformity. X-rays of the normal hip (contralateral x-rays) are important for screening and identification of the native neck shaft angle and hip offset.

Start by tracing the deformed hip on tracing paper. For VITO in femoral neck pseudoarthrosis, it is advisable to use a higher-angled plate fixation device (120° or 130°), which will allow excellent correction without unwanted medial translation of the shaft. An angled blade plate is the preferred implant and provides excellent angle stable fixation even in small femoral heads.[21] Another advantage is that only small amounts of bone are removed compared to other devices. The main limitation of the blade plate is that a rigorous surgical technique is mandatory because of the lack of plate modularity and difficulties with blade insertion. Other implants such as sliding hip screws, prebent 90° dynamic condylar screw (DCS), and locked plates have all been described as showing good results.[3,27]

The below example shows preoperative templating for a femoral neck nonunion treated with a 120° angled blade plate (Figure 18.5). Angles drawn

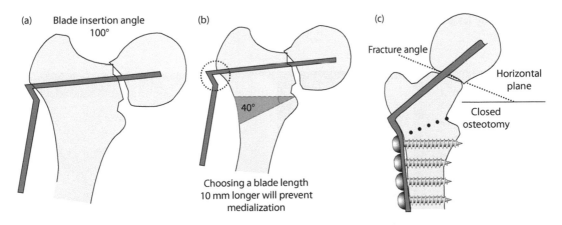

Figure 18.5 Preoperative planning with a 120° blade plate: The blade insertion angle is calculated based on the supplementary angle + the degree of correction (fracture angle: 25°). Tracings are made to calculate the thickness of the lateral wedge and confirm the degree of correction after the planned osteotomy.

from the tracing show that the fracture angle is 65°, and repositioning the fracture perpendicular to the resultant force R would require a correction of 40° (65° − 25°). The starting point for the blade plate is marked A. It should be around 1.5–2 cm above the site of the planned osteotomy to maintain an adequate bone bridge. The insertion angle of the blade plate chisel depends on the angle of correction required. For a 120° blade plate, the angle of insertion into the femoral head would be its supplementary angle, i.e., 60° (180° − 120°) to the femoral shaft if no correction is needed. Since we need a correction of 40°, the angle of insertion would be 100° (60° + 40°).

Preoperative traction to bring the hip down has been described to be useful in cases with high-riding trochanters. However, there is no conclusive evidence to recommend the routine use of preoperative traction to improve results.

Surgical procedure (using a 135° sliding hip screw)

This procedure can be performed on a standard operating table with provision for biplanar fluoroscopy and manual traction, or it can be performed on a fracture table with the lower limb set in traction (Figure 18.6).

A standard vastus-splitting lateral approach is used. The anterolateral Watson-Jones approach can be used if access to the fracture site is required to improve reduction and/or to perform bone grafting.[21]

The site of the transverse limb of the osteotomy at the level of the lesser trochanter is identified under fluoroscopy. A K-wire is then inserted as a reference. Next, the templated starting point for the Richards screw is identified, which is usually 1.5–2 cm above the site of the osteotomy. Drill a guide wire along the intended path of the screw along the axis of the femoral neck, aiming for the inferior or the central portion of the head on AP view and the central on the lateral view. Once the intended trajectory is decided, the entry point for the screw is prepared with the triple reamer and the screw of measured length is inserted. (If a blade plate is used, the entry point for the seating chisel must be in the anterior third of the greater trochanter to obtain a satisfactory direction into the femoral neck and head. Care should be taken not to perforate the posterior cortex in order to protect the capsular blood supply.[28] The sclerotic areas in the neck may require some force to progress the chisel and should be done carefully under fluoroscopy.) After inserting the Richards screw, the transverse limb of the osteotomy is performed using a saw blade under fluoroscopy. The medial cortex is kept intact. The templated wedge thickness is translated onto the lateral cortex and the oblique inferior limb of the osteotomy is now performed. The lateral wedge is removed and can be used as bone graft later. The medial cortex is then broken and the shaft is abducted and clamped to the barrel plate using a Verbrugge clamp to close the osteotomy. Further compression at the osteotomy site can be applied if needed. This can be achieved with the Mueller compression device. Three to four 4.5-mm cortex screws are inserted into the distal fragment, completing the procedure (Figure 18.7). The final correction is confirmed under fluoroscopy and limb length is checked.

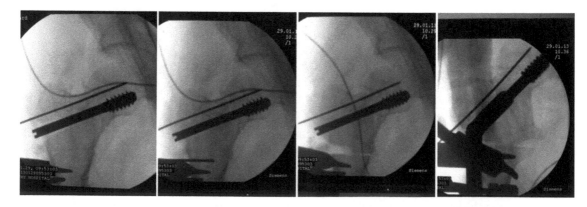

Figure 18.6 Steps of VITO using a 135° sliding hip screw (SHS).

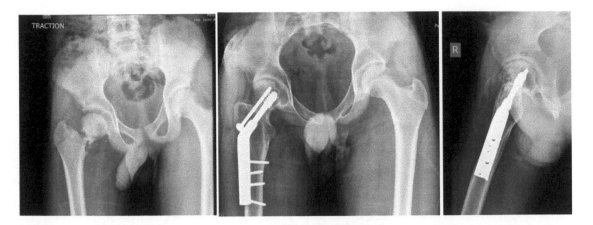

Figure 18.7 Case example of a 17-year-old male with a 9-month-old femoral neck pseudoarthrosis. Valgization was done with a 135° SHS. Union was achieved in 6 months. His Harris Hip Score was 83.

Postoperative Rehabilitation

Postsurgery, patients are mobilized and allowed toe-touch weight bearing from day 1 for a period of 6 weeks.[21] Hip and knee range-of-motion exercises are encouraged. Prophylaxis for preventing deep vein thrombosis is administered. Around 6 weeks, patients should gradually progress to partial weight bearing and transition to full weight bearing when union at the osteotomy site becomes evident. Unrestricted physical activity is permitted after radiological evidence of union.

APPRAISAL OF DIFFERENT TECHNIQUES AND IMPLANTS FOR VALGUS INTERTROCHANTERIC OSTEOTOMY

The technique of valgizing the proximal femur and getting the fracture plane in line with the axis of load transmission can be achieved in different ways. The most common technique is to remove a lateral-based full wedge at the intertrochanteric level. The intertrochanteric level osteotomy achieves excellent bony contact after closure of the osteotomy, and the cancellous bone heals much faster and predictably, minimizing the risks of nonunion at the osteotomy. However, there is risk of failure because of the small bone bridge between the site of entry of the blade/screw and the osteotomy. An adequate bone bridge of 15–20 mm should be preserved. In the case of extracapsular nonunion, the lateral wall may be too thin, causing a high risk for failure. In these cases, the osteotomy can be performed distally at the high subtrochanteric level (Figure 18.8).

Problems with taking a full lateral wedge include limb-length discrepancy and alterations in the mechanical axis.[23,26] Careful preoperative planning is required to avoid this issue.[29] In spite of good planning, limb-length inequality of 1 cm is common in full wedge osteotomies, as reported by Hartford et al.[23] The problem can be minimized by using a half-wedge technique, as shown by Schoenfeld et al.[26] The limitation of the half-wedge technique is less bony contact at the osteotomy, which may increase the possibility of failure. Gavaskar et al. described a no-wedge sliding technique, which relies on sliding of the osteotomy surfaces to bring about valgization of the proximal fragment and can help in limb-length equalization.[30] Sliding of the osteotomy surfaces brings about lateralization of the distal fragment, which restores the mechanical axis (Figures 18.9 and 18.10) and limits lateral compartment overload at the knee joint.

The blade plate is the most common implant used for performing VITO.[31-33] It provides excellent rotational control and only requires very minimal bone removal. The main limitation of the blade plate is the lack of modularity that makes it difficult to use. Risk of malalignment is common unless care is exercised in preventing it. The screw-based devices, the sliding hip screw and the double bent DCS device, are easier to use because of modularity and have been reported to achieve results similar to the blade plate in multiple series.[23,26,34] Screw-based implants lack the rotational stability offered by the

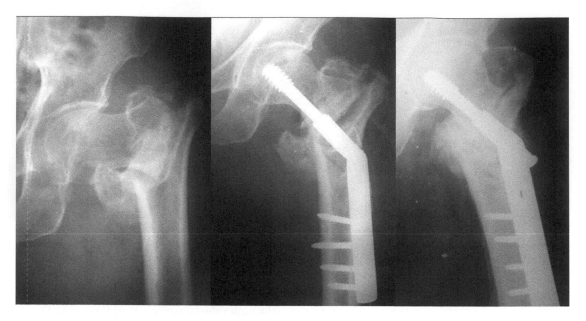

Figure 18.8 For an extracapsular pseudoarthrosis, the osteotomy is performed just below the lesser trochanter to enable an adequate bone bridge laterally.

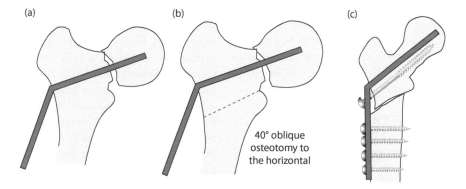

Figure 18.9 Sliding osteotomy: Sliding osteotomy technique relies on an oblique osteotomy made at an angle corresponding to the degree of correction required (fracture angle: 25°). The osteotomy surfaces are slid against each other, achieving necessary valgization with minimal translation.

blade plate and also remove much more cancellous bone compared to the blade plate.[30]

RESULTS OF VALGUS INTERTROCHANTERIC OSTEOTOMY FOR FEMORAL NECK NONUNION

VITO is the single most successful technique for treating femoral neck nonunion.[8,13] The results have been replicated over time and the technique has changed very little from its original description. Multiple authors across the world have reported successful results in different patient populations.[21,29,35–43] Easily reproducible technique, no need for special implants, young patient population, and no need for bone grafting or opening the nonunion site make it an attractive technique with high success rates. Success rates of up to 85–100% have been reported in previous published reports (Table 18.1).

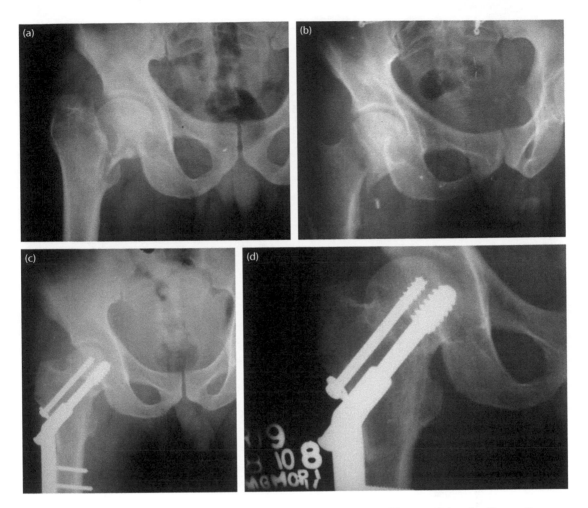

Figure 18.10 Example of a 6-month-old femoral neck nonunion in a 38-year-old male. Correction with a sliding valgus osteotomy with follow-up x-rays show union of both the pseudoarthrosis and osteotomy.

PROBLEMS AND COMPLICATIONS WITH VALGUS INTERTROCHANTERIC OSTEOTOMY

The most common complication reported after a VITO is failure of osteosynthesis (Figure 18.9).

The failure is often seen at the nonunion site while the osteotomy heals predictably. Reasons for failure include poor surgical technique in terms of inadequate valgization, failure of the lateral bone bridge, poor blade/screw position in the femoral head compromising stability, biological failure at the nonunion site, and malalignment in the sagittal plane.[44] Failures are also reported to be more common in cases with severe neck resorption.[29]

Nonunion at the osteotomy site is rare but has been reported in obese patients (BMI > 30) and chronic smokers.[11] Varghese et al. reported failures in patients with a neck resorption ratio (NRR) of <0.52 in their series.[29] NRR was calculated as percentage of intact neck available at the nonunion compared to the normal neck length on the opposite limb (Figure 18.11).

Limb-length discrepancy is another common problem after VITO. Postoperative improvement in limb length is the norm after a VITO, since valgization improves limb length.[23,26] However, achieving equalization in limb length is often a challenge and requires careful preoperative planning.[21] No-wedge and/or half-wedge techniques

Table 18.1 Case series of VITO for femoral neck pseudoarthrosis

Reference	N	Mean follow-up (yr)	Union rate, n/total (%)	AVN, n/total (%)	Implant	Functional outcome
Marti et al.	50	7.1	43/50 (86)	22/50 (44)	DABP	HHS—91
Anglen et al.	13	2	13/13 (100)	2/13 (15)	DABP	HHS—93
Wu et al.	32		32/32 (100)	2/32 (6)	SHS +/− subtrochanteric osteotomy	NA
Kalra et al.	22	2.5	20/22 (85)	2/22 (9)	DABP	75%: good to excellent results
Sringari et al.	20	2	18/20 (90)	Nil	DABP	NA
Magu et al.	48	6	44/48 (94)	2/48 (4)	DABP	HHS—86.7
Khan et al.	16	2.5	14/16 (87)	Nil	SHS: 120°	HHS—88
Said et al.	36	3.5	35/36 (97)	5/36 (13)	Angled blade plate: prebent 130°	NA
Sen et al.	22	3.2	21/22 (97)	5/22 (22)	DABP + nonvascularized fibula	66%: good to excellent results
Gadegone et al.	41	2.75	39/41 (95)	7/41 (17)	SHS (110°–130°) + nonvascularized fibula	HHS—90.9
Gavaskar et al.	11	1	11/11 (100)	Nil	SHS (subtrochanteric osteotomy) no wedge	Oxford—40
Gupta et al.	60	3.5	56/60 (93)	4/60 (6)	SHS, 130° + subtrochanteric osteotomy	HHS—87.5
Varghese et al.	32	5	29/32 (91)	13/32 (44)	DABP	HHS—82

Abbreviations: AVN, avascular necrosis; DABP, double-angled blade plate; SHS, sliding hip screw; HHS, Harris Hip Score; NA, not available.

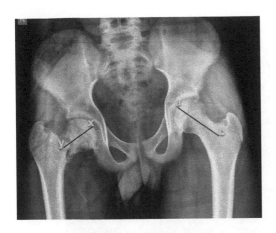

Figure 18.11 The neck resorption ratio (NRR) is calculated by dividing the longest length of the femoral head–neck fragment on the nonunion side (ab) and the length of the intact femoral neck measured to the intertrochanteric line (xy). These measurements help us to calculate the NRR by dividing the longest length of the femoral head–neck fragment on the nonunion side and the length of the intact femoral neck measured to the intertrochanteric line.

when performing VITO have better chances of achieving limb-length equalization.[26,30]

Avascular necrosis of the femoral head (AVNFH) is another reported complication after VITO. This often occurs due to excessive valgization, which increases the joint reaction forces across the hip joint and also affects the blood supply to the femoral head (retinacular arteries).[21,29,42] A valgus angle of >15° compared to the normal side has been shown to increase incidences of AVNFH and should be avoided.[29,45] Avoiding perforation of the blade posteriorly during insertion into the femoral neck is important to prevent iatrogenic injury to the capsular blood vessels. Occurrence of AVNFH can lead to rapid progression and collapse, requiring the need for a total hip arthroplasty (THA).[46] Pre-existing AVNFH before VITO has not been reported to interfere with achieving a successful osteosynthesis. The surgeon should, however, be careful enough to preserve the proximal femur anatomy after VITO so that THA does not pose any technical challenges.[15]

Limp and altered gait after VITO are also relatively common. Mathews reported limp in almost all his patients.[32] The most common cause for limp is valgization itself, which leads to decreased offset (more pronounced in patients with excessive neck resorption) and inefficient abductor lever arm.[21] Decrease in horizontal offset of almost 45% compared to the normal side has been reported after VITO. Limb shortening is another major cause for limp after VITO.[32]

Alteration in mechanical axis is another problem after VITO. This is more evident and possible in higher degrees of correction. A valgus osteotomy at the proximal femur will translate the mechanical axis laterally, resulting in lateral compartment overload and pain (Figure 18.12) due to accelerated degeneration at the knee joint.[47] This can be avoided by translating the shaft (distal fragment) laterally. Lateralization of the distal shaft fragment can be achieved by more easily using a dynamic hip screw (DHS) (Figure 18.13), a no-wedge technique, or a double-angled blade plate of 15 mm more than the measured length of the blade to allow space for lateralization.[30,34]

Since VITO distorts the proximal femur anatomy in the coronal plane, concerns have been raised about difficulties in performing a THA postosteotomy. A take-down or revision osteotomy is often required during a THA, increasing surgical time and complexity of the procedure and requiring the need for more modular and expensive implants.[46] This can be avoided by performing the osteotomy at or slightly above the lesser trochanter since this will preserve the anatomy of the distal segment.[15,29] Excessive translation of the mechanical axis in the coronal plane should also be avoided with careful planning and execution. During the process of preoperative planning, it is useful to template the proximal femur (replicating the postosteotomy situation) to make sure a cemented/uncemented femoral stem can pass through safely without the need for an osteotomy during hip arthroplasty.[48] Finally, any inadvertent malalignments in the sagittal plane should be avoided. Removal of implants should be routinely recommended after 18–24 months. This will help avoid complications during a future arthroplasty if required.

SUMMARY

VITO is the most successful standalone technique for treating femoral neck pseudoarthrosis. The goal is to improve the biomechanical environment at the proximal femur, thereby reorienting the nonunion in line with the axis of load transmission. This supports healing by achieving union

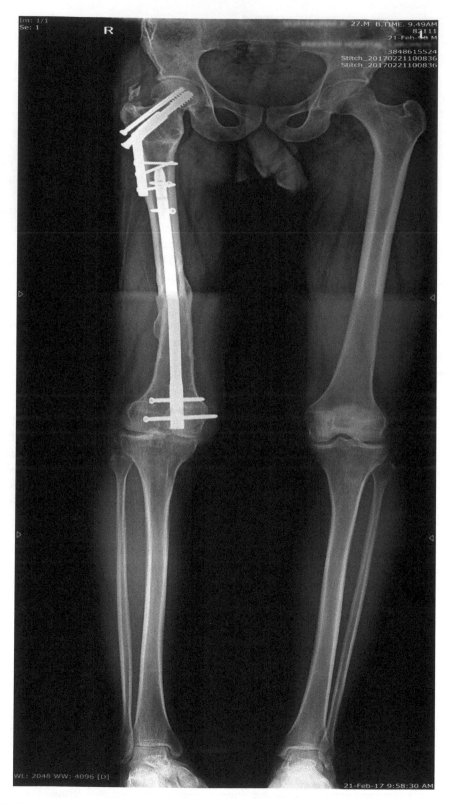

Figure 18.12 Case example in a 26-year-old male shows evidence of knee lateral compartment arthritis 3 years post-VITO.

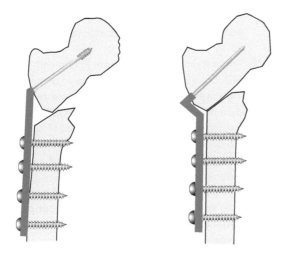

Figure 18.13 How an SHS prevents alteration in the mechanical axis compared to a double-angled blade plate by preventing medialization.

through pure compressive forces without the need of bone grafting procedures. This is a reproducible, relatively simple procedure with high success rates and low complications. Therefore, this has become the procedure of choice for dealing with femoral neck pseudoarthrosis and fixation failures in young patients. Even though failure rates are rare, they can be more frequently seen in the elderly population and patients with severe neck resorption, obesity, and osteoporosis. Smokers should be screened and smoking cessation should be emphasized. Problems of limb-length discrepancy, lateral compartment overloading at the knee, and difficulties with future hip arthroplasty can be avoided with careful planning and a good surgical technique. Excess valgization should always be avoided to prevent or minimize pain and poor functionality and lower incidences of AVNFH.

REFERENCES

1. Jackson M, Learmonth ID. The treatment of nonunion after intracapsular fracture of the proximal femur. *Clin Orthop Relat Res*, 2002; (399): 119–28.
2. Swiontkowski MF, Winquist RA, Hansen ST Jr. Fractures of the femoral neck in patients between the ages of twelve and forty-nine years. *J Bone Joint Surg Am* 1984; 66: 837–46.
3. Liporace F, Gaines R, Collinge C et al. Results of internal fixation of Pauwels type-3 vertical femoral neck fractures. *J Bone Joint Surg Am* 2008; 90: 1654–9.
4. Brandon JY, David WS, David PB, Sean EN. Intertrochanteric osteotomy for femoral neck nonunion: Does "undercorrection" result in an acceptable rate of femoral neck union? *J Orthop Trauma* 2017; 31: 420–6.
5. Prasad KSRK. CORR insights 1: Epiphyseal arterial network and inferior retinacular artery seem critical to femoral head perfusion in adults with femoral neck fractures. *Clin Orthop Relat Res* 2017; 475: 2024–6.
6. LeCroy CM, Rizzo M, Gunneson EE et al. Free vascularized fibular bone grafting in the management of femoral neck nonunion in patients younger than fifty years. *J Orthop Trauma* 2002; 16: 464–72.
7. Nagi ON, Dhillon MS, Goni VG. Open reduction, internal fixation and fibular autografting for neglected fracture of the femoral neck. *J Bone Joint Surg Br* 1998; 80: 798–804.
8. Varghese VD, Boopalan PR, Titus VT, Oommen AT, Jepegnanam TS. Indices affecting outcome of neglected femoral neck fractures after valgus intertrochanteric osteotomy. *J Orthop Trauma* 2014; 28: 410–6.
9. Collinge CA, Mir H, Reddix R. Fracture morphology of high shear angle "vertical" femoral neck fractures in young adult patients. *J Orthop Trauma* 2014; 28: 270–5.
10. Otho CH, William PB, Carl FF. End result study of McMurray osteotomy for acute fractures of the femoral neck. *Am J Surg*, 1951; 81(2).
11. Ballmer FT, Ballmer PM, Baumgaertel F, Ganz R, Mast JW. Pauwels osteotomy for nonunions of the femoral neck. *Orthop Clin North Am* 1990; 21(4): 759–67.
12. Mueller ME. The intertrochanteric osteotomy and pseudoarthrosis of the femoral neck. *Clin Orthop Relat Res* 1999; (363): 5–8.
13. Der Schenkelhalsbruch PF. *Ein Mechanisches Problem*. Stuttgart, Germany: F. Enke, 1935.
14. Alves T, Neal JW, Weinhold PS et al. Biomechanical comparison of 3 possible fixation strategies to resist femoral neck shortening after fracture. *Orthopedics*. 2010; 33: 233–7.

15. Deakin DE, Guy P, O'Brien PJ, Blachut PA, Lefaivre KA. Managing failed fixation: Valgus osteotomy for femoral neck non-union. *Injury* 2015; 3(46): 492–6.

16. Pauwels F. Biomechanical principles of varus/valgus intertrochanteric osteotomy (Pauwels I and II) in the treatment of osteoarthritis of the hip. In: Schatzker J. (ed.) *The Intertrochanteric Osteotomy.* Berlin, Heidelberg: Springer; 1984.

17. Pauwels F. *Biomechanics of the Locomotor Apparatus.* New York: Springer Verlag, 1980.

18. Müller ME. Intertrochanteric osteotomy: Indication, preoperative planning, technique. In: Schatzker J. (ed.) *The Intertrochanteric Osteotomy.* Berlin, Heidelberg: Springer; 1984.

19. Mont MA, Marulanda GA, Jones LC, Saleh KJ, Gordon N, Hungerford DS, Steinberg ME. Systematic analysis of classification systems for osteonecrosis of the femoral head. *J Bone Joint Surg Am* 2006; 88(Suppl 3): 16–26.

20. Raaymakers EL, Marti RK. Nonunion of the femoral neck: Possibilities and limitations of the various treatment modalities. *Indian J Orthop* 2008; 42: 13.

21. Magu NK, Rohilla R, Singh R, Tater R. Modified Pauwels intertrochanteric osteotomy in neglected femoral neck fracture. *Clin Orthop Relat Res* 2009; 467: 1064–73.

22. Mueller ME. The intertrochanteric osteotomy and pseudoarthrosis of the femoral neck. *Clin Orthop* 1999; 363: 5–8.

23. Hartford JM, Patel A, Powell J. Intertrochanteric osteotomy using a dynamic hip screw for femoral neck nonunion. *J Orthop Trauma*, 2005; 19(5): 329–33.

24. Mabry TM, Prpa B, Haidukewych GJ, Harmsen WS, Berry DJ. Long-term results of total hip arthroplasty for femoral neck fracture nonunion. *J Bone Joint Surg Am* 2004; 86-A(10): 2263–7.

25. Yuan BJ, Shearer DW, Barei DP, Nork SE. Intertrochanteric osteotomy for femoral neck nonunion: Does "undercorrection" result in an acceptable rate of femoral neck union? *J Orthop Trauma* 2017; 31(8): 420–6.

26. Schoenfeld AJ, Vrabec GA. Valgus osteotomy of the proximal femur with sliding hip screw for the treatment of femoral neck nonunions: The technique, a case series, and literature review. *J Orthop Trauma* 2006; 20(7): 485–91.

27. Thein R, Herman A, Kedem P, Chechik A MD, Shazar N. Osteosynthesis of unstable intracapsular femoral neck fracture by dynamic locking plate or screw fixation: Early results. *J Orthop Trauma* 2014; 28: 70–6.

28. Sringari T, Jain U, Sharma V. Role of valgus osteotomy and fixation by double-angle blade plate in neglected displaced intracapsular fracture of neck of femur in younger patients. *Injury* 2005; 36: 630–4.

29. Varghese VD, Livingston A, Boopalan PR, Jepegnanam TS. Valgus osteotomy for nonunion and neglected neck of femur fractures. *World J Orthop* 2016; 7(5): 301–7.

30. Gavaskar AS, Chowdary NT. Valgus sliding subtrochanteric osteotomy for neglected fractures of the proximal femur; surgical technique and a retrospective case series. *J Orthop Surg Res* 2013; 8: 4.

31. Jackson M, Learmonth ID. The treatment of nonunion after intracapsular fracture of the proximal femur. *Clin Orthop* 2002; 399: 119–28.

32. Mathews V, Cabanela ME. Femoral neck nonunion treatment. *Clin Orthop* 2004; 419: 57–64.

33. Bartonicek J, Skala-Rosenbaum J, Dousa P. Valgus intertrochanteric osteotomy for malunion and nonunion of trochanteric fractures. *J Orthop Trauma* 2003; 17: 606–12.

34. Kulkarni SG, Kulkarni GS, Babhulkar S, Kulkarni MG, Kulkarni RM. Accuracy of valgus osteotomy using dynamic hip screw. *Injury* 2017; 48(Suppl 2): S2–7.

35. Marti RK, Schüller HM, Raaymakers EL. Intertrochanteric osteotomy for non-union of the femoral neck. *J Bone Joint Surg Br* 1989; 71: 782–7.

36. Anglen JO, Intertrochanteric osteotomy for failed internal fixation of femoral neck fracture. *Clin Orthop Relat Res* 1997; (341): 175–82.

37. Kalra M, Anand S. Valgus intertrochanteric osteotomy for neglected femoral neck fractures in young adults. *Int Orthop* 2001; 25: 363–6.

38. Wu CC, Shih CH, Chen WJ, Tai CL. Treatment of femoral neck nonunions with a sliding compression screw: Comparison with and without subtrochanteric valgus osteotomy. *J Trauma* 1999; 46: 312–7.

39. Gupta S, Kukreja S, Singh V. Valgus osteotomy and repositioning and fixation with a dynamic hip screw and a 135° single-angled barrel plate for un-united and neglected femoral neck fractures. *J Orthop Surg (Hong Kong)* 2014; 22: 13–7.

40. Khan AQ, Khan MS, Sherwani MK, Agarwal R. Role of valgus osteotomy and fixation with dynamic hip screw and 120° double angle barrel plate in the management of neglected and ununited femoral neck fracture in young patients. *J Orthop Traumatol* 2009; 10: 71–8.

41. Said GZ, Farouk O, Said HG. Valgus intertrochanteric osteotomy with single-angled 130° plate fixation for fractures and non-unions of the femoral neck. *Int Orthop* 2010; 34: 1291–5.

42. Sen RK, Tripathy SK, Goyal T, Aggarwal S, Tahasildar N, Singh D, Singh AK. Osteosynthesis of femoral-neck nonunion with angle blade plate and autogenous fibular graft. *Int Orthop* 2012; 36: 827–32.

43. Gadegone WM, Ramteke AA, Lokhande V, Salphade Y. Valgus intertrochanteric osteotomy and fibular strut graft in the management of neglected femoral neck fracture. *Injury* 2013; 44: 763–8.

44. Barrack RL, Rosenberg AG. *The Hip.* 2nd ed., Philadelphia: Lippincott Williams & Wilkins; 2006. pp. 107–123.

45. Brown TE, Cui Q, Mihalko WM, Saleh KJ. *Arthritis & Arthroplasty: The Hip.* Philadelphia: Saunders–Elsevier; 2009: pp. 70–75.

46. Ferguson GM, Cabanela ME, Ilstrup DM. Total hip arthroplasty after failed intertrochanteric osteotomy. *J Bone Joint Surg Br* 1994; 76: 252–7.

47. Browner BD, Jupiter JB, Krettek C et al. *Skeletal Trauma: Basic Science, Management, and Reconstruction.* Philadelphia, PA: Elsevier/Saunders, 2015.

48. Breusch SJ, Lukoschek M, Thomsen M, Mau H, Ewerbeck V, Aldinger PR. Ten-year results of uncemented hip stems for failed intertrochanteric osteotomy. *Arch Orthop Trauma Surg* 2005; 125: 304–9.

19

McMurray's osteotomy: A forgotten procedure of the hip

RAJU VAISHYA AND ABHISHEK VAISH

INTRODUCTION

Thomas Porter McMurray (1887–1949), a disciple of Sir Robert Jones of Liverpool, UK, became famous for introducing an osteotomy of the proximal femur to treat nonunion of the fractured neck of the femur. McMurray was the first professor of orthopedics in Liverpool and was credited to have started the world-famous postgraduate course of MCh (Orth.).

Until recently, the problem of the nonunion of the fractured neck of the femur remained a significant challenge for surgeons to manage. Although McMurray's osteotomy might be a "forgotten osteotomy" now, it was indeed one of the most popular surgical treatments for various hip pathologies for almost 5–6 decades after its first introduction by McMurray in 1936.[1] Initially, McMurray described it for the nonunion of the fractured neck of the femur, but later on, he also advocated for it for fresh femoral neck fractures and osteoarthritis of the hip.[2,3]

Before the popularity of osteotomy around the hips, most hip pathology used to be treated surgically by hip arthrodesis, which was not an easy procedure to perform and led to severe morbidity. However, as patients were followed for a long duration, it became clear that there was indeed a lacuna between arthrodesis and arthroplasty. This lacuna was appropriately filled by the various osteotomies around the hip. Although various osteotomies around the hip were described as early as the nineteenth century, the real use and popularity of these procedures must be credited to McMurray, who described a medial displacement intertrochanteric osteotomy in the 1930s.

CHARACTERISTICS OF McMURRAY'S OSTEOTOMY

It is an intertrochanteric, oblique osteotomy of the hip, where the distal osteotomized femoral shaft is displaced medially, under the fractured neck and femoral head.[4] This osteotomy starts from the lateral femoral cortex, just below the level of the lesser trochanter, and extends medially in an oblique fashion to cut the femoral neck just above the level of the lesser trochanter, leaving the attached iliopsoas tendon to the lesser trochanter in the distal fragment (Figure 19.1).[5]

The initially described McMurray's osteotomy was not fixed with any metallic implants, and it was held in position using the 11/2 hip spica until union. However, several implants have been used to fix this osteotomy using cancellous screws,

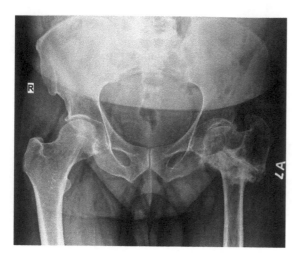

Figure 19.1 McMurray's osteotomy of the left hip, showing an oblique osteotomy pattern with medial displacement.

Smith-Petersen nail (with or without plate), and Wainwright's plate (Figure 19.2). These fixation devices helped in preventing the displacement of the osteotomy in the spica and maintaining the osteotomy in the desired position.

Indications

1. Nonunion of fractured neck of femur
2. Displaced, fresh subcapital fractured neck of femur (in younger individuals)
3. Osteoarthritis of the hip

Mechanism of action

A. *In fractures*
   1. It makes the fracture line more horizontal and therefore converts the shearing forces to compressive forces, which helps in promoting the union of the fracture.
   2. It acts as a "defunctioning osteotomy," by facilitating transmission of weight from the femoral head to the distal shaft, thereby bypassing the fracture site. That is also popularly known as the "armchair effect" of this osteotomy (Figures 19.1 through 19.3). Hence, even if the fracture fails to unite after this osteotomy, painless weight-bearing is possible.
   3. Since this osteotomy brings the cut surface of the femur underneath the femoral neck

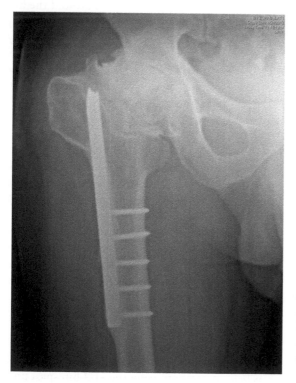

Figure 19.2 McMurray's osteotomy fixed with a Wainwright plate.

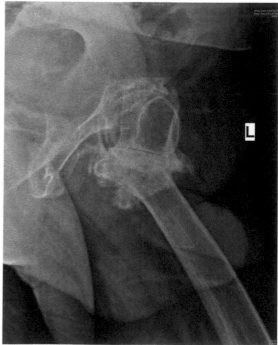

Figure 19.3 "Armchair effect" of McMurray's osteotomy.

fracture, it acts to provide bone graft to the fractured neck of femur and there promotes its healing.

B. *In osteoarthritis of the hip*: McMurray's osteotomy became a popular alternative surgical option (to hip arthrodesis) for the treatment of hip osteoarthritis in the late 1930s. Its proposed mechanism of action was:

1. The altered thrust of weight-bearing.
2. The adducted position of the femoral head brought a different articular surface of the femoral head in contract with the weight-bearing area of the acetabulum.

Surgical procedure

A. *Preoperative planning*

1. *Radiography*
   a. *Plain radiographs*: Good-quality true anteroposterior (AP) and lateral radiographs of the hip are mandatory to assess the hip and identify the bony landmarks and hip pathology.
   b. *Computed tomography (CT) and magnetic resonance imaging (MRI)*: These investigations are often not required to diagnose the fracture. However, these investigations may be useful in the following situations:
      i. In doubtful fracture patterns
      ii. The uncertainty of union of the fracture
      iii. Assessment of vascularity of the femoral head
      iv. Early diagnosis of the hip osteoarthritis
      v. Excluding other hip pathology in complex cases

2. *Limb traction*: In established femoral neck nonunion with severe overriding of the femoral shaft, preoperative skin or skeletal traction is helpful in stretching the soft tissue contractures and making the surgical procedure easier.

3. *Preoperative planning*: A preoperative drawing is essential to determine the level and localization of the osteotomy. Planning regarding how to fix the osteotomy should also be done well in advance and all necessary implant inventory should be checked beforehand.

B. *Intraoperative*

1. *Positioning*: Supine over a fracture table. Intraoperative fluoroscopy is recommended. The radiolucent table and positioning of C-arm and image intensifier should be checked before washing and draping.

2. *Approach*: A standard lateral approach, with about a 6–7-cm incision. Expose the lateral femoral shaft in the inter- and subtrochanteric area. Make an osteotomy starting below the level of the lesser trochanter and proceed obliquely to finish medially proximal to the lesser trochanter under image intensifier control. The obliqueness of this osteotomy helps in an easier medial displacement. It is critical that the osteotomy exit above the lesser trochanter so as to bring the distal fragment in direct contact with the fracture site. The inward pull of the psoas major muscle, which is inserted at the lesser trochanter, further helps in maintaining the displacement.

3. *Intraoperative tips and tricks*: In this osteotomy, the displacement of the distal fragment is done by manual pressure and by abducting the limb so as to bring it under the head of the femur. It is now recommended to avoid displacement of the shaft greater than 50% of the width to minimize the distortion of proximal femoral anatomy and to avoid complexity in future total hip joint replacement.

   The fracture can be fixed along with maintaining the displacement at the osteotomy site by using implants such as cancellous screws or a Smith-Petersen nail (with or without plate) or using special plates like those of Wainwright or Tupman.

C. *Postoperative care*: The leg is positioned on a splint with the hip in slight abduction and flexion. As per pain tolerance, active and passive knee flexion should commence on day 1. Non-weight-bearing walking is suggested until bony union is confirmed on x-ray at 6 weeks duration. At 6 weeks, abductor strengthening exercises can begin. Final radiological follow-up is done at 1 year after surgery. Implant removal is not advisable unless it causes trouble or another hip procedure is warranted.

Outcomes

Published studies have documented good medium- and long-term results in achieving union in the established nonunion and fresh fractures of the femoral neck. It can also provide satisfactory pain relief in osteoarthritis of the hip. However, with the availability of excellent fracture fixation devices like cannulated cancellous screws (CCSs), the dynamic hip screw (DHS), and proximal femoral nail (PFN), fracture fixation for the femoral neck can be done satisfactorily, and the need for such an osteotomy is rare. Similarly, with the advent of total hip replacement (THR), end-stage hip arthritis is now universally managed by it and osteotomy around the hip is rarely used. This procedure is suitable for osteoarthritis of the hip and ununited fracture but not for avascular necrosis (AVN) after the fractured neck of the femur.

TOTAL HIP REPLACEMENT AFTER McMURRAY'S OSTEOTOMY

In the long term, McMurray's osteotomy patients may develop secondary osteoarthritis due to the altered biomechanics of the hip and may require total hip replacement. These cases are not straightforward and are often quite complicated to execute (Figures 19.4 and 19.5). There are several technical challenges posed by the previous osteotomy while executing a total hip replacement.[6] These include:

A. *Soft tissue contractures*: Various muscles around the hips are severely contracted and must be adequately released during the surgery. These muscles include iliopsoas, adductors, glutei, and short external rotators.
B. *Bony abnormalities*: There is a severe distortion of the anatomy of the proximal femur with blockage of the medullary canal by the bone formed at the previously done osteotomy site. There may also be a deficiency of medial bone stock if the calcar was previously involved wholly or partially in the osteotomy.
C. *Surgical problems*: It may be quite difficult to restore the hip center and fully correct the limb-length discrepancy in these cases.

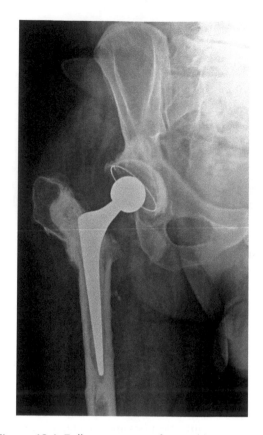

Figure 19.4 Follow-up x-ray of a total hip replacement done after McMurray's osteotomy.

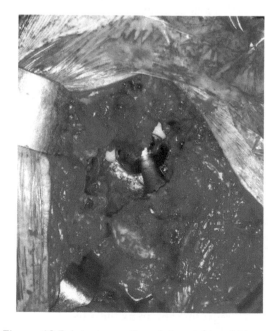

Figure 19.5 Intraoperative picture of total hip replacement in a case of a previously done McMurray's osteotomy.

Advantages of McMurray's osteotomy

- It promotes union across the fracture site, since it makes the fracture line more horizontal and converts the shearing forces into compressive forces.
- Due to the "armchair effect," this defunctioning osteotomy may provide painless weight-bearing even if the fracture is not united. It is possible because the distal fragment is placed directly under the head of the femur and therefore the weight transmission occurs from the femoral head to the distal shaft fragment, bypassing the fracture site.

Disadvantages of McMurray's osteotomy

McMurray's osteotomy, although a good salvage procedure for some of the difficult problems of the hip, is still associated with several disadvantages that have led to its decreased popularity. The various shortcomings of this procedure include:

- Altered biomechanics of the hip, leading to secondary osteoarthritis of the hip.
- Complexity in future THR due to distortion of proximal femoral anatomy.
- Limb-length discrepancy (significant shortening).
- Displacement of the osteotomy if not internally fixed.

Complications

McMurray's osteotomy is not an entirely benign procedure. It may be associated with the following problems:

- Delayed union or nonunion of the osteotomy site
- Heterotopic ossification
- Neurovascular injuries
- Stiffness of the ipsilateral hip and knee joints

REFERENCES

1. McMurray TP. Ununited fractures of the neck of the femur. *J Bone Joint Surg* 1936; 18: 319.
2. McMurray TP. Fracture of the neck of the femur treated by oblique osteotomy. *Br Med J* 1938; 1: 330.
3. McMurray TP. Osteoarthritis of the hip joint. *Br J Surg* 1935; 22: 716–27.
4. Mishra US. Intertrochanteric displacement osteotomy in the treatment of femoral neck fractures. *Injury* 1979; 10: 183–9.
5. Phaltankar PM, Bhavnani K, Kale S, Sejale S, Patel BR. Is McMurray's osteotomy obsolete? *J Postgrad Med* 1995; 41: 102–3.
6. Nagi ON, Dhillon MS. Total hip arthroplasty after McMurray's osteotomy. *J Arthroplasty* 1991: 6; S17–22.

20

Pauwels osteotomy of the hip

RAJU VAISHYA AND ABHISHEK VAISH

INTRODUCTION

Friedrich Pauwels (1885–1980) was born and brought up in Germany. He was the son of a machine manufacturer, which influenced him to study natural sciences apart from medicine. Pauwels is also known as the founder of modern biomechanics.

Intracapsular fractures of the neck of femur remain a significant management challenge to most orthopedic surgeons all over the world and therefore are considered an unsolved fracture. It is, indeed, always preferable to preserve the head of the femur rather than to bring in problems associated with the replaced head, specifically in younger individuals. It is known that the fractured femoral neck has a substantially high incidence of nonunion (10%–20%); hence, many hip preservation techniques like osteotomy around the hip have been described to save the involved hip, especially in young individuals.

Principles of Pauwels osteotomy

Pauwels (1940) proved various biomechanical principles about the fractured neck of the femur[1]:

1. Pure compressive stress encourages the formation of bony callus.
2. Tensile stress retards bone formation.
3. Shearing stresses are harmful and prevent the formation of bony callus.

In the normal neck-shaft angle, shearing, tensile, and compressive stresses are exerted equally on the femoral neck, whereas in varus positions, all the forces are increased, and in valgus positions, these forces are decreased.

According to Pauwels's calculation, in coxa valga with a neck-shaft angle of 150–155°, compressive forces are high, but shearing forces are absent or minimal. Therefore, with a valgus osteotomy, the shearing and tensile stresses are converted into pure compressive forces.

Pauwels demonstrated from his biomechanical research work that the femoral neck nonunion was often due to abnormal shear forces acting across the fracture site, and that converting these into compressive forces with an osteotomy can increase the incidence of union and avoid the need for arthroplasty.[2]

INDICATIONS

Pauwels femoral osteotomy in adults is of two types: (A) varus and (B) valgus osteotomy. The lateral closed-wedge valgus osteotomy has many more indications than the medial closed-wedge varus osteotomy; hence, the valgus osteotomy is much more commonly used.[3] The primary indications for this osteotomy include:

A. *Varus osteotomy*
   - Coxa valga

- Excessive femoral anteversion, with hip dysplasia
- Avascular necrosis (AVN) of the femoral head (to rotate the area of weight-bearing)

B. *Valgus osteotomy*
- Nonunion of femoral neck fracture (Figure 20.1)
- Intertrochanteric femoral deformities:
    a. Rotational deformities (e.g., slipped capital femoral epiphysis)
    b. Frontal plane deformities (e.g., coxa vara, malunion of fractures with varus, and fibrous dysplasia with shepherd's crook deformity)
    c. Sagittal deformities (e.g., malunited fractures, flexion contracture of hip)
    d. Significant bone loss of the distal femur and femoral shortening (which requires proximal femoral lengthening)
- Total hip arthroplasty requiring femoral osteotomy (e.g., in developmental dysplasia of hip [DDH] or for other causes of high-riding dislocated hip)
- Hip osteoarthritis or avascular necrosis in young and active individuals

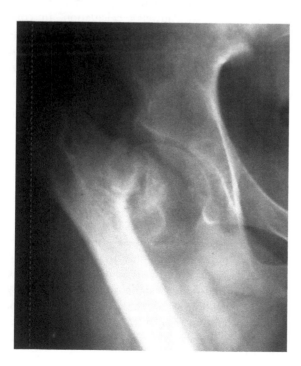

Figure 20.1 A ununited intracapsular fractured neck of femur in a young adult with absorption of the neck and severe coxa vara.

Contraindications

- Infection at the site of the surgical field
- Limitations of hip motion (stiffness)
- Advanced osteoarthritis or osteonecrosis
- Inflammatory arthritis
- Severe osteoporosis (which may not allow stable internal fixation)

Surgical procedure

A. *Preoperative planning*
1. *Radiography*
    a. *Plain radiographs*: Good-quality true anteroposterior (AP) and lateral radiographs of the hip are mandatory to assess the hip and identify bony landmarks and hip pathology.
    b. *Computed tomography (CT) and magnetic resonance imaging (MRI)*: These investigations are often not required to diagnose the fracture. However, these investigations may be useful in the following situations:
        i. In doubtful fracture patterns
        ii. Uncertainty of union of the fracture
        iii. Assessment of vascularity of the femoral head
        iv. Early diagnosis of hip osteoarthritis
        v. Excluding other hip pathology in complex cases
2. *Limb traction*: In established femoral neck nonunion with severe overriding of the femoral shaft, preoperative skin or skeletal traction is helpful in stretching the soft tissue contractures and making the surgical procedure more comfortable.[4]
3. *Preoperative planning*: A preoperative drawing is essential to determine the level and localization of the osteotomy. Planning regarding how to fix the osteotomy should also be done well in advance, and all necessary implant inventory should be checked beforehand. A templating of the normal hip is crucial, as it provides valuable information about the size of the wedge required to correct the deformity and the position of the implant. First, an angle that the fracture line makes with the

horizontal should be measured. The angle of the wedge is then measured to remove the bone from the intertrochanteric region and ensure that a physiological orientation of the fracture line is achieved.

B. *Intraoperative*:

Step 1: Positioning

The patient is positioned supine on a fracture table, and intraoperative fluoroscopy is recommended. The radiolucent table and positioning of C-arm and image intensifier should be checked before washing and draping.

It is often difficult to calculate the corrective angle in chronic nonunion. The exact measurement of the angle is possible only after the fracture has been reduced on a fracture table. It is important to realize that in patients with a resorbed neck that a retroversion could be caused while impacting the fracture during internal fixation.

Step 2: Reduction and stabilization

It is often difficult to reduce the fracture by closed manipulation in ununited and neglected fractures, and it should only be attempted on a fracture table. However, it is important to realize that excessive traction in the zeal to achieve reduction may injure the scarred retinaculum and its vasculature. Sometimes, the inferior spike in the proximal fractured fragment may prevent reduction and would require osteotomy to achieve an acceptable alignment. Pen reduction of the fractured neck of the femur should be reserved as a last resort, when the fracture is irreducible by all closed means, as it could further compromise the blood supply to the femoral head. Once the reduction is achieved, it should be maintained with K-wires, and then the fracture can be stabilized with an appropriate implant (e.g., screw, plate, or angled blade plate).

Step 3: Lateral closed-wedge osteotomy and fixation

A desired lateral closing wedge is taken from the intertrochanteric region, after which the osteotomy is closed by moving the limb into valgus position. Sometimes, to correct a substantial deformity, the calculated wedge may be significant (40° or so). However, it has been realized that the desired effect can

be achieved with a smaller wedge (25–30°), even in such situations. It has been seen that in cases where an osteotomy is not indicated to achieve valgus, the osteotomy, if done, can help improve the blood supply of the femoral head. A sliding or dynamic hip screw can help in compressing the fracture site. Several implants have been used to fix this osteotomy using a screw and barrel plate, like the dynamic hip screw (Figure 20.2). These fixation devices help in preventing displacement of the osteotomy and maintaining the osteotomy in the desired position of correction.[5] When a double-angled blade plate is used, the length of the blade should be 5–10 mm shorter than the measured length. While inserting the blade plate, a firm impaction often achieves compression at the fracture site and is the most crucial factor in attaining union (Figure 20.3).

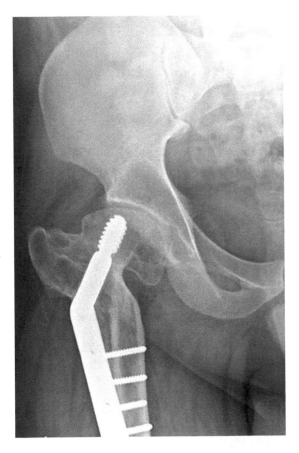

Figure 20.2 Pauwels valgus osteotomy fixed with a dynamic hip screw and plate.

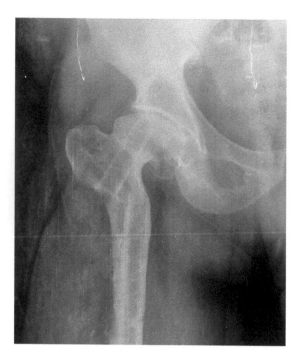

Figure 20.3 Healed valgus osteotomy of Pauwels.

Pitfalls to be avoided during surgery include the following.

Excessive valgus: To convert a grade-III Pauwels fracture pattern to grade-I pattern would require a wedge correction of about 40–50°. To obtain the right inclination of the fracture line in these cases, a large wedge needs to be removed, which is associated with several problems:

a. It can cause the osteotomy to extend from the intertrochanteric into the subtrochanteric region.
b. It may also produce severe distortion of the proximal femoral anatomy and deformity (abduction and external rotation).
c. It may damage the blood supply to the femoral head and increase the risk of AVN.
d. It makes future total hip replacement complex and challenging.

Total hip replacement after a Pauwels osteotomy: Total hip replacement after a Pauwels osteotomy is quite challenging, due to distorted femoral anatomy. Several technical modifications and tricks need to be considered:

a. The entry point for the reaming should be carefully planned to avoid reaming a false passage.
b. While broaching the femoral canal, an abnormal bridge of bone is often encountered, which should be carefully negotiated.
c. If an uncemented stem is being used, a longer distal fitting stem is preferred, which must bypass the last screw hole to avoid any stress riser and possible periprosthetic fracture in the future.
d. The trochanteric fragment may remain as an ununited fragment and needs to be reattached separately.
e. When the proximal femoral anatomy is grossly distorted, an additional corrective osteotomy may be required.
f. To negotiate defects in the posteromedial cortex, use of special modular or calcar-replacing stem is recommended.
g. If cemented arthroplasty is performed, avoid leakage of the bone cement by plugging the screw holes from outside the femoral shaft.

C. *Postoperative care*: The leg is positioned on a splint with the hip in slight abduction and flexion. As per pain tolerance, active and passive knee flexion can commence on day 1. Non-weight-bearing walking until bony union is confirmed on x-ray at 6 weeks duration. At 6 weeks, abductor strengthening exercises can begin. Final radiological follow-up is done at 1 year after surgery. Implant removal is not advisable unless it causes trouble or another hip procedure is warranted.

Modification of Pauwels osteotomy

Magu et al. (2009) described a modification of Pauwels osteotomy of the hip for fractured neck of the femur.[6] They performed the surgery through a two-stage incision, using the Watson-Jones approach. In the first stage, using the proximal part of the incision, the nonunion was fixed with 6.5-mm cancellous screws after reducing the fracture. In the second stage, the intertrochanteric valgus osteotomy was performed and fixed with a double-angled osteotomy blade plate. They claimed good results in more than 90% of their 46 reported cases.

OUTCOMES

Published studies have documented good medium- and long-term results in achieving union in the established nonunion and fresh fractures of the femoral neck. It can also provide satisfactory pain relief in osteoarthritis of the hip. Although with the availability of excellent fracture fixation devices like the dynamic hip screw (DHS), fracture fixation of the femoral neck can be done satisfactorily; hence, the need for such an osteotomy is rare. Similarly, with the advent of total hip arthroplasty (THA), end-stage hip arthritis is now universally managed by it and osteotomy around the hip is rarely used. This procedure is suitable for osteoarthritis of the hip and ununited fracture but not for avascular necrosis after the fractured neck of the femur.

DISADVANTAGES

In this osteotomy, the hip biomechanics and anatomy of the fracture line are restored indirectly and not at the site of the fracture. An alternative option to overcome this drawback could be to correct the deformity at the nonunion site through a surgical dislocation and internal fixation of the fracture. This technique corrects the deformity directly but presents with a high risk of avascular necrosis of the femoral head.

Complications

Pauwels osteotomy is not an entirely benign procedure. It may be associated with the following complications:

- Residual shortening of the limb (1–2 inches)
- Cutout of the implant and loss of fixation of the osteotomy (Figure 20.4)
- AVN (10%–40%)
- Delayed union or nonunion of the osteotomy site
- Heterotopic ossification
- Neurovascular injuries
- Stiffness of the ipsilateral hip and knee joints
- Conversion to THA (5%–10%)

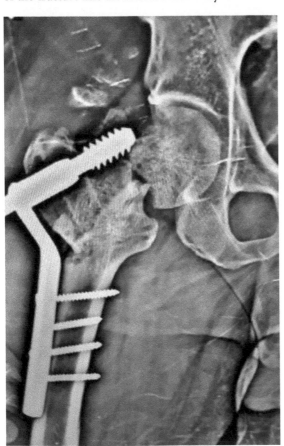

Figure 20.4 Loss of fixation of the osteotomy with cutting out of the dynamic hip screw.

REFERENCES

1. Pauwels F. Osteoarthritis. In: *Biomechanics of the Normal and Diseased Hip: Theoretical Foundation, Technique and Results of Treatment: An Atlas.* New York: Springer; 1976. p. 129–271.
2. Pauwels F. The fractures of the femoral neck. A mechanical problem. In: *Biomechanics of the Locomotor Apparatus.* Berlin: Springer-Verlag; 1980. p. 1–105.
3. Aparto A, Pellegrino P, Kain MSH, Masse A. Do osteotomies of the proximal femur still have a role? *Curr Rev Musculoskelet Med* 2014; 7: 323–9.
4. Said GZ, Farouk O, Said HGZ. Valgus intertrochanteric osteotomy with single-angled 130° plate fixation for fractures and non-unions of the femoral neck. *Int Orthop (SICOT)* 2010; 34: 1291–5.
5. Varghese VD, Livingston A, Boopalan PR, Jepegnanam TS. Valgus osteotomy for nonunion and neglected neck of femur fractures. *World J Orthop* 2016; 7(5): 301–7.
6. Magu NK, Rohilla R, Singh R, Tater R. Modified Pauwels' intertrochanteric osteotomy in neglected femoral neck fracture. *Clin Orthop Relat Res* 2009; 467(4): 1064–73.

21

Dickson's high geometric osteotomy

K. MOHAN IYER

Intracapsular fractures of the neck of the femur end up in nonunion due to two factors, mainly because of (1) the neck being absorbed due to the shearing forces at the fracture site and (2) avascularity of the femoral head. In the young, perfect anatomical restoration of the femoral head and neck is preferable and osteosynthesis is achieved by osteotomy. Osteosynthesis was advocated by Dickson in 1953 if the fracture remained painful with an unsatisfactory function. Dickson used a cancellous bone graft and reported that, when combined with an abduction osteotomy, the results with delayed union were encouraging if the fracture was impacted to ensure a rapid and complete take of the graft. He also observed that irreversible changes occur with the onset of avascular necrosis.

Here, the line of osteotomy is changed from vertical (shearing) force to a horizontal (impacting) force. The osteotomy is done just below the greater trochanter, and the distal fragment is abducted 60° and fixed with a plate (Figure 21.1).

INDICATIONS

Nonunion with viable femoral neck and varus displacement.

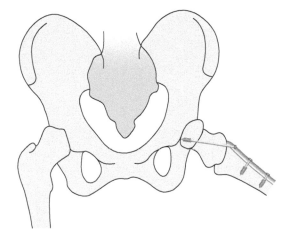

Figure 21.1 Fixation of the osteotomy.

ADVANTAGES

1. Easy to perform
2. Immediate stability can be provided
3. Converts sheer force into compressive force
4. Gives a high rate of union
5. Improves abductor strength
6. Increases limb length

22

Girdlestone resection arthroplasty

K. MOHAN IYER

Girdlestone resection arthroplasty is a salvage procedure aimed at pain relief and control of infection, which results in approximately 2 to 3 inches of limb shortening.

Gathorne Girdlestone was born in Oxford, UK and he later joined Sir Robert Jones to set up the Robert Jones and Agnes Hunt Orthopedic Hospital in Oswestry. William and Charles Mayo met Sir Jones in 1906, and William thereafter published an article titled "Present-Day Surgery in England and Scotland" in the *Journal of the Minnesota Medical Association*. William also observed that Sir Jones's ability to use splints, plaster, and alternative means for immobilization was particularly skillful. He was impressed with Sir Jones's decisiveness, details of operation, and treatment and thus considered it an ideal model of practice, which it is even today. Sir Jones visited the Mayo Clinic in the United States in 1928 to establish guidelines for orthopedic education.

Modern technological advancements in primary and revision hip arthroplasty have revolutionized the treatment of failed primary total hip replacements, hence the decision to undertake a Girdlestone procedure is taken as a last resort, as such patients have a very high anesthetic and operative risk.

Aspiration of hips postoperatively treated by Girdlestone arthroplasty for culture is particularly difficult, whereby surgeons can reassess for residual infection, which plays a very important part before revision.

This operation was originally used by Girdlestone (1945) to promote healing in cases of septic arthritis of the hip, thus allowing free drainage and gradual obliteration of the cavity from below by granulation from its depths.

Later, the operation was used in noninfective cases as a primary treatment for osteoarthritis of the hip. With the evolution of total hip arthroplasty, this procedure has mainly remained as a last-resort salvage procedure.

In a nutshell, the operation entails removal of the head and neck of the femur, along with excision of the superior lip of the acetabulum and interposition of soft tissue, essentially the gluteus medius muscle between the raw bones.

INDICATIONS

1. Tuberculosis of the hip joint
2. Pyogenic hip joint
3. Nonunion of fractured neck of femur in an elderly patient
4. Avascular necrosis (AVN) of the femoral head

ADVANTAGE

Painless mobile hip joint

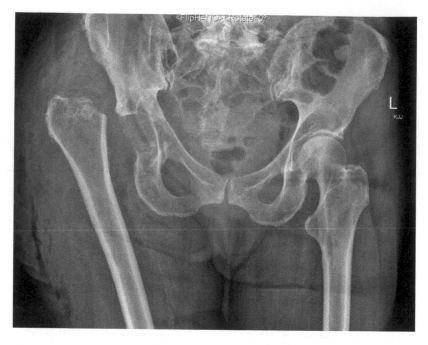

Figure 22.1 Girdlestone resection arthroplasty. (Courtesy: Dr Rajesh Botchu, Consultant MSK Radiologist, Royal Orthopaedic Hospital, Birmingham, UK.)

TECHNIQUE OF OPERATION

1. *Position of the patient*: The patient is in the lateral position, with the affected hip uppermost. The patient is made more comfortable with the leg resting on a soft platform, just as in a total hip arthroplasty.

2. *Exposure*: The hip is then opened up by a Gibson's posterolateral incision, followed by splitting the gluteal aponeurosis and the fascia lata below, through the gluteus maximus proximally to the level of the greater trochanter (Figure 22.1).

   The hip joint is then exposed by detaching the gluteus medius and short lateral rotators from the trochanter. Once the hip joint is exposed, all affected pathologies, such as the infected prosthesis from the femoral cavity and the acetabulum, the bone cement from the femoral canal, and the head and neck of the femur, resection of the upper lip of the acetabulum, implantation of soft tissues, and closure of the wound in layers are carried out. In certain cases, the wound is closed with deep tension sutures and the skin with interrupted skin sutures, or in certain selected cases, it may be preferable to leave a small polyethylene tube beneath the muscle for drainage.

3. *Postoperative management*: Normally, dressings are given in a spica fashion and the limb then rested in a Thomas splint, or the lower limb is maintained in an upper tibial skeletal traction with a weight of 8–10 lbs with the knee held in 5–10° of flexion. This is carried on for 4 weeks, after which the traction and splint are removed, with the patient left free in bed for hip and knee exercises. Later, graduated weight-bearing is carried out.

   The thing of greatest importance in this procedure is to not leave any spikes in the bone but to leave a smooth, sloping surface to avoid this complication.

   Another problem faced is the tendency of the leg to lie in external rotation. Should this become troublesome, then a transfer of the psoas may be considered.

   In many cases, weight-bearing may be delayed for 2–3 months, when a weight-relieving caliper may be considered along with a heel raise.

23

Sugioka's transtrochanteric anterior rotational osteotomy

K. MOHAN IYER

This procedure is done in avascular necrosis (AVN) of the hip joint to prevent progressive collapse of the articular surface so that it improves the congruity of the hip joint. This method was first described by Sugioka[1] and called transtrochanteric anterior rotational osteotomy of the femoral head in the treatment of osteonecrosis affecting the hip: a new osteotomy operation. This operation may be extremely useful, particularly in young patients who have been selected carefully when the lesion is in stage II or early stage III with involvement of less than 30% and depression less than 2 mm.

This method can also be used in the treatment of slipped capital femoral epiphysis, partial defects of the femoral head in the weight-bearing area due to trauma and tumor, and osteoarthritis of the hip with localized changes in weight-bearing area, and it does not prevent any prosthetic replacement at a later date.[1] In order to achieve this, the femoral head and neck segment is rotated anteriorly around its long axis through a transtrochanteric osteotomy so that the weight-bearing surface is transmitted to the posterior articular surface of the femoral head, which is not involved in the ischemic process. A modified transtrochanteric rotational osteotomy is an effective method for delaying the progression of collapse in the treatment of selected cases of osteonecrosis of the femoral head.[2] The extent of necrosis was determined by the method described by Kerboul et al.,[3] and the exact location of the lesion

was determined by magnetic resonance imaging (MRI), which is then used to determine the rotation angle required for the modified transtrochanteric rotational osteotomy. They concluded that an anterior rotational osteotomy was indicated if the lesion involved less than the posterior third of the entire femoral head on a true lateral radiograph, while a posterior rotational osteotomy was indicated if the lesion involved more than the posterior third of the entire femoral head but the anterior portion of the head was still intact. They also coined the term used for this procedure: modified transtrochanteric rotational osteotomy (MTRO), and muscle-pedicle-bone graft (MPBG) in another study undertaken to assess the long-term outcomes of transtrochanteric rotational osteotomy for nontraumatic osteonecrosis of the femoral head.

Morita et al.[4] concluded that 15-year outcomes after transtrochanteric rotational osteotomy (TRO) for osteonecrosis of the femoral head (ONFH) are unfavorable because osteoarthritic changes occur after 5 years postoperation.

TECHNIQUE

Through a lateral approach, the capsule is exposed to reach the greater trochanter, which is then osteotomized and reflected proximally along with the attached tendons of the gluteus medius and minimus, and piriformis (Figure 23.1).

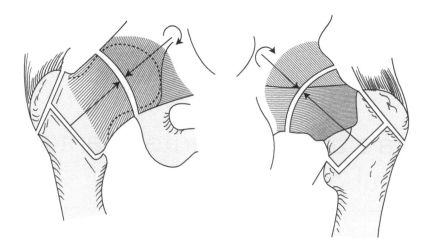

Figure 23.1 Osteotomy of the greater trochanter along with the attached tendons of gluteus medius and minimus, and piriformis.

Thereafter, the hip joint capsule is incised circumferentially while carefully protecting the posterior branch of the medial circumflex artery, which is located at the inferior edge of the quadratus femoris. Two pins are placed laterally to medially in the greater trochanter in a plane perpendicular to the femoral neck. Then, a transtrochanteric osteotomy is made, followed by a second osteotomy at right angles to the first osteotomy, roughly at the superior edge of the lesser trochanter such that the

greater trochanter is left with the distal fragment (Figure 23.2).

After completing the second osteotomy, use the proximal pin to rotate the proximal fragment about 45–90°, the exact degree depending on the size of the necrotic area (Figure 23.3).

Thereafter, the osteotomy is fixed internally with large screws and a washer.

Radiographs (Figure 23.4) are done immediately and after 1 year.

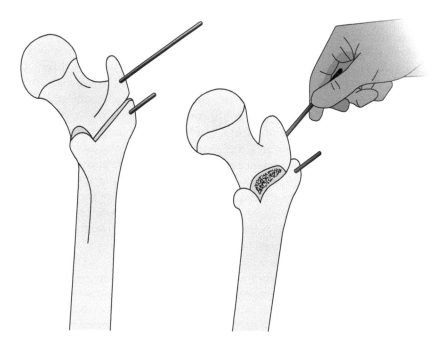

Figure 23.2 Transtrochanteric osteotomy at right angles to the first osteotomy.

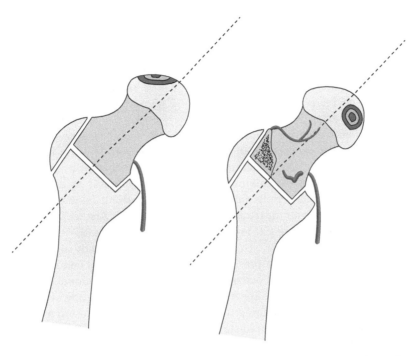

Figure 23.3 Rotation of the proximal fragment to bring the necrotic area away from the weight-bearing region.

Postoperative skin traction may be given for 2–3 weeks, during which time an active range of exercises may be started at around 10–14 days.

In addition, in the literature there have been reports to suggest that good postoperative repair of the necrotic lesion can be expected for young patients with extensive post-traumatic femoral head osteonecrosis despite extensive necrotic lesion. The primary principle of femoral head rotational osteotomy is to move the residual viable region to the

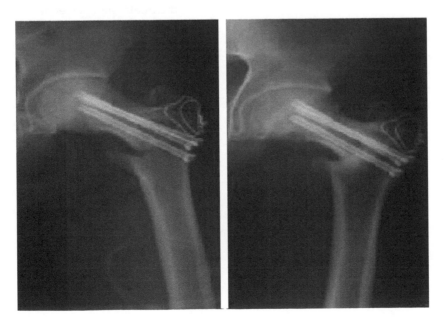

Figure 23.4 Postoperative radiographs done immediately (left) and after 1 year (right).

weight-bearing area through rotation and to move the necrotic lesion away from the main weight-bearing area. The secondary principle is to achieve joint stability by reducing the femoral head from its subluxed position to its centripetal position.

The results of high-degree posterior rotational osteotomy (HDPRO) for extensive femoral head osteonecrosis are excellent.[5] Another study demonstrated that the absence of progression of collapse and a sufficient postoperative intact ratio without the need for marked varus realignment may be associated with favorable results following anterior rotational osteotomy for the treatment of subchondral insufficiency fracture (SIF) of the femoral head in young adults.[6]

There is also a suggestion that joint preservation treatment may improve the clinical outcomes for small lesions at the precollapse stage. The finding of a crescent sign, femoral head flattening, and acetabular involvement suggest an advanced stage of AVN in which joint preservation options are less effective than total hip arthroplasty (THA).[7]

In unstable slipped upper femoral epiphysis, although some joint degeneration is inevitable in the long term, TRO is an effective salvage procedure for treating AVN after unstable slipped capital femoral epiphysis (SCFE).[8] Finally, it may be concluded with certainty that the results of transtrochanteric rotational osteotomy can be improved by criteria based on the use of MRI.

REFERENCES

1. Sugioka Y. Transtrochanteric anterior rotational osteotomy of the femoral head in the treatment of osteonecrosis affecting the hip: A new osteotomy operation. *Clin Orthop Relat Res* 1978; (130): 191–201.
2. Yoon TR, Abbas AA, Hur CI, Cho SG, Lee JH. Modified transtrochanteric rotational osteotomy for femoral head osteonecrosis. *Clin Orthop Relat Res* 2008; 466(5): 1110–6.
3. Kerboul M, Thomine J, Postel M, D'Aubigne RM. The conservative surgical treatment of idiopathic aseptic necrosis of the femoral head. *J Bone Joint Surg Br* 1974; 56: 291–6.
4. Morita D, Hasegawa Y, Okura T, Osawa Y, Ishiguro N. Long-term outcomes of transtrochanteric rotational osteotomy for non-traumatic osteonecrosis of the femoral head. *Bone Joint J* 2017; 99–B: 175–83.
5. Ishikwa T, Atsumi T, Tamaoki S, Nakanishi R, Watanabe M, Kobayashi Y, Tanabe S, Kajiwara T. Early repair of necrotic lesion of the femoral head after high-degree posterior rotational osteotomy in young patients—A study evaluated by volume measurement using magnetic resonance imaging. *J Hip Preserv Surg* 2015; 2(2): 145–51.
6. Sonoda K, Motomura G, Ikemura S, Kubo Y, Yamamoto T, Nakashima Y. Favorable clinical and radiographic results of transtrochanteric anterior rotational osteotomy for collapsed subchondral insufficiency fracture of the femoral head in young adults. *JBJS Open Access* 2017; 2(1): e0013.
7. Gasbarra E, Perrone FL, Baldi J, Moretti VBA, Tarantino U. Conservative surgery for the treatment of osteonecrosis of the femoral head: Current options. *Clin Cases Miner Bone Metab* 2015; 12(Suppl 1): 43–50.
8. Yamamoto T, Fukushi Jun-ichi, Motomura G, Hamai S, Kohno Y, Iwamoto Y. Transtrochanteric rotational osteotomy for avascular necrosis of the femoral head after unstable slipped capital femoral epiphysis: 10-year clinical results. *J Orthop Sci* 2016; 21(6): 831–5.

24

Hip reconstruction osteotomy by Ilizarov method as a salvage option for abnormal hip joints

MASOOD UMER, YASIR MOHIB, TALAL AQEEL QADRI,
AND HAROON RASHID

INTRODUCTION

Chronic hip instability with pain and limp is a challenging orthopedic clinical situation to handle. The problem is further complicated in younger individuals. The gold-standard treatment, which restores joint mechanics most optimally, is a total hip replacement,[1,2] yet a hip arthroplasty in the younger population presents with issues such as earlier need for revision arthroplasty and higher chances of dislocation due to their active lifestyle.[3] Another viable option, especially in males, is hip arthrodesis, yet it comes with concerns of decreased range of motion, limp, and early degeneration in the spine, knee, and contralateral hip.[4,5]

Pelvic support osteotomies, introduced as early as 1936, presented an alternative solution to such problems, where a medial displacement of the anatomical axis was shown to provide greater stability.[6] After initially being introduced by Lance, numerous other variations were published by other authors,[7,8] yet these subtrochanteric medial displacement osteotomies disregarded the excessive valgus displacement of the mechanical axis as well as the gross limb-length discrepancy. Gavriil Ilizarov was the first to combine the pelvic support osteotomy with a second, more distal varus osteotomy for correction of mechanical axis as well as for limb-length restoration[9,10]; in addition, he emphasized the importance of securing the proximal osteotomy in extension for improved stability of the hip. Essential to the procedure described by Ilizarov was the need for compliance with the Ilizarov principles of distraction osteogenesis and stability and guided lengthening provided by a circular fixator, hence the name Ilizarov hip reconstruction.[9-11] Various studies have been published since then, presenting the procedure as a viable and reproducible solution, as well as highlighting its complications.

INDICATIONS AND CONTRAINDICATIONS

Indications and contraindications include chronic unstable hip joint secondary to infective processes,

Table 24.1 Indications in chronic unstable hip joint

Indications	Details
Neglected developmental dysplasia of hip (DDH)	Neglected or unsuccessfully treated
Femoral neck pseudoarthrosis	Not satisfactorily treated with classic techniques
Osteoarthritis in young	
Avascular necrosis (AVN) of femoral head in young	
Girdlestone due to failed previous reconstructive surgery or arthroplasty	Complete destruction of head and neck
Chronic hip dislocation in young	
Early septic arthritis or proximal femur osteomyelitis	Hunka types IV or V
Proximal focal femoral deficiency	Aitken types C and D

Table 24.2 Contraindications in chronic unstable hip

Contraindications	Relative contraindications
Poor patient compliance	Patient younger than 12
Nonambulating patients	Elderly patients
	Chronic paralytic hip dislocation

developmental dysplasia, and traumatic injury or neoplastic process. Tables 24.1 and 24.2 represent a few indications and contraindications.

PLANNING

Preoperative evaluation should always start with a detailed history and general physical and local examination. The history needs particular emphasis on the cause of hip instability and any previous treatments. A past history of delayed bone healing, infection, and multiple surgical procedures may require strict adherence to preservation of as much biology as possible, especially when performing osteotomies. An understanding of prolonged treatment, external fixation, and need for regular follow-up with radiographs should be explained to the patient. In addition, the surgeon needs to be sure of the patient's needs and his/her primary complaints, including the need for squatting and difficulty in hip abduction causing restriction in activities of hygiene and procreation. The examination needs to document hip and knee range of motion, presence of contractures, limb-length discrepancy, and Trendelenburg sign and gait; a record of a functional score of the patient is helpful for follow-up and research purposes.

Radiographic assessment is essential and includes a pelvic anteroposterior (AP) in neutral position and a maximum adduction crosslegged AP view of the pelvis made with the patient supine and the involved hip flexed and maximally adducted over the opposite leg (Figure 24.1);[13] this helps determine the level of proximal osteotomy. An idea of leg length discrepancy is gained with an AP scannogram, as well as assessing the presence of deformities in the femur and tibia. The presence of contractures may obscure AP views and lead to underestimation of limb-length discrepancy (LLD); in such cases, a lateral scannogram may be obtained. The level of the second osteotomy may be estimated by first drawing the proximal osteotomy in maximal abduction and then drawing a straight line perpendicular to the highest points on the pelvis (Figure 24.2).[13] The point where the

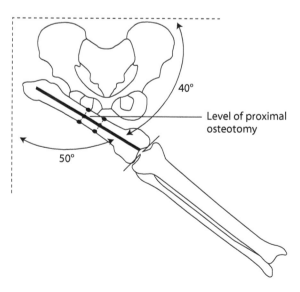

Figure 24.1 Measuring the level of proximal osteotomy.

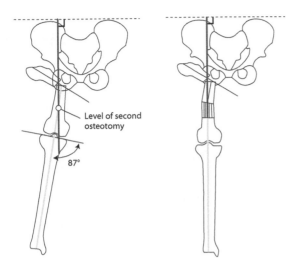

Figure 24.2 The level of second osteotomy.

perpendicular line transects the femur is the point of the second osteotomy.

TECHNIQUE

The patient is placed supine on a regular radiolucent or traction table. If placed on a traction table, a transepicondylar wire is passed and

tensioned over a half-ring, which is then connected to the traction apparatus with the knee suspended and flexed 90° (Figure 24.3); this allows the quadriceps to be completely stretched during pin insertion, theoretically causing a lower chance of knee contracture postoperatively. The assembly consists of proximal, middle, and distal segments. Three (6- or 7.5-mm) Schanz screws are passed proximal to the osteotomy site. It is important to place these pins in abduction and extension so that when the arch is attached, the osteotomy made, and proximal assembly attached to the middle segment, it should be perpendicular to the floor, yet the segment should be in flexion and adduction.

An alternative technique is to intraoperatively maximally adduct and slightly flex the affected limb over the other limb; this is the final pelvis support position of the proximal fragment. While it is held in adduction, the first Schanz pin is passed parallel to the horizontal line of the pelvis as well as to the floor, and an arch is connected perpendicular to the floor. The second and third Schanz pins are passed into the proximal fragment and secured to the arch (Figure 24.4). After performing the proximal osteotomy, the final position would automatically assume a flexed, adducted, and externally rotated position once

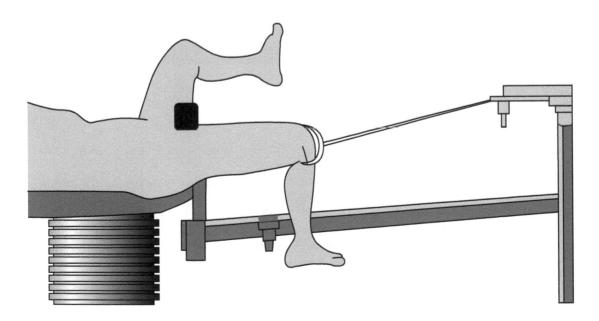

Figure 24.3 The assembly on a regular radiolucent or traction table for pin insertions in abduction and extension.

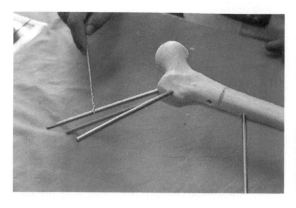

Figure 24.4 The upper femur stabilized part with 2–3 Schanz pins in different directions.

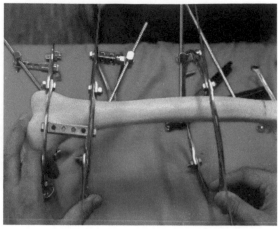

Figure 24.6 The proximal osteotomy site.

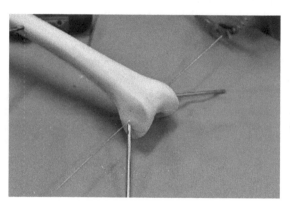

Figure 24.5 The distal assembly with pins through the distal femur, which is ready for the planned osteotomies.

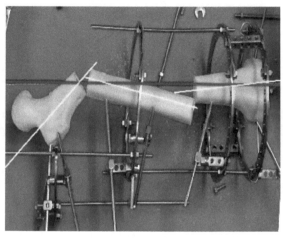

Figure 24.7 The second osteotomy site.

made parallel to the distal assembly. The middle segment valgus should be equivalent to the femoropelvic adduction, or with addition of 15° of overcorrection; it is stabilized with 2–3 Schanz pins in different directions and connected to a complete ring or a ring and arch, perpendicular to the mechanical axis. For the distal assembly, a 1.8-mm Ilizarov wire is passed parallel to the knee joint and tensioned over a full ring, and additional wires and pins are passed and secured to the distal assembly (Figure 24.5).

Finally, the proximal and distal osteotomies are made at the preplanned levels and all

three assemblies are locked to each other with rods.

At the second osteotomy site, the middle and distal assemblies are connected to each other with motors on the lateral side and hinges on the medial side. The level of the distal osteotomy is placed such that after varus correction, the center of the knee joint is the same distance from the midline of the body as compared with the contralateral side. The ankle and knee joint inclinations in the coronal plane should be horizontal and parallel to the pelvis (Figures 24.6 and 24.7).

CASE EXAMPLES

CASE 1

Young female presented with bilateral neglected dysplastic hip causing pain was treated with staged Ilizarov hip reconstruction. Postoperatively, the patient's mechanical axis and limb length were restored, and clinically the patient was pain free (Figure 24.8).

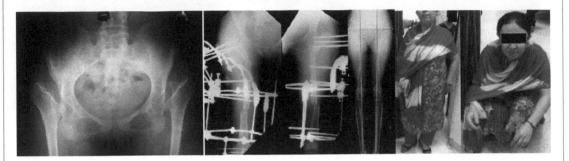

Figure 24.8 Postoperatively, patient's mechanical axis and limb length were restored, clinically patient was pain free.

CASE 2

Young man with spondyloepiphyseal dysplasia treated with one-stage bilateral Ilizarov hip reconstruction. Leg length restoration is not an issue in such cases (Figure 24.9).

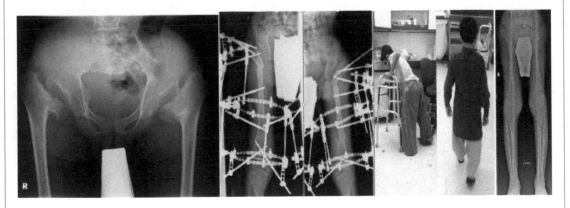

Figure 24.9 Patient with spondyloepiphyseal dysplasia treated with one-stage bilateral Ilizarov hip reconstruction.

CASE 3

Fourteen-year-old boy with destruction of right hip resulting from septic arthritis presented with painful range of motion and limp. He was managed by Ilizarov hip reconstruction; the figure demonstrates 1-year post-op restoration of alignment (Figure 24.10).

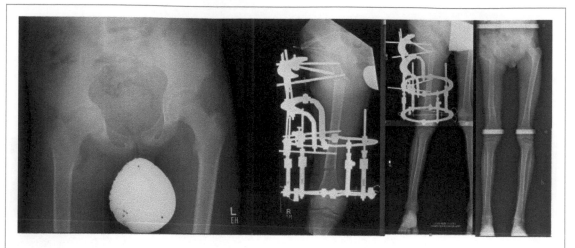

Figure 24.10 Destruction of right hip as a result of septic arthritis was managed by Ilizarov hip reconstruction.

CASE 4

An 18-year-old man with destruction of hip joint resulting from septic arthritis; right hip presented with Trendelenburg gait. One-year postoperative x-ray showed restoration of the mechanical axis (Figure 24.11).

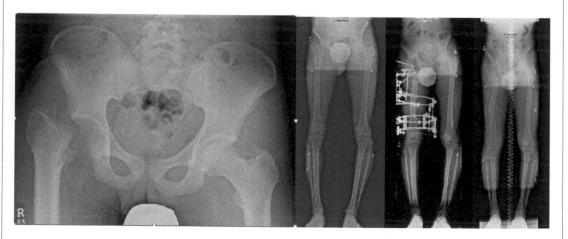

Figure 24.11 Destruction of hip joint as a result of septic arthritis is shown preoperatively at left; a 1-year postoperative x-ray at right shows restoration of the mechanical axis.

COMPLICATIONS

Knee extension contracture is usually the result of multiple pins being passed through the extensor mechanism, causing pain in flexion of the knee postoperatively. Due to the prolonged duration of treatment, soon enough patients develop adhesions and arthrofibrosis. Some preventive measures to avoid a knee contracture include flexing the knee before application of Ilizarov, as shown earlier; encouraging early range-of-motion exercises; attaching a half-ring near the joint to allow knee bending; gentle handling of tissue during surgery to decrease fibrosis; and preventing infection.

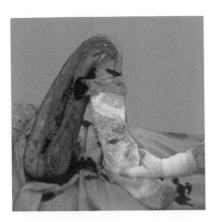

Figure 24.12 A young lady with Judet quadricepsplasty after removal of Ilizarov.

Figure 24.12 presents a 20-year-old woman treated for right dysplastic hip with Ilizarov hip reconstruction, unable to flex knee beyond 15°, who required Judet quadricepsplasty after removal of Ilizarov.

Pin tract infection remains one of the commonest complications encountered with an external fixator. Risk factors for pin tract infection include patient's intrinsic medical status, surgical technique, and postoperative care of pin tracts. A decreased immune status, poor skin conditions, and smoking are factors that may increase risk for pin tract infection.[12] Intraoperatively, minimizing necrosis is the key to avoiding pin tract infection, including careful soft tissue handling, no tenting of skin, and predrilling to avoid bone necrosis.[12] Postoperatively, daily cleaning of pin tracts with an antiseptic solution (chlorhexidine, Pyodine) is suggested. Pin tract infection is further classified according to the severity of infection into minor and major, requiring treatment ranging from local wound care to removal of pins and antibiotic coverage, and sometimes a formal wound debridement.

Early consolidation of osteotomy is especially common in noncompliant patients, and usually requires a revisit to the operating room (OR) for osteotomy. A close follow-up is required with radiographs to monitor healing of the second osteotomy site especially, and distraction may need to be tapered according to patient healing potential.

Other less common complications reported include refracture, nonunion,[13] and bone remodeling in young patients, causing loss of desired extension or valgus angulation at the proximal osteotomy site.

Figure 24.13 presents a 33-year-old woman with neglected developmental dysplasia of hip (DDH) causing pain and limp, treated with Ilizarov hip reconstruction 6 years back. Restoration of length was less than normal, and there is also proximal migration of the proximal femur. She required revision of the Ilizarov hip reconstruction due to impingement and pain.

NEWER TECHNIQUES

Recent advances in Ilizarov hip reconstruction have mainly focused on reducing rates of complications. For pin tract infection and loosening, hydroxyapatite-coated pins have been shown to have reduced rates of infection, though their effect on deep infection, malunion, or loosening secondary to infection

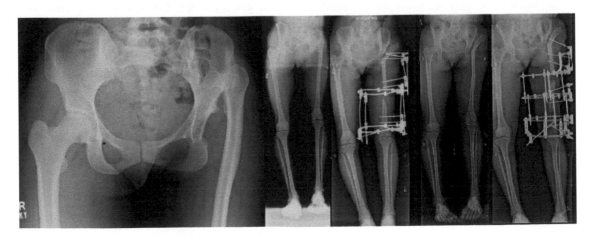

Figure 24.13 A young lady with neglected DDH treated with Ilizarov hip reconstruction 6 years back.

seems to be questionable.[15] Other recent findings by Chou et al. reported that application of topical pexiganan acetate to pin sites caused 75% decreased rates of infection in rabbits.[16] Dejong et al. reported significantly decreased rates of infection with addition of a lipid, hydroxyapatite, and chlorhexidine to pins implanted in goat tibia.[17]

A newer technique published by Krieg et al. addressed dealing with the compliance issues associated with prolonged external fixation.[14] Using principles of Ilizarov hip reconstruction, the proximal valgus extension osteotomy was fixed with a locking compression plate and the distal, lengthening varisation osteotomy stabilized with a motorized intramedullary distraction nail. A healing index of 33 days/cm and full weight-bearing after 6 months was seen, and at a 1-year follow-up, they reported improved Trendelenburg gait and limb equalization with no complications.[14]

REFERENCES

1. Kim Y.-H, Oh S.-H, Kim J.-S. Primary total hip arthroplasty with a second-generation cementless total hip prosthesis in patients younger than fifty years of age. *J Bone Joint Surg A* 2003; 85(1): 109–14.
2. Paavilainen T, Hoikka V, Paavolainen P. Cementless total hip arthroplasty for congenitally dislocated or dysplastic hips: Technique for replacement with a straight femoral component. *Clin Orthop Relat Res* 1993; 466(297): 71–81.
3. Garvin KL, Bowen MK, Salvati EA, Ranawat CS. Long-term results of total hip arthroplasty in congenital dislocation and dysplasia of the hip. A follow-up note. *J Bone Joint Surg A* 1991; 73(9): 1348–54.
4. Callaghan JJ, Brand RA, Pedersen DR. Hip arthrodesis. A long-term follow-up. *J Bone Joint Surg A* 1985; 67(9): 1328–35.
5. Sponseller PD, McBeath AA, Perpich M. Hip arthrodesis in young patients. A long-term follow-up study. *J Bone Joint Surg A* 1984; 66(6): 853–9.
6. Milch H. The 'pelvic support' osteotomy. *J Bone Joint Surg Am* 1941; 23(3): 581–95.
7. Lance PM. *Osteotomies sous-trochanterienne dans le traitement des luxations congenitales inveterees de la hanche.* Masson & Cie: Paris; 1936.
8. Pafilas D, Nayagam S. The pelvic support osteotomy: Indications and preoperative planning. *Strat Traum Limb Recon* 2008; 3(2): 83–92.
9. Ilizarov GA. *Transosseous Osteosynthesis.* New York: Springer; 1983.
10. Ilizarov GA, Samchukov ML. Reconstruction of femur by Ilizarov method in the treatment of arthrosis deformans of the hip joint. *Ortop Travmatol Protez* 1988; 6: 10.
11. Samchukov ML, Birch JG. Pelvic support femoral reconstruction using the method of Ilizarov: A case report. *Bull Hosp JT Dis* 1992; 52(1): 7.
12. Kazmers N, Fragomen A, Rozbruch S. Prevention of pin site infection in external fixation: A review of the literature. *Strat Traum Limb Recon* 2016; 11(2): 75–85.
13. Umer M, Rashid H, Umer H, Raza H. Hip reconstruction osteotomy by Ilizarov method as a salvage option for abnormal hip joints. *Biomed Res Int* 2014; 2014: 1–6.
14. Krieg A, Lenze U, Hasler C. Ilizarov hip reconstruction without external fixation: A new technique. *J Child Orthop* 2010; 4(3): 259–66.
15. Saithna A. The influence of hydroxyapatite coating of external fixator pins on pin loosening and pin track infection: A systematic review. *Injury* 2010; 41(2): 128–32.
16. Chou TG, Petti CA, Szakacs J, Bloebaum RD. Evaluating antimicrobials and implant materials for infection prevention around transcutaneous osseointegrated implants in a rabbit model. *J Biomed Mater Res A* 2010; 92(3): 942–52.
17. DeJong ES et al. Antimicrobial efficacy of external fixator pins coated with a lipid stabilized hydroxyapatite/chlorhexidine complex to prevent pin site infection in a goat model. *J Trauma* 2001; 50(6): 1008–14.

25

Ilizarov hip reconstruction osteotomy for neglected dislocation of the hip in young adults

OSMAN A. E. MOHAMED

INTRODUCTION

Neglected dislocation of the hip joint in young adults is a difficult problem. Patients with an unstable hip secondary to any etiology usually have loss of bone from the proximal femur, shortening of the limb, or both. The two main complaints of patients with a neglected dislocation of the hip joint are pain and leg length inequality. Leg length inequality associated with a unilateral neglected dislocation of the hip usually results in shorter step length, lower pelvis, a lateral shift of the ground reaction force, decreased maximum adduction moments of the hip and knee on the affected side, and increased maximum adduction moments of the hip and knee on the unaffected side.[1] Patients with an untreated or unsuccessfully treated congenital dislocation of the hip, septic arthritis of the hip, avascular necrosis of the femoral head with or without hardware, and paralytic dislocation or subluxation of the hip joint due to poliomyelitis usually have loss of bone from the proximal femur, shortening of the limb, or both.[2] Numerous salvage procedures have been proposed for the treatment of neglected dislocation of the hip. The two popular treatment options for a neglected dislocation of the hip are total joint replacement and pelvic support osteotomy.[3] Many authors have claimed that a total hip arthroplasty (THA) affords significant clinical improvement and significantly reduces pain and leg length inequality.[4,5] Others insist that joint replacement is exposed to high mechanical stresses and a high risk for failure, especially in young patients.[6–9] In addition, revision of a THA in a patient with congenital hip dysplasia or dislocation is often more difficult than a standard revision operation.[10] Schanz pointed out that in congenital dislocation of the hip, the pelvis tilts on weight-bearing until the femur on the dislocated side impinges on the lower border of the pelvis. If the femur is angled to align the upper fragment with the sidewall of the pelvis and the lower fragment parallel with the axis of weight-bearing, the lurching gait will be diminished because the stable position is reached earlier. Depression of the trochanter also improves the leverage of the glutei.[11] The lower femoral fragment should also be extended backward at the osteotomy site to decrease pelvic tilt and diminish lumbar lordosis. Many authors have described a proximal femoral valgus osteotomy for treatment of a neglected dislocation of the hip joint. This method provides hip stability and improved hip function.[2,12–14] The drawbacks of this approach are further leg shortening and disturbance of the mechanical axis of the leg.[2] Ilizarov developed the technique of pelvic support osteotomy using his apparatus and biologic principles. He described a double osteotomy: a proximal femoral valgus extension osteotomy for correction of stability and a distal femoral osteotomy for lengthening and correction of the mechanical axis of the leg.[13]

BASIC PRINCIPLES

It is important to choose the right patient for this procedure. This is an extra-articular procedure, and a patient with a stiff, painful, and damaged but located femoral head is not a suitable candidate. In cases of developmental dysplasia of hip (DDH), the procedure is only suitable if the hip is painful and dislocated, the acetabulum is severely dysplastic, and there is sufficient adduction to move the femoral head away from the sidewall of the pelvis where impingement is judged to be the source of pain. The patient described here has many of the suitable features for Ilizarov hip reconstruction, principally a mobile, albeit flail hip, and shortening and instability with little pain. The destroyed femoral head is the classic indication.[15] The steps of the procedure are to carry out a percutaneous subtrochanteric valgus femoral osteotomy, stabilized with an Ilizarov external fixator, and then a more distal femoral osteotomy for correction of valgus and for lengthening. The distal osteotomy can be stabilized with a standard Ilizarov fixator, but it is easier to use a Taylor spatial frame, which will be the method described here.[16]

INDICATIONS OF PELVIC SUPPORT OSTEOTOMY (PSO)

- Neglected congenital hip dislocation
- Infantile and early childhood septic arthritis or osteomyelitis of the proximal femur
- Girdlestone resection arthroplasty due to failed previous reconstructive surgery or arthroplasty
- Traumatic hip dislocation with hip instability irretrievable by open reduction or total joint replacement
- Femoral neck pseudarthrosis[17]

PREOPERATIVE PLANNING FROM CLINICAL ASSESSMENT[18]

Refer to Figures 25.1 through 25.10.

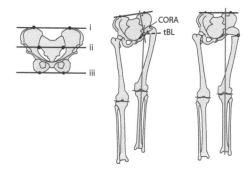

Figure 25.1 Preoperative planning taking the highest point on the iliac crests as an indicator. (Redrawn from Paley D. Hip joint considerations. In Paley D (ed): *Principle of Deformity Correction*. Heidelberg: Springer Verlag; 2003.)

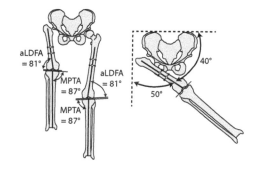

Figure 25.2 Preoperative planning taking into consideration the level of the anterior iliac spines as an indicator. (Redrawn from Paley D. Hip joint considerations. In Paley D (ed): *Principle of Deformity Correction*. Heidelberg: Springer Verlag; 2003.)

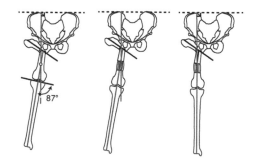

Figure 25.3 Preoperative planning taking into consideration the level of the Ischial tuberosity as an indicator. (Redrawn from Paley D. Hip joint considerations. In Paley D (ed): *Principle of Deformity Correction*. Heidelberg: Springer Verlag; 2003.)

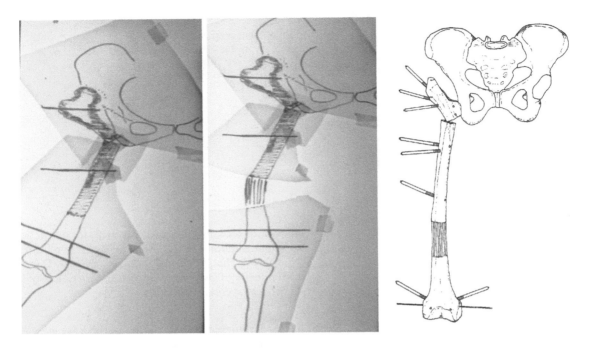

Figure 25.4 Preoperative planning on actual x-rays and site of pin insertion.

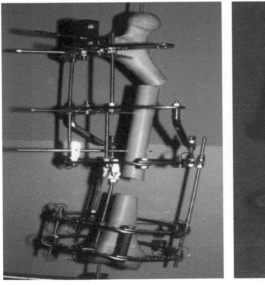
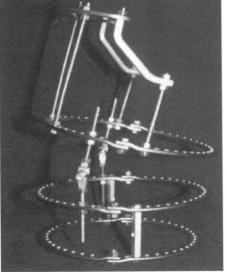

Figure 25.5 Preoperative planning for frame.

TECHNICAL PEARLS

Correct patient positioning is important, bearing in mind the conflicting demands of having a level pelvis and free access to the gluteal area for both the surgeon and the image intensifier (Figure 25.9). A semilateral position is practical. As for any femoral frame, there has to be free access underneath the femur, which can be achieved by supporting the leg on a frame or bolster.[19]

i. *Level and degree of the proximal femoral osteotomy*: Opinions differ; I place the leg into maximum adduction, and the level of the

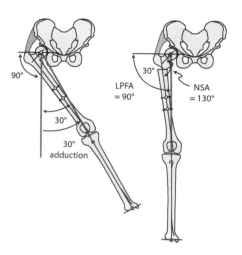

Figure 25.6 Preoperative planning for proximal osteotomy. LPFA, lateral proximal femoral angle; NSA, neck shaft angle. (Redrawn from Paley D. Hip joint considerations. In Paley D (ed): *Principle of Deformity Correction*. Heidelberg: Springer Verlag; 2003.)

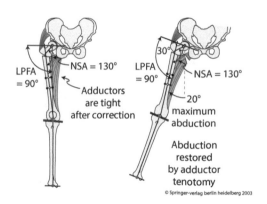

Figure 25.7 Preoperative planning for correction proximal osteotomy. (Redrawn from Paley D. Hip joint considerations. In Paley D (ed): *Principle of Deformity Correction*. Heidelberg: Springer Verlag; 2003.)

osteotomy is a little proximal to the level of the ischial tuberosity. Figure 25.9 shows the pre-placed drill holes for the osteotomy in the bone at this level. The degree of angulation is determined by the amount of adduction possible. If a deformed femoral head is present and causing impingement pain, adequate adduction must be present to move the femoral head sufficiently away from the pelvis. If this is not possible, then a Girdlestone procedure may be required in addition. It is therefore advisable to obtain maximum adduction x-rays prior to surgery.[20]

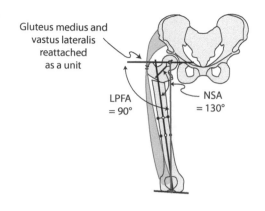

Figure 25.8 Preoperative planning for correction gluteus medius muscle tension. (Redrawn from Paley D. Hip joint considerations. In Paley D (ed): *Principle of Deformity Correction*. Heidelberg: Springer Verlag; 2003.)

ii. *Stabilizing the osteotomy*: In this case, a Russian arch was used for proximal fixation after predrilling the osteotomy with many drill holes to facilitate the osteotomy. In the AP plane, the ring is aligned at the desired angle of correction to the shaft and to the shaft in the lateral (sagittal) plane. Be careful not to angulate it into flexion or extension unless correction of significant fixed flexion is desired. A threaded rod with a simple hinge is run down from the arch with the hinge at the medial edge of the osteotomy. A 5/8 spatial frame ring of the same diameter as the proximal ring of the spatial frame ring for the distal correction is attached to this hinge orthogonal to the shaft (Figure 25.9). If some extension is desired at the osteotomy to correct a fixed flexion deformity, then a Russian-style multiaxial hinge can be used to permit this. Lock the hinge. Attach the proximal ring of the distal spatial frame to the femur and join to the 5/8 ring, as this makes for better stability.[21,22]

iii. *Osteotomy*: This should be carried out percutaneously under x-ray control. Complete division of the bone will be accompanied by some displacement, but the hinge (Figure 25.14) will control this. Unlock the hinge and angulate the osteotomy the desired amount—usually to align the Russian arch to the 5/8 ring. Lock the hinge and then stabilize by placing threaded rods between the

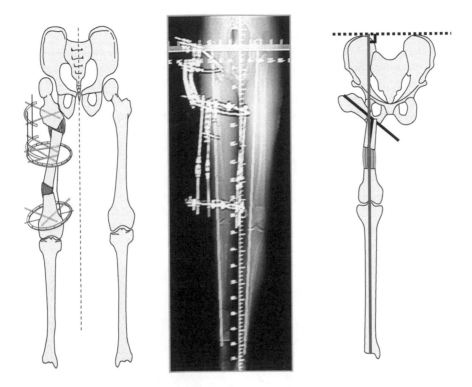

Figure 25.9 Preoperative planning for correction. (Redrawn from Paley D. Hip joint considerations. In Paley D (ed): *Principle of Deformity Correction*. Heidelberg: Springer Verlag; 2003, and follow-up x-ray.)

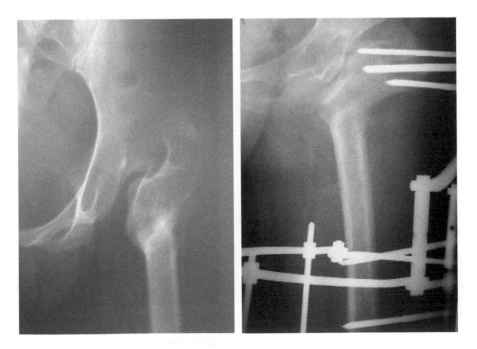

Figure 25.10 Follow-up x-rays before (right) and after (left) removal.

two rings. Ideally, the distal fragment should translate medially by about 1/3 to 1/2 of the diameter of the bone for correct alignment. Using this technique, the osteotomy can be easily controlled.[23]

iv. *Distal deformity correction*: The distal spatial frame is then completed and a distal osteotomy carried out.

IMAGES DURING TREATMENT

Intraoperative x-rays

See Figures 25.11 through 25.16.

AVOIDING AND MANAGING PROBLEMS

- Obtain the requisite preoperative radiographs to plan the level and degree of proximal osteotomy correction.
- Place enough hip extension proximally to allow the hip to lock.
- Consider removing and replacing the proximal pins one at a time through a new skin incision to release tethered soft tissues after the acute correction.
- Flex and extend the hip and knee fully after the fixator is applied to release tight soft tissue (e.g., iliotibial band).

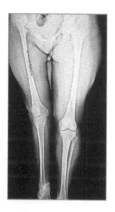
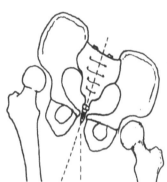
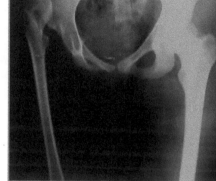

Figure 25.11 Follow-up x-rays, preoperative.

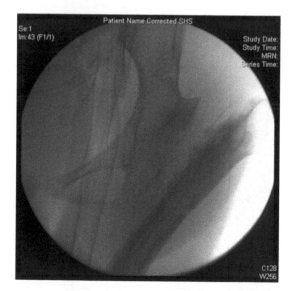

Figure 25.12 Maximum adduction view in theater. Drill holes.

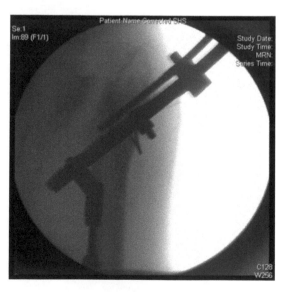

Figure 25.13 Proximal fixation with Russian arch marks the site of proposed proximal femoral osteotomy. Note hinge position.

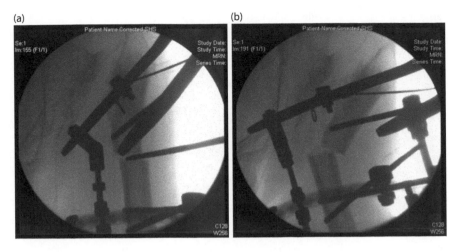

Figure 25.14 **(a, b)** Completing the osteotomy as per preoperative planning.

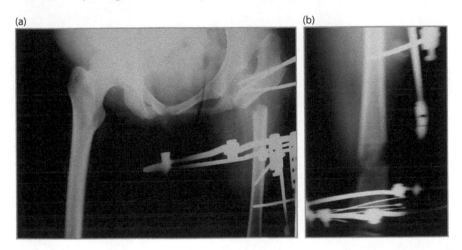

Figure 25.15 **(a, b)** Hinge to angulate desired amount as per preoperative planning.

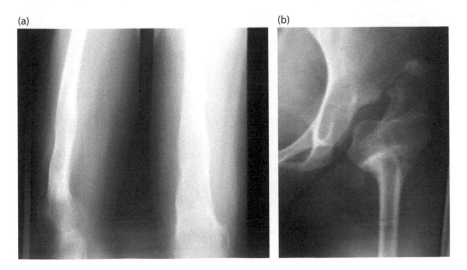

Figure 25.16 **(a, b)** Completed osteotomy and desired hinge.

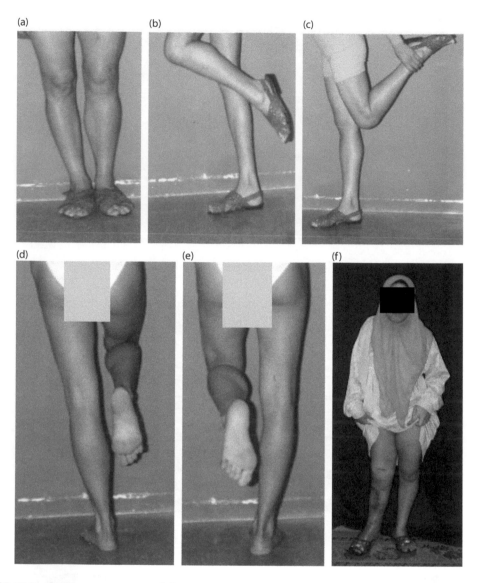

Figure 25.17 **(a–f)** Hip movement at follow-up.

ADVANTAGES

By combining an angular proximal femoral osteotomy and a distal femoral lengthening, hip instability and limb-length discrepancy can be corrected concurrently, avoiding the need for multiple surgical procedures (Figures 25.16 and 25.17). The effect of the proximal osteotomy is to place the femur under the pelvis and as a result to support the pelvis. In addition, the gluteal muscles are stretched maximally and the pelvis is stabilized during the single-limb stance phase of gait. This results in resolution of the Trendelenburg gait and sign. Angulation of the proximal femur is well marked by the soft tissue bulk of the proximal thigh and displaces the large soft tissue mass laterally, which provides a more normal appearance to the limb. The functional abduction obtained on the surgically-treated side aids perineal hygiene and sexual function in women.

DISADVANTAGES

1. Time in the fixator.
2. A subsequent total hip arthroplasty would be much more difficult after this hip reconstruction and leg-lengthening procedure.

3. The possibility of loss of angulation due to remodeling.
4. Short follow-up period in the literature.

CONCLUSIONS

Early results of Ilizarov modification of pelvic support osteotomy may be encouraging. However, the possibility of deterioration with time and unpredictability of improvement of Trendelenburg gait should be considered.

REFERENCES

1. Aksoy MC, Musdal Y. Subtrochanteric valgus-extension osteotomy for neglected congenital dislocation of the hip in young adults. *Acta Orthop Belg* 2000; 66: 181–6.
2. Bombelli R. Structure and function in normal and abnormal hips. *Hip Joint Considerations*. 3rd ed., Berlin, Heidelberg: Springer Verlag; 1993, pp. 1–55.
3. Catagni MA, Malzev V, Kirienko A. Treatment of disorders of the hip joint. In: Maiocchi AB (ed): *Advances in Ilizarov Apparatus Assembly*. Medi Surgical Video, Milan; Springer Verlag; 1998, pp. 119–22.
4. Dearborn JT, Harris WH. Acetabular revision after failed total hip arthroplasty in patients with congenital hip dislocation and dysplasia. Results after a mean of 8.6 years. *J Bone Joint Surg* 2000; 82-A: 1146–53.
5. Decking J et al. Cementless total hip replacement with subtrochanteric femoral shortening for severe developmental dysplasia of the hip. *Arch Orthop Trauma Surg* 2003; 123: 357–62.
6. Davlin LB et al. Treatment of osteoarthrosis secondary to congenital dislocation of the hip. Primary cemented surface replacement compared with conventional total hip replacement. *J Bone Joint Surg* 1990; 72; 1035–42.
7. Garvin KL, Bowen MK, Salvati EA, Ranawat CS. Long-term results of total hip arthroplasty in congenital dislocation and dysplasia of the hip. A follow-up note. *J Bone Joint Surg* 1991; 73-A: 1348–54.
8. Ilizarov GA. *Transosseous Osteosynthesis*. 1st ed., New York: Springer Verlag; 1983, pp. 701–27.
9. Inan M, Bomar JD, Kucukkaya M, Harma A. A comparison between the use of a monolateral external fixator and the Ilizarov technique for pelvic support osteotomies. *Acta Orthop Traumatol Turc* 2004; 38: 252–60.
10. Kim YH, Oh SH, Kim JS. Primary total hip arthroplasty with a second-generation cementless total hip prosthesis in patients younger than fifty years of age. *J Bone Joint Surg* 2003; 85: 109–14.
11. Kocaoglu M, Eralp L, Sen C, Dincyurek H. The Ilizarov hip reconstruction osteotomy for hip dislocation: Outcome after 4–7 years in 14 young patients. *Acta Orthop Scand* 2002; 73: 432–8.
12. Lai KA, Lin CJ, Jou IM, Su FC. Gait analysis after total hip arthroplasty with leg-length equalization in women with unilateral congenital complete dislocation of the hip: A comparison with untreated patients. *J Orthop Res* 2001; 19: 1147–52.
13. Lai KA, Lin CJ, Su FC. Gait analysis of adult patients with complete congenital dislocation of the hip. *J Formos Med Assoc* 1997; 96: 740–4.
14. Lai KA, Liu J, Liu TK. Use of iliofemoral distraction in reducing high congenital dislocation of the hip before total hip arthroplasty. *J Arthroplasty* 1996; 11: 588–93.
15. McQueary FG, Johnston RC. Coxarthrosis after congenital dysplasia. Treatment by total hip arthroplasty without acetabular bone-grafting. *J Bone Joint Surg* 1988; 70-A: 1140–4.
16. Milch H. The "pelvic support" osteotomy. *Clin Orthop* 1989; 249: 4–11.
17. Paavilainen T, Hoikka V, Solonen KA. Cementless total replacement for severely dysplastic or dislocated hips. *J Bone Joint Surg* 1990; 72-B: 205–11.
18. Paley D. Hip joint considerations. In Paley D (ed): *Principle of Deformity Correction*. Heidelberg: Springer Verlag; 2003.

19. Parvizi J et al. Surgical treatment of limb-length discrepancy following total hip arthroplasty. *J Bone Joint Surg* 2003; 85-A: 2310–7.

20. Samchukov ML, Birch JG. Pelvic support femoral reconstruction using the method of Ilizarov: A case report. *Bull Hosp Jt Dis* 1992; 52: 7–11.

21. Schanz A. Zur Behandlung der veralteten Angeborenen Huftverrenkung. *Munchen Med Wschr* 1922; 69: 930–41.

22. E-M mowafi H. Outcome of pelvic support osteotomy with the Ilizarov method in the treatment of the unstable hip joint. *Acta Orthop Belg* 2005; 71: 686–91.

23. Emara KM. Pelvic support osteotomy in the treatment of patients with excision arthroplasty. *Clin Orthop Relat Res* 2008; 466: 708–13.

26

Arthroscopic hip preservation surgery

PRAKASH CHANDRAN

INTRODUCTION

Improvement in arthroscopic techniques with improved instrumentation supplemented with advances in imaging techniques allows surgeons to diagnose and manage a wide range of intra-articular and periarticular hip derangement, where until recently, a major open procedure including surgical dislocation of the hip would have been required. The arthroscopic technique on the hip joint was first demonstrated on cadaveric hips by Dr. Michael Burman in 1931, and the procedure was first clinically performed for infection by Dr. Kenji Takagi in 1939. In the past decade, arthroscopic techniques have advanced significantly and are now being used to deal with various hip pathologies.

Structurally, the hip joint has the femoral head deeply recessed in the bony acetabulum, and the fibrocapsular and muscular envelopes pose a significant challenge for arthroscopic examination of the hip. Restraint of the hip joint requires a significant distraction force to allow safe instrumentation. The proximity of the sciatic nerve, lateral femoral cutaneous nerve, and femoral neurovascular structures requires good understanding of the surface anatomy to ensure safe portal placement. Technical advances in distraction of the hip, intraoperative imaging, needle positioning, and appropriate portal placement have helped to improve the accessibility and visualization of the hip joint.

The common hip pathologies now routinely managed arthroscopically are acetabular labral tears, femoroacetabular impingement (FAI), chondral injuries, loose bodies, joint infection, capsular laxity, and injuries to the ligamentum teres. Some extra-articular conditions, including internal and external snapping hip, synovial chondromatosis and other synovial abnormalities, crystalline hip arthropathy (gout and pseudogout), post-traumatic intra-articular debris, osteonecrosis of the femoral head, and mild to moderate hip osteoarthritis with mechanical symptoms, are also being managed arthroscopically. Advanced arthroscopic techniques, in conjunction with open femoral and/or periacetabular osteotomy, are used in the management of dysplasia and complex hip deformities. Advances in techniques also allow for reconstruction of the acetabular labrum, ligamentum teres, and capsulorrhaphy in cases of instability, and repair of injuries to the gluteal tendons are being considered.[1,2]

In the presence of infected open wounds, skin ulceration, or cellulite in and around the hip area and acute osteomyelitis of the femur or acetabulum, hip arthroscopy is contraindicated to deal with other pathologies; some also consider

Table 26.1 Indications and contraindications for hip arthroscopy

Indications	Contraindications
Labral tears	Infected open wounds or cellulite in and around the hip area
Femoroacetabular impingement	Protrusio
Chondral injuries	Heterotopic ossification
Loose bodies	Ankylosis, advanced hip arthritis, severe dysplasia
Capsular laxity	
Ligamentum teres injuries	
Synovial chondromatosis	
Synovial abnormalities	
Crystalline hip arthropathy (gout and pseudogout)	
Infection	
Management of post-traumatic intra-articular debris	
Osteonecrosis of the femoral head	
Mild to moderate hip osteoarthritis with mechanical symptoms	
Long-standing, unresolved hip joint pain with positive physical findings	
Internal and external snapping hip	

heterotopic ossification, advanced osteoarthritis, protrusio, and ankylosis contraindications to perform hip arthroscopy (Table 26.1).

SURGICAL ANATOMY OF THE HIP

The hip is a ball-and-socket type of diarthrodial joint, formed between the femoral head and the acetabulum. The femoral head sits deep into the acetabular socket and the acetabulum is further deepened by the fibrocartilaginous labrum, providing stability to the hip joint. The capsule, along with the ligamentum teres and extra-articular ligaments, adds to the stability. The hip joint has a triplanar motion; however, the inherent stability of the hip restricts the terminal range of hip movement. Muscles around the hip joint (Table 26.2) contribute to stability and help with mobility. The muscles can be compartmentalized into the gluteal muscles and the muscles of the anterior, medial, and posterior aspects of the thigh. Innervation to the hip is primarily by the obturator nerve and by the branches of the femoral and sciatic nerves. The primary source of blood supply to the hip joint is the medial femoral circumflex artery with supplementation from the femoral and gluteal vessels. Knowledge of the surgical anatomy and surface markings is of great importance while considering arthroscopic intervention of the hip joint.

Table 26.2 Hip muscles and movements

Hip movements	Muscles
Hip flexion	Iliopsoas, rectus femoris, and sartorius
Hip extension	Gluteus maximus and hamstrings (semitendinosus, semimembranosus, and long head of biceps femoris)
Hip abduction	Gluteus medius and minimus The tensor fascia lata also helps with abduction in a flexed hip
Hip adduction	Adductor brevis, longus and magnus; pectineus; and gracilis
Hip external rotation	Obturator internus, obturator externus, superior and inferior gemellus, quadratus femoris, and piriformis
Hip internal rotation	Secondary actions of the anterior fibers of the gluteus medius and minimus, tensor fascia lata, semimembranosus, semitendinosus, pectineus, and posterior part of the adductor magnus

Femoroacetabular impingement, acetabular labrum, and articular cartilage pathology constitute the majority of the conditions that can be managed preserving the hip joint. The acetabular labrum is a fibrocartilaginous tissue attached to the rim of the acetabulum and continues as the transverse acetabular ligament inferiorly bridging the cotyloid fossa. The labrum increases the depth, surface area, volume, congruity, and stability of the hip joint. The labrum adds 33% to the acetabular volume and contributes an average of 22% to articulating surface area.[3] It provides a seal around the osseous acetabulum and femoral head. This fluid seal produces a negative intra-articular pressure, significantly adding to hip joint stability.[4]

Microscopically, the collagen fibers in the anterior aspect of the labrum are arranged parallel to the labral-chondral junction, but in the posterior aspect, they are aligned perpendicular to the junction. The orientation of the collagen fibers parallel to the labral-chondral junction in the anterior labrum may render it more prone to damage compared to the posterior labrum, where the collagen fibers are directly anchored in the acetabular cartilage. Sensory fibers, mechanoreceptors, and free nerve fibers densely populate the acetabular labrum, capsule, and transverse acetabular ligament, suggesting their potential roles as source of hip pain. It has been found that the anterior zone of the labrum contains the highest relative concentration of sensory fibers.[5–7] The acetabular labrum receives its blood supply from radial branches of a periacetabular periosteal vascular ring that traverses the osseolabral junction on its capsular side and continues toward the labrum's free edge.[8,9]

Acetabular labrum tears have been implicated as a cause of hip pain in adult patients; 74% of the tears are located in the anterosuperior quadrant. Two distinct types of tears of the labrum have been identified histologically. The first consists of a detachment of the fibrocartilaginous labrum from the articular hyaline cartilage at the transition zone. The second consists of one or more cleavage planes of variable depth within the substance of the labrum. Labral tears can occur early in the arthritic process of the hip and may be one of the initial derangements of degenerative hip disease.[6]

Loss of labral function, either via tear or debridement, may induce hip microinstability, subluxation, or dislocation. Breakage of the labral fluid seal is the rationale behind loss of joint stability.[9,10] Labral preservation, particularly with larger tears, may be important for maintaining hip stability.[11] The ligamentum teres connects the center of the femoral head to the acetabular fossa, and lesions of the ligamentum teres are being increasingly recognized as a cause of persistent hip pain, particularly due to microinstability.

The approach to arriving at a diagnosis would be to differentiate the various structures starting from the bony anatomy of the hip joint, proximal femur and pelvis, lumbar and sacral spine, and cartilage structures, which include the articular cartilage and acetabular labrum, synovial tissue, capsule including the ligaments, muscles, tendons, bursas, and surrounding neurovascular structure.

IMAGING

Imaging helps in defining and confirming the pathoanatomy; routinely, plain radiographs, magnetic resonance (MR) arthrograms, and computed tomography (CT) with 3D reconstruction are employed.

Radiography

Anteroposterior and lateral hip radiographs are usually performed; other views in the oblique plane and also in varying degrees of rotation of the hip can be taken as indicated. A standard anteroposterior hip radiograph includes images of both sides of the hip on the same film and projects toward the middle of the lines connecting the upper symphysis pubis and anterior-superior iliac spine; lower extremities should be internally rotated by 15–20° and the distance from the x-ray tube to the film should be 1.2 meters. There are multiple imaging techniques for lateral hip radiography, including frog-leg lateral view, Löwenstein view, and cross-table lateral view. Studies have observed that 87% of patients with labral tears had an identifiable underlying structural abnormality that could be seen on plain radiographs. Plain radiographic evaluation of the hip is dependent on patient positioning and subject to inconsistencies in radiographic technique; image quality limits its reliability.[4,11]

Evaluation of images

In order to evaluate an image, it is critical to confirm that the x-ray was properly taken and the patient was in an appropriate position. Generally, anteroposterior and false-profile views provide information on the shape of the acetabulum, whereas other lateral images provide information on proximal femoral parts, including the femoral head. The following specific information can be obtained from anteroposterior hip radiographs: (1) leg length, (2) neck-shaft angle, (3) acetabular coverage: the lateral center-edge (CE) angle and femoral head extrusion index, (4) acetabular depth, (5) acetabular inclination, (6) acetabular version, (7) head sphericity, and (8) joint space width. The lateral view helps evaluate the sphericity of the femoral head, joint congruency, and shape and offset of the head–neck junction. In the false-profile view, the anterior coverage of the femoral head can be assessed.

In lateral hip radiographs, the shape and offset of the femoral head–neck junction and the offset alpha angle are assessed; axial computed tomography or magnetic resonance imaging is used for more accuracy. A cam deformity is diagnosed if the alpha angle exceeds 50–55° (Figure 26.1).

Computed tomography scan of the hip and pelvis

Both computed tomography (CT) and magnetic resonance imaging (MRI), with and without intra-articular contrast medium, are now routinely performed to define hip pathological anatomy. CT allows accurate evaluation of the bony anatomy of the hip, and also the anatomic relationships between the femoral head and the acetabulum, independent of patient position. Femoral and acetabular version, femoral head coverage, asphericity, and the relationship between abnormal anatomy and mechanical causes of cartilage and labrum degeneration in preosteoarthritic hips can be defined.[6,10,12] On the femur, the CT scan helps to measure the alpha angle, femoral neck version angles, coxa valga, and coxa vara. On the acetabular side, CT scan helps in quantifying anteversion/retroversion and inclination. CT scan also helps in identifying a combination of these abnormalities. Ninety percent of patients with labral pathology show structural abnormalities that can be identified on CT scans.

Ultrasound of the hip

Advancement in the ultrasonographic technique has improved accuracy in evaluating pathologies of both intra-articular and extra-articular soft tissues in and around the hip joint; this includes the muscles, tendons, and bursae. It is becoming increasingly popular due to its easy accessibility, availability, lack of radiation exposure, and low costs. The distinct advantage of the ultrasound (US) is that it allows for dynamic evaluation, wherein the joint and soft tissues can be visualized while taking the joint through the motions. It is also a valuable tool in guiding infiltrations/intervention around the hip joint for both diagnostic and therapeutic purposes.[12]

The high-frequency linear transducer, typically with frequencies at approximately 7–12 MHz, may have adequate penetration for hip examination, and a lower-frequency sector transducer may be required if the patient is obese. For US examination, the hip area is divided into four quadrants: the anterior, medial, lateral, and posterior.

The ultrasound examination is performed sequentially, starting in a supine position from the anterior quadrant and working around to the lateral, posterior, and medial sides. In the anterior aspect, the iliopsoas tendinopathy, bursitis, and snapping iliopsoas tendon can be evaluated; on the lateral side, evaluation focuses on the iliotibial band, tensor fasciae latae, rectus femoris, and gluteus medius tendon for hip abductor tendinopathy or tear. Posteriorly, hamstring tendons and muscles, ischiogluteal bursitis and piriformis, and on

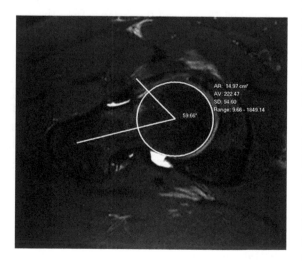

Figure 26.1 Alpha angle.

the medial side the adductor longus and the gracilis can be visualized.

Magnetic resonance

Magnetic resonance (MR) imaging is becoming increasingly essential in the workup of bone and soft tissue abnormalities of the hip. Intra-articular injection of a contrast medium is required to obtain a precise diagnosis of intra-articular pathology such as labral tears, cartilaginous lesions, femoroacetabular impingement, and intra-articular foreign bodies, and while evaluating for developmental dysplasia of the hip. Evaluation of the labrum and cartilage is better with a 3T magnetic field. MR arthrography of the hip sequences includes fat-saturated T1-weighted 3-mm slices in axial oblique, coronal, and sagittal planes; fat-saturated T2-weighted 4-mm slices in the coronal plane; and fat-saturated three-dimensional (3D) gradient echo T1-weighted 1-mm slices allowing for multiplanar and radial reconstructions. This helps in the detection of acetabular labrum lesions (Figure 26.2).[13–15]

Labral tears

Imaging of the labrum and studies of path anatomy lead to classification of labral lesions. In 1996, Czerny et al.[16] proposed an MR imaging classification (Table 26.3) of acetabular labrum lesions with reference to increasing stages of

severity, and Blankenbaker et al. [17] classified based on the location of the tear (Table 26.4). Lage et al.[18] described an arthroscopic classification based on the morphology of labral tears (Table 26.5). However, further studies did not find a good correlation between these classifications and resorted to morphological description of the tear. A linear or curvilinear increased signal at the insertion of the labrum suggests a partial tear (Figure 26.3a,b).

This needs to be correlated clinically, as it can sometimes be found in asymptomatic patients. The presence of a paralabral cyst suggests a complete labral tear.[19]

Femoroacetabular impingement

Cam-type FAI shows signs of flattening or a convexity of the anterosuperior part of the normally concave femoral head–neck junction[22,23] and an alpha angle exceeding 55°.[24] The alpha angle is measured on an axial-oblique image between the axis of the femoral neck and a line connecting the femoral head center with the point of change in the radius of the curvature on the anterior part of the femoral head. Cam deformity is diagnosed if the alpha angle exceeds 50–55° (Figure 26.4a,b).

In more severe cases, there may be an associated subchondral edema, subchondral microcyst, or fibrocystic changes in the anterosuperior part of the femoral neck. As a consequence, there is extensive anterosuperior labral injury.[21,23]

Pincer-type FAI causes direct contact between the anterior acetabular border and the femoral head–neck junction. In this type of FAI, there is a morphological anomaly of the acetabulum that causes excessive coverage of the femoral head, such as coxa profunda, acetabular protrusion, or acetabular retroversion.[24–26] In long-standing cases, lesions to the posteroinferior cartilage by a contrecoup mechanism may appear.[20]

Articular cartilage

MR arthrogram can help assess the presence and severity of cartilage loss.[27,28] The articular cartilage in the hip is thin, and due to the direct apposition of the femur and acetabulum, it is difficult to differentiate femoral from acetabular cartilage with standard MR imaging. Sensitivity and specificity of MR arthrography in the detection

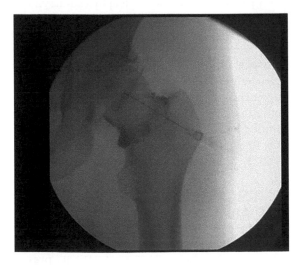

Figure 26.2 Hip arthrogram (intra-articular contrast).

Table 26.3 Czerny et al.'s magnetic resonance arthrography classification of labral tears

Stage 0	Homogeneous low signal intensity, triangular shape, continuous attachment to the lateral margins of the acetabulum without a notch or a sulcus. A recess between the joint capsule and the labrum, which consists of a linear collection of the contrast material extending between the cranial margin of the acetabular labrum and the joint capsule
Stage 1A	Labral tears have an area of increased signal intensity in the center that does not extend to the margins, a triangular shape, and a continuous attachment to the lateral margin of the acetabulum without the sulcus. A normal labral recess is also present
Stage 1B	Similar to stage 1A but thickened, and no labral recess is present
Stage 2A	An extension of contrast into the labrum without detachment from the acetabulum, are triangular, and have a labral recess
Stage 2B	Like stage 2A but thickened, and the labral recess is not present
Stage 3A	Labrum is detached from the acetabulum but triangular in shape
Stage 3B	Like stage 3A but thickened

Table 26.4 Blankenbaker et al.'s magnetic resonance arthrography classification of labral tears

Type 1	Frayed: Irregular margins of the labrum without a discrete tear
Type 2	Flap tear: Contrast extending into or through the labral substance
Type 3	Peripheral longitudinal: Contrast partially or completely between the labral base and acetabulum labral detachment
Type 4	Thickened and distorted and thus likely unstable

Table 26.5 Lage et al.'s arthroscopic classification of labral tears

Radial flap	Disruption of the free margin of the labrum with subsequent formation of discrete flap
Radial fibrillated	Appearance of a shaving brush; hairy appearance at the free margin
Longitudinal peripheral	Of variable length along the acetabular insertion of the labrum
Unstable	Subluxing labrum

of chondral lesions using T1-weighted spin-echo sequence are estimated to be about 62%–79% and 77%–94%. Cartilage is categorized into normal, signal heterogeneity, fissuring, thinning to <50% of the normal thickness, thinning to >50% of the normal thickness, and full thickness cartilage loss (Figure 26.5).

Cartilage lesions are also correlated with bone marrow edema, subchondral cyst formation, and subchondral osteosclerosis.

Intra-articular foreign bodies

MR and multidetector computed tomography (MDCT) arthrography help differentiate intra-articular foreign bodies from osteophytes, synovial folds, or hypertrophic synovitis. Intra-articular foreign bodies are seen surrounded by contrast medium and only partially in the case of osteophytes and synovial.

Abnormality of the ligamentum teres

Abnormality of the ligamentum teres, such as complete or partial tear, can be identified. Degenerated ligamentum teres can be seen in young patients, often associated with avascular osteonecrosis of the femoral head or slipped capital femoral epiphysis. Recently, studies have demonstrated microinstability with deficient ligamentum teres.

PHYSICAL EXAMINATION OF THE HIP AND PELVIS

A history followed by physical examination of the hip is key for evaluation of patients presenting with hip pain. A comprehensive history and detailed physical examination of the hip are key

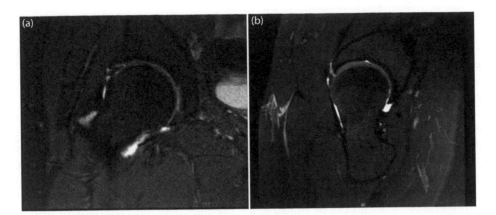

Figure 26.3 **(a, b)** Labral tear.

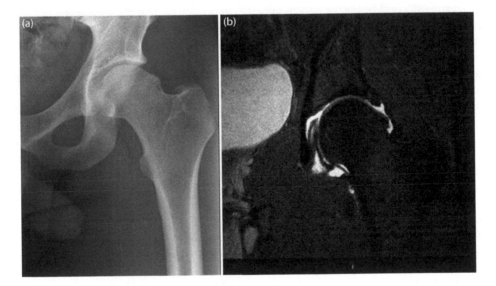

Figure 26.4 **(a, b)** Cam lesion.

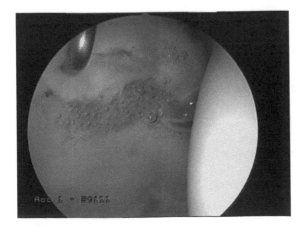

Figure 26.5 Labrum and articular cartilage.

to identifying the pathology. A systematic assessment of the hip and surrounding structures that includes osteochondral, capsulolabral, musculotendinous, and neurovascular structures should be performed. Hip examination should be performed in a systematic and orderly approach with clear understanding of the principles of each test used. The findings during the examination will direct toward special tests and other areas to be examined in detail.

Typically, a femoroacetabular impingement will present with groin pain on sitting or deep flexion of the hip (squatting), pain during certain movement/position (during sporting activities), or clicking/popping at hip (e.g. golf swing). Pain is usually insidious onset and progressive and typically demonstrates the C sign (the patient will hold his or her hand in the shape of a C and place it above the greater trochanter, with the thumb positioned posterior to the trochanter and fingers extending into the groin). The pain will increase on flexion, adduction, and internal rotation movements at the hip. The pain is typically intermittent and activity-related. The nature of the pain can also give clues to the diagnosis; if the pain is sharp and acute with associated symptoms of "locking" or giving way, consider labral pathology. Pain associated with specific movements can be related to a single musculotendinous unit, tendinitis, or bursitis. A history of sports and recreational activities can help determine the type of injury and also guide the treatment, considering the patient's goals and expectations.

Assessment of the anterior femoroacetabular impingement or apprehension test is performed in a supine position by passive flexion, internal rotation, and adduction of the hip. This can be supplemented by the dynamic internal rotatory impingement (DIRI) test. The McCarthy test assesses for posterior impingement. The test is performed with the patient in a supine position, with the patient's hips at the end of the couch and the contralateral hip and knee held flexed by the patient. A positive test is indicated by pain as the affected hip is moved into extension and external rotation. The dynamic external rotatory impingement test (DEXRIT) assesses for superolateral and posterior femoroacetabular impingement.

It is important to be able to differentiate extra-articular from intra-articular pathology. A comprehensive assessment algorithm provides a rational approach to patient evaluation and improves clinical decision-making and treatment plans.

SURGICAL TECHNIQUE

Arthroscopic access to the hip joint is more challenging because of the anatomical constraints; the femoral head is deeply placed in the bony acetabular socket. The thick fibrocapsular and muscular envelopes around the hip joint increase the amount of force required for distraction of the hip.[30] The limited space of the hip joint, despite distraction with traction, can add to the complexity of the procedure. The proximity of the sciatic nerve, lateral femoral cutaneous nerve, and femoral neurovascular structures requires precise portal placement.

The arthroscopic surgical anatomy of the hip joint is divided into the central compartment, peripheral compartment, and extra-articular structures (Table 26.6). To access the central compartment, distraction of the joint surfaces by traction is required. Different designs of hip distracters are available to achieve distraction at the hip joint; distracters can be conveniently attached to the existing operating table and distraction can be effectively achieved at the beginning of the surgery. A systematic sequential approach is followed to visualize the structures; depending on personal preferences, the central or peripheral compartment can be approached first. If the hip joint is tight, one could start with the peripheral compartment and then proceed to the central compartment.

Table 26.6 Arthroscopic access to the hip

Central compartment (With traction)	Peripheral compartment (No traction)	Periarticular/extra-articular structures (No traction)
Anterior labrum	Peripheral femoral head and its articular cartilage	Gluteal musculature
Anterolateral labrum		Iliotibial band
Posterior labrum	Femoral neck	Iliopsoas
Acetabular facets	Joint capsule	Fascia lata
Acetabular articular cartilage	Capsular portion of the labrum	Piriformis muscles
Femoral articular cartilage	Medial synovial plica	External rotators
Ligamentum teres	Articular recess (medial, anterior, posterior recesses)	Sciatic nerve
Transverse ligament		Greater sciatic foramen exploration
	Zona orbicularis	
	Dynamic evaluation of hip articulation	

Flexible instruments are now available that allow for improved access to most structures within the hip joint.

Patient position

Supine and lateral positions are widely used to access the hip joint arthroscopically; the choice of position depends on one's understanding of the orientation of structures, familiarity with the position, and training. Both supine and lateral positions have been shown to give good access to the hip joint and the extra-articular structures.

Arthroscopic access to the hip joint in a supine position was described by Byrd in 1994. The patient is positioned on the traction table with the foot secured in a traction boot. The leg is positioned in adduction, the hip joint is flexed to 10°, and the femur is in slight internal rotation. A well-padded perineal support is required to ensure good countertraction. The lateral position was described by Glick in 1987; special table attachments allow for adequate pelvic stabilization, and a well-padded perineal post provides the countertraction in a lateral position when the traction is applied.

Theater layout and equipment

The layout of the theater equipment depends on the surgeon's preference for supine or lateral positioning of the patient. The equipment should be positioned such that monitor screens are within visual range and minimal movement of equipment is needed during the procedure. The arthroscopic monitor placed right opposite across the table and the fluoroscopic monitor placed at the foot end work well. All other kit, including shavers and pump, can be placed between these two monitors (Figure 26.6).

A standard traction table or additional traction extension attachments are used to achieve traction; a well-padded perineal post (at least 9 cm of perineal padding) is used for distraction of the hip. The foot is wrapped in wool, placed in a foam boot, and firmly secured and attached to the distraction device. While in lateral position, care must be taken not to crush the contralateral thigh between the post and the operating table when the traction is applied. The perineum is checked before and after traction has been

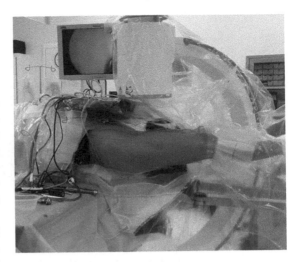

Figure 26.6 Theater equipment layout.

applied. Traction is cautiously applied under image intensifier guidance and the hip's distractibility is confirmed prior to draping. General anesthesia with good muscle relaxation or regional anesthesia is necessary for safe distraction of the hip. Hypotensive anesthesia helps the surgeon minimize pump pressure and decrease fluid extravasation. It is safer to keep the distraction time under 2 hours.

Portals

The standard portals commonly used are anterolateral, posterolateral, anterior, and modified anterior. Other portals described are proximal transgluteal, superolateral, modified anterior portal proximal, and distal (Figure 26.7).

Portal placement

Following preparation and draping, traction is reapplied to distract the joint. A fluoroscope is used to guide the initial portal placement. A spinal needle can be passed into the hip joint at this stage and an air arthrogram can be performed; this allows for loss of vacuum, and the joint can be distracted further. A 14-gauge needle and Nitinol guide wire are used to create an anterolateral portal. The needle is advanced into the hip joint under image intensifier control with the bevel surface facing the femoral head. Once in the joint, the Nitinol guide wire is inserted and the needle is removed, the portal is dilated,

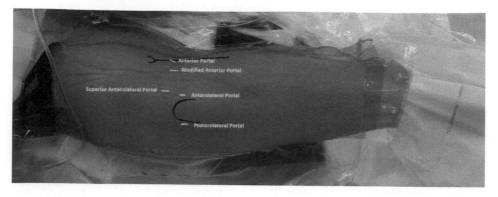

Figure 26.7 Portal placement.

and the arthroscope is introduced. Under direct vision, the modified anterior portal (MAP) is placed at an approximately 30° angle anterior to the anterolateral portal using a 14-gauge spinal needle and Nitinol wire. Depending on the location of the pathology and the interventions required, additional portals may be necessary. Care should be taken to avoid damage to the intra-articular structures, particularly the femoral articular surface and labrum. An interportal capsulotomy is then created with a curved Beaver Blade; a satisfactory cuff of capsular tissue is left adjacent to the labrum and acetabular rim. A systematic sequential approach is followed to visualize and evaluate the structures and deal with the pathology. Capsulotomy can be further extended as required.

A 4-mm 70° arthroscope is used for the duration of the procedure. Intra-articular visualization is optimized with appropriate fluid flow (a medium flow rate of approximately 0.7 L/min) and fluid pressure balanced with mean arterial pressure; usually, fluid pressure with pump-assisted flow is kept at 40 mmHg.

Central compartment

The anterior, superior, and posterior chondrolabral complex are visualized and assessed using an arthroscopic probe/hook. The acetabular articular surface is visualized and evaluated. The ligamentum teres is viewed and dynamically assessed while rotating the limb into maximum internal and then external rotation. The femoral head surface is then assessed. Additional portals may be placed depending on the location pathology that needs addressing.

Peripheral compartment

Multiple techniques are described to access the peripheral compartment. The anterior capsule is relaxed by releasing the traction and flexing the hip 20–30°. Some surgeons recommend a superolateral viewing portal. A 14-gauge × 6-inch spinal needle is directed under image intensifier control to the superior head–neck junction. The bevel is rotated such that it is opposed to the bony surface. The spinal needle is then advanced with the bevel sliding along the anterior surface of the femoral neck. The portal is then established in the usual manner. Care must be taken to prevent the guide wire penetrating the medial capsule. Also, care should be taken against breakage of the guide wire.

Alternatively, some surgeons use a swing-over technique to move from the central compartment to the peripheral compartment. Here, the existing central compartment portals are used. The traction is released and the hip flexed during this process. This technique is especially useful in the management of superior and posterosuperior peripheral compartment pathology.

The peripheral compartment is systematically assessed and an image intensifier used to ensure a complete assessment of the peripheral compartment. Dynamic examination of the hip joint is performed and femoroacetabular impingement and adequacy of surgery can be assessed.

The choice of instruments available continues to increase. Newer instruments are being designed to ease access and help with intervention. The initial capsulotomy is done using a Beaver Blade; graspers are available for removing loose bodies. A wide range of suture-passing instruments are used for labral repair and capsular placation; a microfracture awl is used to treat a full thickness acetabular chondral defect. Powered instruments such as soft tissue shavers and a variety of bone burrs are used. Radiofrequency probes are increasingly being used. Repair of labral tears is usually done by use of bone anchors and knot or knotless systems.

COMPLICATIONS

Risks and complications specifically associated with the hip arthroscopic procedure include traction injury and perineal pressure sores, which can be significantly reduced by using a large perineal post that is well padded and greater than 9 cm in diameter. Use traction force as minimally as necessary to distract the joint adequately and also keep the traction time to a minimum (not to exceed 2 hours). Testicular and labial injury, including vaginal tears, have been reported. Perineal nerve neuropraxia is the commonest nerve injury reported. Traction injuries to pudendal, femoral, or sciatic nerves can also occur. Most traction injuries recover fully within hours of surgery. Traction injuries are shown to be directly related to the traction force and duration of traction. Direct injury to the lateral femoral cutaneous nerve has been reported during anterior or modified anterior portal placement, and it is important to have detailed knowledge of surface anatomy. Other structures at risk from portal placement are the femoral neurovascular bundle, which is in close proximity to the anterior portal, and the sciatic nerve, which is close to the posterolateral portal.

Iatrogenic chondral and labral injuries are usually underreported. Adequate distraction, careful initial cannulation, and gentle technique can minimize articular scuffing, gouging, and labral damage. To minimize iatrogenic injuries, some surgeons access the peripheral compartment first and place the guide wire into the central compartment under direct vision. Broken guide wires and instruments, though infrequent, can be a challenge to retrieve. Careful retraction of the guide wire and controlled cannula insertion minimize the risk of wire breakage.

Postoperative hip instability and subluxation have been reported, particularly following acetabular rim recession in dysplastic hips; care must be taken not to recede the acetabular rim to the point of destabilizing the hip. Femoral neck fractures have been associated following femoral cam excision. Intra-abdominal or retroperitoneal fluid extravasation and abdominal compartment syndrome can be life threatening and are a particular risk when the procedure is performed following an acetabular fracture.

Postoperative infection is rare; one has to be vigilant of aseptic techniques to prevent infection. Intraoperative bleeding can obscure the surgeon's view; it can be overcome by increase in fluid pressure and radiofrequency (RF) coagulation of bleeding points. Postoperative bleeding is rare; however, it has been reported following damage to branches of major vessels, particularly the branch of the superior gluteal artery. Other rare complications reported are osteonecrosis, impotence, trochanteric bursitis, and chronic regional pain syndrome (CRPS).

Failure to improve the symptoms, and on occasion make them worse, should be discussed with the patient prior to undertaking the procedure. Failure to gain access to the hip may also be regarded as a complication since it is not always possible to enter the hip arthroscopically.

SPECIFIC CONDITIONS

Acetabular labral tears

Independent of the etiology, labral tears are more common in the anterosuperior quadrant (Figure 26.8).

In this location, the mechanical resistance of the labrum to traction (associated with instability) and compression (associated with femoroacetabular impingement) is less compared to all other regions. Acetabular labral tears are usually a consequence

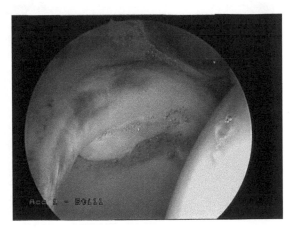

Figure 26.8 Labral tear with bruising of the labrum.

of bone deformity, femoroacetabular impingement (FAI), trauma, degeneration, dysplasia, capsular laxity, instability, and supraphysiological movements of the hip. It is believed that labral tears rarely occur in the absence of bony abnormalities. Labral lesions are associated with chondropathy with delamination of the acetabular cartilage; the cartilage sheet appears like a wave when separated from the underlying bone, described as a wave sign (Figure 26.9).

An unstable labrum can cause mechanical impingement and sharp pain with locking episodes and with time leads to loss of articular cartilage, progressively evolving into osteoarthritis.

The goal of arthroscopic intervention is to retain as much healthy labrum as possible and remove non-salvageable, loose, and devitalized labrum, mainly to stabilize and relieve symptoms for mechanical reasons. It is believed that arthroscopic surgical management of the labral tear, in conjunction with complete correction of any osseous pathomorphology, could influence the progression of osteoarthritis in the hip joint. Therefore, early restoration of the normal morphology of the hip joint is advised before the setting in of chondropathy and osteoarthritis. The labrum has the capacity to heal after refixation. At 1 year following surgery, labral fixation is shown to achieve better results than resection and has a lower reoperation rate. A poor prognosis is associated with the presence of cartilage thinning or cartilage injuries of Outerbridge grade IV or Tönnis grade III or IV. If the joint space is less than 2 mm, progression to arthroplasty occurs in 80% of such cases in an average of 2 years.

Most of the vascular supply to the labrum comes from the capsular contribution;[29] the articular surface of the labrum has decreased vascularity and limited synovial covering. The labrum is thinner in the anterior inferior section and thicker and slightly rounded posteriorly. During repair, the labral tear is identified and the margins defined. A motorized shaver is then used to debride and remove the torn portion of the labrum. A high-speed burr is used to decorticate the acetabular rim. This provides a bleeding surface for the graft to heal. The labrum is repaired by using a bioabsorbable suture anchor, which is placed on the rim of the acetabulum between the labrum and the capsule. Once the anchor is placed, the suture material is passed through the split in the labrum in a vertical mattress suture technique. The suture is tied down by using standard arthroscopic knot-tying techniques or knotless methods (Figure 26.10).

For an intrasubstance split in the labrum, a bioabsorbable suture is passed around the split by using a suture lasso or similar suture-passing instrument. The suture is tied, thus reapproximating the split labral tissue. It is vital that the associated pathology be dealt with to minimize recurrence and improve outcome. In cases where a significant portion of the labrum is deficient or removed, the labrum can be reconstructed with rectus autograft, iliotibial band, hamstrings, and auto- or allograft.

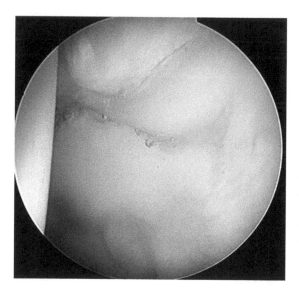

Figure 26.9 Wave sign.

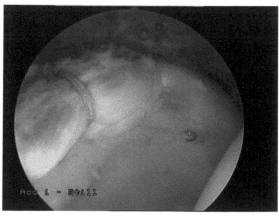

Figure 26.10 Labral tear repair.

Femoroacetabular impingement

Femoroacetabular impingement is a mechanical mismatch between the femoral head and the acetabulam; the impingement of the femoral head–neck junction occurs against the rim of the acetabulum in the position of flexion and internal rotation. As a consequence, labral tears occur with associated injuries to the adjacent cartilage on the rim of the acetabulum, which predisposes toward arthritis. The estimated prevalence of asymptomatic FAI in the general population is 10%–15%. Ganz described two clinical types, cam and pincer lesions. The cam impingement type is where the anterosuperior part of the anatomical neck of the femur is hypertrophied and convex in shape and impinges on the labrum and acetabulum. The pincer type is where there is excessive coverage of the femoral head by the acetabulum. The cam type is more frequent compared to the pincer type. In more than 70% of cases, both acetabular and femoral lesions are found, and these are described as "mixed" impingement. The deformity may also be secondary to previously undiagnosed silent slips of the femoral epiphysis or from other congenital reasons, e.g. acetabular retroversion. In some cases, cartilage injury may occur in atypical locations, particularly in ballet dancers, where the impingement is due to overloading above the physiological level without secondary structural causes identified.

Surgical intervention in cases of femoroacetabular deformities before irreversible cartilage injuries occur can possibly delay the evolution of hip arthrosis. Conventionally, an open surgical dislocation technique for removal of excessive bone at the head–neck junction was performed and popularized by Ganz. The procedure is now effectively performed arthroscopically by using appropriate hip distraction techniques, portals, and instruments. Arthroscopic management comes with the advantages of a smaller incision, shorter recovery time, and potentially fewer complications than open surgery.

On accessing the peripheral compartment as described earlier, the head–neck recess is visualized and the location of the head–neck junction identified. The surgery involves sequential management of the pathology; the sequence may vary between surgeons. It must be ensured that all underlying pathology is addressed. Depending on the surgeon's preference, the peripheral or central compartment can be accessed first. Surgical treatment involves correction of the deformities on both sides of the joint by means of osteochondroplasty. The author's choice would be to excise the pincer lesion and perform the labral repair/reconstruction first, followed by excision of the cam lesion (Figure 26.11).

In cases of retroversion, anterior acetabular osteoplasty, and in case of protrusion, circumferential osteoplasty is performed. Significant acetabular retroversion may require periacetabular osteotomy. The nonsalvageable labral tissue is debrided and the salvageable labral tissue should be preserved and repaired. If there is significant loss of labral tissue, reconstruction can be done with capsular tissue, gracilis, iliotibial band (ITB), or allograft. The capsule over the anterosuperior acetabulum is elevated from the bony rim by use of cautery. The acetabuloplasty is performed with a high-speed burr. The pincer lesion is defined and excised. The acetabular rim adjacent to the labral damage is decorticated to expose bleeding bone for repair/reconstruction. Repair is performed as described above. Smaller labral deficiencies can be reconstructed using capsular autograft. Capsular tissue is a less robust graft source; it is locally available and can be used to fill small segmental defects. The femoral head-neck recess is visualized, head and neck osteoplasty is performed to remove cam deformity, and the aim is to recreate the normal alpha angle

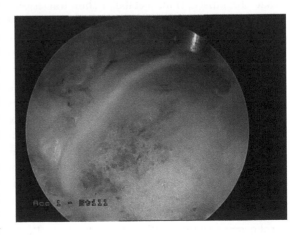

Figure 26.11 Cam excision (osteochondroplasty).

as measured on standard plain films to allow for FAI-free motion of the hip. In cases with acetabular dysplasia or borderline dysplasia, e.g. lateral center-edge angle less than 25° or in cases of ligamentous laxity, patients benefit from capsular closure or capsular plication to restore hip stability. Capsular tissue reconstruction in itself would be inadequate and is likely to leave these patients with persistent instability.

Studies comparing open and arthroscopic surgical techniques showed that there were no significant differences in the precision of osteochondroplasty of the femoral head in cases of camlike impingement. Significant improvements in the Western Ontario and McMaster Universities (WOMAC) arthritis score and Harris Hip Score (HHS) have been published. Conversion to arthroplasty has been reported from 3% to 9% at 2 years following the procedure. With minimum complications reported, 76% of athletes treated for FAI had fully returned to their sports after an arthroscopic FAI surgery. The factors that predicted improvements were preoperative HHS > 80, previous joint space larger than 2 mm, and labral repair rather than resection during the arthroscopy procedure.

Articular cartilage

Articular cartilage defects can occur on both the femoral head and the acetabular surface. Labral tears occurring at the watershed zone may destabilize the adjacent acetabular conditions. Arthroscopic observations support the concept that labral disruption, acetabular chondral lesions, or both frequently are part of a continuum of degenerative joint disease. Chondral injuries may occur in association with a multitude of hip conditions including labral tears, loose bodies, osteonecrosis, slipped capital femoral epiphysis, dysplasia, and degenerative arthritis. Cartilage integrity is evaluated and various restoration techniques like fibrin glue for cartilage delamination, microfracture in cartilage loss, stem cell therapy for cartilage lesions, autologous chondrocyte implantation, mosaicplasty, osteochondral autograft, and osteochondral allograft are described. Although good results have been reported, most studies lack a control group and the small number of patients limits these studies.

Hip septic arthritis

Arthroscopy has been successfully used to assess the hip joint for draining infective collection, washout of the joint, and debridement, and to obtain synovial tissue samples. It is minimally invasive compared to conventional open arthrotomy. Numerous studies have looked at the outcome of arthroscopic washout in both children and adults and have reported a superior outcome by the arthroscopic method (90% good results with the arthroscopic technique compared to 70% good results with the open technique).

Pigmented villonodular synovitis

Pigmented villonodular synovitis presents as a focal or diffuse lesion. Both of these presentations can be addressed using arthroscopic excision. The prognosis is poorer in diffuse cases, with early progression to arthritis.

Synovial chondromatosis

Synovial chondromatosis and loose bodies can be managed arthroscopically; studies have observed that some patients recovered well without the need for further treatments. Due to difficulties in accessing posteromedial and posterolateral areas in the peripheral compartment, recurrences can be higher.

Irrigation and debridement of the inflammatory tissue in autoimmune diseases, ankylosing spondylitis, rheumatoid arthritis, and psoriatic arthritis have been shown to improve the range of motion and diminished synovitis on magnetic resonance imaging; studies show that 75% of patients were satisfied with the outcome.

Arthroscopy in hip trauma

Hip arthroscopy can be useful in post-traumatic cases, both in traumatic hip dislocation and fractures. Most commonly, arthroscopy can be used to deal with post-traumatic bony or cartilaginous free bodies in the joint; to assess the state of the articular cartilage, fractured acetabular border or femoral head, teres ligament injuries, and joint instability; and in arthroscopic-assisted fracture fixation. Bleeding obscuring the arthroscopic view and fluid extravasation are the added risks.

Osteonecrosis of the femoral head

Hip arthroscopy can be used to evaluate the joint cartilage and its integrity in osteonecrosis. Studies have found damage to the femoral cartilage that had not been detected through magnetic resonance imaging in up to 36% of patients. Arthroscopy is usually performed together with decompression of the femoral head in Ficat stages I or IIa of osteonecrosis. With minimal risk to the circulation of the femoral head, Ellenrieder et al. demonstrated that, in patients with Steinberg stages II and III, without head collapse or chondral lesions, decompression could be performed in association with grafting using autologous graft cylinders. In cases of collapse (Steinberg IV), reduction of the collapsed portion was performed with fluoroscopy control and the articular surface checked with arthroscopy.

Painful hip arthroplasty

Evaluation of painful hip arthroplasty by means of arthroscopy is helpful for collection of synovial fluid and tissue samples for analysis and microbiological studies. Other sources of pain can also be evaluated, such as joint instability, aseptic loosening, impingement between components, and adhesions. Extra-articular causes can be evaluated and addressed, e.g. iliopsoas tendinitis, interposition of foreign bodies, etc.

Hip dysplasia

Arthroscopy in cases of dysplasia has limited indications and should be considered cautiously. Some studies report good results from arthroscopic procedures in borderline dysplastic hips. However, others studies have found acceleration of the degenerative process that evolved into severe arthritis, lateral migration of the femoral head with instability, and persisting pain symptoms following the arthroscopic procedure. Some authors consider the presence of dysplasia a contraindication to perform hip arthroscopy.

Arthroscopy and labral repair together with or after periacetabular osteotomy have shown good results. The acetabular reorientation provides a better environment and altered stress, allowing the repaired labrum to heal.

Slipped capital femoral epiphysis and Perthes sequelae

Slipped capital femoral epiphysis and Perthes sequelae cause camlike femoroacetabular impingement. Careful evaluation of the deformities by radiographs and computed tomography reconstructions is necessary to plan intervention. In cases of alteration of the femoral offset, i.e. significant posterior slippage, realignment of the proximal femur by means of intra-articular or subtrochanteric osteotomy may be needed along with osteochondroplasty to correct the femoroacetabular impingement. Arthroscopic procedures have been shown not to affect the natural history of Perthes disease; however, they help to improve quality of life.

Teres ligament injuries and capsule repair in cases of instability

The function of the ligamentum teres is not entirely clear; it can be tensioned with flexion, abduction, and external rotation, or by extension in external rotation of the hip. Injuries to the ligamentum teres are divided into three groups: I—partial traumatic, II—total traumatic, and III—degenerative rupture. After initial description by Philippon et al., reconstruction of the ligamentum teres was reported in a selected group of patients with complaints of instability and supraphysiological movements. The capsule-ligament stabilizers of the hip continue to be studied, and their role has still not been fully defined. Techniques for capsule repair have been described; however, the long-term outcome remains unknown.[30]

Extra-articular pathological conditions around the hip

The commonest indications for extra-articular arthroscopy are trochanteric bursitis, external snapping, and tendinopathy of the gluteus minimus and gluteus maximus, which together cover the concept of the painful syndrome of the greater trochanter, internal snapping, and piriformis syndrome (deep gluteal pain).

External snapping

External snapping is produced due to friction between the greater trochanter and the thickened posterior portion of the iliotibial band or the thickened anterior fibers of the gluteus maximus during flexion or extension. It may or may not be painful. The primary management relies on physiotherapy and stretching. Release of the structures can be performed as an open or arthroscopic procedure to diminish tension in the iliotibial band. The techniques described also include half-releasing the gluteal tendon at its femoral insertion, on the linea aspera, to release the tension.

Trochanteric bursitis and injuries of the gluteal muscles

As the etiology is varied, there are many therapeutic options for trochanteric bursitis. The management relies principally on physiotherapy and stretching. In cases that are refractory to conservative treatment, surgical interventions by means of arthroscopic debridement and release of tight iliotibial band have been shown to be safe and efficient.

Incomplete or complete tears of the gluteal muscle insertions have been shown to be associated with chronic trochanteric bursitis with a positive Trendelenburg sign. These injuries are often underdiagnosed. There is paucity of literature on the long-term prognosis of these tears with or without interventions.

Internal snapping

Internal snapping generally occurs when the tendon of the iliopsoas rubs against the iliopectineal eminence or femoral head. Arthroscopically, tenotomy can be performed at the level of the lesser trochanter or through the anterior capsular region of the hip. Studies have shown no significant difference in the outcome between these two techniques. However, arthroscopic release had a lower complication rate and less postoperative pain than the open technique. Iliopsoas pressure symptoms and pain have been reported post-hip arthroplasty; arthroscopic release of the iliopsoas tendon has been shown to improve symptoms.

Piriformis syndrome

Also known as deep gluteal pain, this is a pathological condition diagnosed by ruling out other causes and is hypothesized to be due to muscle spasms or compression by the piriformis muscle, fibrous bands, vascular malformations, and adherences to the obturator muscles and the quadratus femoris muscle. It manifests as pain in the gluteal region, with or without accompanying sciatic pain. It worsens with local deep pressure and generally continues for years.

The management is mainly conservative. Surgery is indicated in refractory cases. Classically, open decompression is described. Proximity to the sciatic nerve and the risk of potential nerve injury warrant extreme caution. Endoscopic exploration of the sciatic nerve accompanied by tenotomy of the piriformis and neurolysis of the sciatic nerve, with intraoperative neural monitoring (evoked potential and electroneuromyography), achieved significant improvement after surgery, without recurrences and without neurological injuries.

REHABILITATION

The postoperative recovery period is mainly focused on early physical therapy and a structured, progressive rehabilitation program. Rehabilitation depends on the operative findings and the procedure performed; it should be tailored to individual needs. Postoperative rehabilitation progresses through the stages starting initially from regaining joint motion, strengthening of muscles, development of proprioception, advanced strengthening, and development of agility. The final stages of rehabilitation should be sports-specific.

In general, for patients following FAI surgery/labral reconstruction, toe-touch weight to partial weight-bearing is maintained for 6 weeks. Range of motion is allowed within a pain-free range during this period. The patient subsequently progresses to full weight-bearing and full range of motion, and therapy is sequentially advanced as shown in Table 26.7. When range of motion and strength are satisfactory, progression is made to sport-specific training.

OUTCOME ASSESSMENT

For assessing the outcome following hip arthroscopy, numerous patient-reported outcome measures are in use. The commonly used outcome measures look at either the general well-being of the person, e.g. SF-12, or can look at specific improvement with the hip symptoms and function, e.g. Hip Outcome

Table 26.7 Rehabilitation program

Week	Exercises
Week 1	• Isometrics—gluteal, quads, trans abs, hip abduction • Passive stretching, piriformis stretch (side-lying), quad stretch (prone), adductor stretch (sitting) • Stationary bike—high seat, no resistance
Week 2	• Week 1 exercises • Quadruped rocking • Standing internal hip rotation exercises
Weeks 3–4	• Gait re-education • ROM exercises (cont. week 1 and 2 exercises) • Stretching calf, hamstring, and ITB • Bike—no resistance, increase time • Leg press, cross-trainer, Swiss ball • Core stability • Hydrotherapy
Weeks 5–6	• Continue with previous exercises • Bike—with resistance • Balance work—e.g. wobble board • Core stability—progress as able • Lunges, lateral side steps, knee bends, jog/walk
Week 7+	• Increase hydrotherapy exercises (squats, step-ups/downs, 1/4–1/2 lunges) • Running—progress from straight line to multidirectional • Sports-specific

Score. The most recommended tools for assessment of young adults with hip pain and undergoing non-surgical treatment or hip arthroscopy are the Hip and Groin Outcome Score (HAGOS), Hip Outcome Score (HOS), International Hip Outcome Tool-12 (iHOT-12), and iHOT-33. These patient-reported outcomes are validated and contain adequate measurement qualities. They are all checked for test-retest reliability, construct validity, responsiveness, and interpretability.[31]

Various scoring systems are available for quantification of hip pain, function, and severity of symptoms. The Harris Hip Score, Modified Harris Hip Score, Merle d'Aubigné score, Non-Arthritic Hip Score, Musculoskeletal Function Assessment (MFA), and Western Ontario and McMaster Universities Osteoarthritis Index are in use. The use of a visual analog score is also useful for the quantification of pain at rest and pain with activities.

REFERENCES

1. Kelly BT, Buly RL. Hip arthroscopy update. *HSS J.* 2005; 1(1): 40–8.
2. Edwards DJ, Lomas D, Villar RN. Diagnosis of the painful hip by magnetic resonance imaging and arthroscopy. *J Bone Joint Surg Br* 1995; 77(3): 374–6.
3. Seldes RM, Tan V, Hunt J, Katz M, Winiarsky R, Fitzgerald RH Jr. Anatomy, histologic features, and vascularity of the adult acetabular labrum. *Clin Orthop Relat Res* 2001; (382): 232–40.
4. Philippon MJ, Nepple JJ, Campbell KJ, Dornan GJ, Jansson KS, LaPrade RF, Wijdicks CA. The hip fluid seal—Part I: The effect of an acetabular labral tear, repair, resection, and reconstruction on hip fluid pressurization. *Knee Surg Sports Traumatol Arthrosc* 2014; 22(4): 722–9.
5. Cashin M, Uhthoff H, O'Neill M, Beaulé PE. Embryology of the acetabular labral-chondral complex. *J Bone Joint Surg Br* 2008; 90(8): 1019–24.
6. Kılıçarslan K, Kılıçarslan A, Demirkale İ, Aytekin MN, Aksekili MA, Uğurlu M. Immunohistochemical analysis of mechanoreceptors in transverse acetabular ligament and labrum: A prospective analysis of 35 cases. *Acta Orthop Traumatol Turc* 2015; 49(4): 394–8.
7. Gerhardt M, Johnson K, Atkinson R, Snow B, Shaw C, Brown A, Vangsness CT Jr. Characterisation and classification of the neural anatomy in the human hip joint. *Hip Int* 2012; 22(1): 75–81.
8. Kalhor M, Horowitz K, Beck M, Nazparvar B, Ganz R. Vascular supply to the acetabular labrum. *J Bone Joint Surg Am* 2010; 92(15): 2570–5.
9. Petersen W, Petersen F, Tillmann B. Structure and vascularization of the acetabular labrum with regard to the pathogenesis and healing of labral lesions. *Arch Orthop Trauma Surg* 2003; 123(6): 283–8.

10. Smith MV, Panchal HB, Ruberte Thiele RA, Sekiya JK. Effect of acetabular labrum tears on hip stability and labral strain in a joint compression model. *Am J Sports Med* 2011; 39(Suppl): 103S–S.

11. Lim S-J, Park Y-S. Plain radiography of the hip: A review of radiographic techniques and image features. *Hip & Pelvis* 2015; 27(3): 125–34.

12. Lin Y-T, Wang T-G. Ultrasonographic examination of the adult hip. *J Med Ultrasound* 2012; 20(4): 201–9.

13. Aubry S, Bélanger D, Giguère C, Lavigne M. Magnetic resonance arthrography of the hip: Technique and spectrum of findings in younger patients. *Insights Imaging* 2010; 1(2): 72–82.

14. Plotz GM, Brossmann J, von Knoch M, Muhle C, Heller M, Hassenpflug J. Magnetic resonance arthrography of the acetabular labrum: Value of radial reconstructions. *Arch Orthop Trauma Surg* 2001; 121(8): 450–7.

15. Kubo T, Horii M, Harada Y, Noguchi Y, Yutani Y, Ohashi H, Hachiya Y, Miyaoka H, Naruse S, Hirasawa Y. Radial-sequence magnetic resonance imaging in evaluation of acetabular labrum. *J Orthop Sci* 1999; 4(5): 328–32.

16. Czerny C, Hofmann S, Neuhold A, Tschauner C, Engel A, Recht MP, Kramer J. Lesions of the acetabular labrum: Accuracy of MR imaging and MR arthrography in detection and staging. *Radiology* 1996; 200(1): 225–30.

17. Blankenbaker DG, DeSmet AA, Keene JS, Fine JP. Classification and localization of acetabular labral tears. *Skeletal Radiol* 2007; 36(5): 391–7.

18. Lage LA, Patel JV, Villar RN. The acetabular labral tear: An arthroscopic classification. *Arthroscopy* 1996; 12(3): 269–72.

19. Magee T, Hinson G. Association of paralabral cysts with acetabular disorders. *AJR Am J Roentgenol* 2000; 174(5): 1381–4.

20. Bredella MA, Stoller DW. MR imaging of femoroacetabular impingement. *Magn Reson Imaging Clin N Am* 2005; 13(4): 653–64.

21. Ganz R, Parvizi J, Beck M, Leunig M, Notzli H, Siebenrock KA. Femoroacetabular impingement: A cause for osteoarthritis of the hip. *Clin Orthop Relat Res* 2003; (417): 112–20.

22. Tanzer M, Noiseux N. Osseous abnormalities and early osteoarthritis: The role of hip impingement. *Clin Orthop Relat Res* 2004; 429: 170–7.

23. Kassarjian A, Yoon LS, Belzile E, Connolly SA, Millis MB, Palmer WE. Triad of MR arthrographic findings in patients with cam-type femoroacetabular impingement. *Radiology* 2005; 236(2): 588–92.

24. Notzli HP, Wyss TF, Stoecklin CH, Schmid MR, Treiber K, Hodler J. The contour of the femoral head–neck junction as a predictor for the risk of anterior impingement. *J Bone Joint Surg Br* 2002; 84(4): 556–60.

25. Beck M, Kalhor M, Leunig M, Ganz R. Hip morphology influences the pattern of damage to the acetabular cartilage: Femoroacetabular impingement as a cause of early osteoarthritis of the hip. *J Bone Joint Surg Br* 2005; 87(7): 1012–8.

26. Siebenrock KA, Schoeniger R, Ganz R. Anterior femoroacetabular impingement due to acetabular retroversion. Treatment with periacetabular osteotomy. *J Bone Joint Surg Am* 2003; 85-A(2): 278–86.

27. Nishii T, Tanaka H, Nakanishi K, Sugano N, Miki H, Yoshikawa H. Fat-suppressed 3D spoiled gradient-echo MRI and MDCT arthrography of articular cartilage in patients with hip dysplasia. *AJR Am J Roentgenol* 2005; 185(2): 379–85.

28. Neumann G, Menduiti AD, Zou KH, Minas T, Coblyn J, Winalski CS, Lang P. Prevalence of labral tears and cartilage loss in patients with mechanical symptoms of the hip: Evaluation using MR arthrography. *Osteoarthr Cartil* 2007; 15(8): 909–17.

29. Shetty VD, Villar RN. Hip arthroscopy: Current concepts and review of literature. *Br J Sports Med* 2007; 41: 64–8.

30. Beaule PE, Zaragoza E, Copelan N. Magnetic resonance imaging with gadolinium arthrography to assess acetabular cartilage delamination. A report of four cases. *J Bone Joint Surg Am* 2004; 86-A(10): 2294–8.

31. Cerezal L, Arnaiz J, Canga A, Piedra T, Altónaga JR, Munafo R, Pérez-Carro L. Emerging topics on the hip: Ligamentum teres and hip microinstability. *Eur J Radiol* 2012; 81(12): 3745–54.

27

Emerging concepts in arthroscopic hip preservation surgery: Labral reconstruction and capsular preservation

VICTORIA DAS, MICHAEL B. ELLMAN, AND SANJEEV BHATIA

INTRODUCTION

Over the past two decades, understanding of the anatomy and function of the hip joint has rapidly evolved, and surgical treatment options have followed suit. Increased focus has been placed on maintenance and preservation of native hip anatomy, with minimally invasive techniques such as arthroscopic labral repair and femoroacetabular impingement (FAI) correction. Clinical outcomes following arthroscopic labral repair with femoroplasty and/or acetabuloplasty are well established in the literature, with excellent short-, mid-, and long-term outcomes in terms of pain reduction, improved function, and ability to return to activities.[11,20,25,27,33] Indeed, these procedures remain the mainstay of treatment for arthroscopic hip treatment of labral pathology and FAI.

Recent advancements in the hip preservation literature with regards to the anatomy and biomechanical function of two important hip structures, the labrum and fibrous hip capsule, have inspired novel interest in preserving or reconstructing these two structures when necessary. Labral reconstruction is a treatment option that uses a graft to reconstruct the native labrum. The technique and outcomes of labral reconstruction have been described relatively recently, and labral reconstruction is a cutting-edge procedure that has shown promising early outcomes in properly indicated patients.[4,6,9,42,43,45] Equally important, the hip capsule acts as a fibrous mesh composed of multiple ligaments that support and stabilize the joint throughout motion. There are several studies demonstrating the importance of maintaining capsular integrity during hip arthroscopy,[3,14,39] and various capsular preservation techniques have been developed to optimize clinical outcomes.

The aim of this chapter is to review two emerging concepts in hip arthroscopy: (i) labral reconstruction and (ii) capsular preservation. We will elucidate the important biomechanical evidence for and against each procedure, pertinent clinical outcomes, and the authors' current indications for the aforementioned techniques.

LABRAL RECONSTRUCTION

Labral pathology is one of the most common diagnoses among adolescent and adult patients who present for treatment of hip pain.[20] The estimated prevalence of labral pathology is not well understood, but previous reports range from 39% to 85% of the general population.[7,37,40] In recent years, understanding of the biomechanical function and role of the acetabular labrum has improved significantly. The labrum plays a crucial role in the stability, lubrication, proprioception, and kinematics of the hip[2,18,32,36] and helps to prevent dynamic micro- and macroinstability of the hip joint via formation of a suction seal with the femoral head. Consequently, surgical procedures that maintain and preserve proper hip anatomy, such as labral repair, have shown superior results to labral debridement or excision.[11,25,26]

Labral reconstruction was first described in 2009 by Philippon et al.[35] as a treatment option for patients with an irreparable labrum. The technique is a cutting-edge procedure that involves the use of a graft to reconstruct the native labrum and has increased in popularity over the past several years (Figure 27.1).

Recent biomechanical evidence suggests that labral reconstruction may play a pivotal role when the native labrum is of poor quality or has previously been debrided/excised. For example, a cadaveric study revealed that partial labral resection results in dramatic loss of fluid pressurization and change of the hip seal.[36] Labral reconstruction not only improved fluid pressurization, almost to the normal state, but maintained it over time, similar to labral repair. In contrast, another study suggests that labral reconstruction may not prevent fluid efflux compared to labral repair or the intact labral state.[8]

The acetabular labrum also plays an important role in stabilization of the joint to distraction forces secondary to the suction seal effect.[32] Similar to the study of hip fluid pressurization, labral reconstruction was found to significantly improve stability to distractive forces compared to partial and complete labral resection, though not to the extent of labral repair.[32] Further, cadaveric models have assessed the contact area, contact pressure, and peak force in hips with labral pathology compared to hips with a reconstructed acetabular labrum.[28] In one investigation, hip contact pressure increased in the presence of labral resection but was significantly reduced following labral reconstruction.[28] In addition, labral reconstruction reduced peak forces in the hip compared to labral resection. These studies demonstrate that certain types of labral pathology, particularly complex intrasubstance labral tears or inflamed, adhesed labral tissue seen in revision surgery, may be indicated for labral reconstruction.

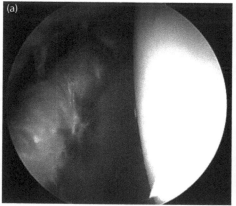 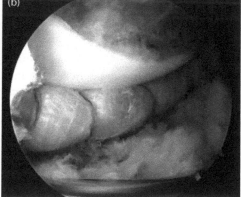

Figure 27.1 Labral reconstruction was first described in 2009 by Philippon et al.[35] as a treatment option for patients with an irreparable labrum. The technique is a cutting-edge procedure that involves the use of a graft to reconstruct the native labrum and has increased in popularity over the past several years. Here we see a completed labral reconstruction with iliotibial band allograft in the distracted (a) position and reduced position (b). Note the suction seal has been restored.

Clinically, promising short-term patient-reported outcomes have been reported with arthroscopic labral reconstruction. The existing literature reveals success rates of approximately 75%–90% with 2- to 3-year follow-up following arthroscopic labral reconstruction with allograft or autograft.[6,10,19,31] White et al. have published several recent studies on arthroscopic labral reconstruction using a front-to-back technique with fascia lata allograft.[41,43,46] In one study,[46] 131 hips underwent labral reconstruction (the majority of these primary reconstructions), with significant improvements in multiple patient-reported outcomes at 2 years. However, the authors also reported a 13.7% revision rate at 2 years, with 10% conversion to total hip arthroplasty. When compared to primary labral repair, these results are inferior to findings published by Cvetanovich et al., who reported a 1.2% revision rate and 1.7% conversion to total hip arthroplasty (THA) at 2 years following 386 labral repairs.[11] Further, the return-to-play rate following primary labral repair has been reported to be >92%,[30,34] compared to 85% in one study following reconstruction.[6]

More recently, White et al. published an interesting study comparing primary labral repair on one hip to primary labral reconstruction on the contralateral hip in patients undergoing bilateral staged hip arthroscopy.[44] The authors reported a 31% failure rate for the primary labral repair and a 0% failure rate following primary labral reconstruction and concluded that primary labral reconstruction may be a better procedure than primary labral repair. However, this study has attracted significant controversy within the hip community, with two separate letters to the editor elucidating various levels of bias that may confound the results.[5,12] Further, it should be noted that there are currently no mid- or long-term outcomes on labral reconstruction. Therefore, future studies are necessary to clarify the aforementioned findings before drawing significant conclusions.

INDICATIONS FOR LABRAL RECONSTRUCTION

Decision-making for the labrum during arthroscopic hip surgery can be a challenge, but certain guidelines have been developed (Figure 27.2).

While arthroscopic labral repair has shown promising patient outcomes,[11,25] there exists a population of patients in which labral repair is less optimal. The authors' indications for labral reconstruction include: (i) irreparable labral tears or insufficient labral tissue in a primary setting (i.e., labral hypoplasia or labral ossification), (ii) failed

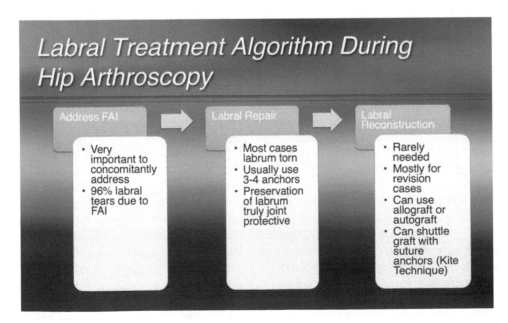

Figure 27.2 Labral treatment algorithm. (Adapted from Domb BG et al. *J Am Acad Orthop Surg* 2017; 25(3): e53–e62.)

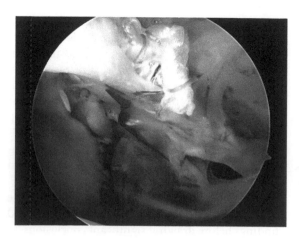

Figure 27.3 An example of a failed labral repair with poor quality labral tissue in a revision hip arthroscopy setting. Note the numerous adhesions and erythema at the capsulolabral junction.

labral repairs with poor quality labral tissue in a revision setting (Figure 27.3), and (iii) previous labral debridements in a revision setting.

In select cases, a labral repair may not be feasible or adequate to restore the suction seal of the hip joint.[19,35,42,45] When the tissue is too small or ossified, it lacks surface area to heal and can fail to provide an adequate seal with the femoral head.[32,36] For this reason, a labrum <2 mm or with significant intralabral ossification is considered an indication for primary labral reconstruction.[13] Of note, this situation is rare in the authors' high-volume hip arthroscopy practices, with <1% of primary cases requiring primary reconstruction. Revision procedures, on the other hand, more frequently require reconstruction. Revision cases provide a challenging situation, as these patients may present with poor-quality labral tissue following previous labral debridement, resection, or failed repair.[45] In these cases, labral reconstruction may provide a viable alternative for maintaining and preserving labral function.

Importantly, it must be noted that labral reconstruction is not without significant risk, especially in a primary setting. Biomechanically, there are inherent disadvantages to labral reconstruction compared to labral repair. First, at time zero, a labral reconstruction construct inherently reproduces only 66% of the normal distractive stability of a native hip.[36] This predisposition to instability may be compounded by the circumstances that labral reconstruction frequently requires: (i) significant

acetabular rim resection, which may iatrogenically create a setting of borderline or frank dysplasia from a previously normal acetabular socket; and (ii) more capsular disruption than typical labral repair procedures, thereby preventing or limiting adequate capsular repair.[42] Additionally, labral reconstruction is a technically difficult procedure that requires longer operative times and traction times compared to labral repair, thereby predisposing patients to possible traction-related complications and neuropraxias at a greater rate than labral repair procedures.[21] Last, it is notable that patients undergoing labral reconstruction in the primary setting often have poor options short of total hip arthroplasty in the revision setting, particularly due to extensive disruption of the native labrum and capsule. Unfortunately, this can create a significant problem in younger patients, one that may become more evident in the future as many of these short-term outcome cohorts reach mid and long term.

CAPSULE AND FUNCTION

Although much attention has been directed toward the labrum during the explosive growth of hip arthroscopy in recent years, the capsule is now known to be equally important to hip stability.[36] Much like the shoulder capsule, the human hip capsule is notable for having multiple confluent ligaments that aid in hip stability (Figure 27.4).

Most notable is the iliofemoral ligament anteriorly that functions to restrain the femoroacetabular joint from anterior translation during leg extension. The function of the iliofemoral ligament is aided only by the zona orbicularis, a fibrous ring that tightens during hip extension and loosens during hip flexion.[14,24] The result is a "screw home" mechanism that provides tremendous stability to the femoroacetabular joint during human movement.

Similar to the shoulder, the hip joint receives stability from both static and dynamic factors. Static factors contributing to hip stability include the labrum and the bony architecture—particularly acetabular socket depth. Dynamically, hip stability is aided by muscular contraction but also the hip capsule's screw home mechanism, as previously noted. Each individual may have a differing set of host factors that may or may not predispose their hip to iatrogenic microinstability following

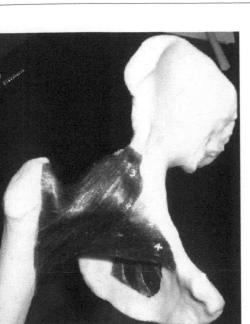

Figure 27.4 Although much attention has been directed toward the labrum during the explosive growth of hip arthroscopy in recent years, the capsule is now known to be equally important to hip stability.[36] Much like the shoulder capsule, the human hip capsule is notable for having multiple confluent ligaments that aid in hip stability.[23]

hip arthroscopy.[23] For instance, borderline dysplasia (lateral center edge angle 20–25°) is a condition where the acetabulum has a shallower architecture, thereby increasing the role dynamic stabilizers play in providing hip stability. In this scenario, appropriate capsular preservation is paramount for reducing the risk of iatrogenic postoperative hip microinstability following surgery.[16] Routine capsular closure during hip arthroscopy is generally recommended for these reasons according to most authors.[3,11,15,16,22,29]

CAPSULAR DECISION-MAKING

Although the hip capsule is an important stabilizer of the hip and generally requires closure or plication, there are some scenarios in which routine capsular closure or plication is unwarranted. Clinically, if the hip is noted to have significant preoperative stiffness, adhesive capsulitis, or a synovial proliferative disorder, a capsulotomy may actually be therapeutic.[14] Intraoperative factors that may suggest a reduced need for capsular repair

or plication include capsular hypertrophy or thickening, limited pliability, or hyperemic capsular tissue consistent with adhesive capsulitis.[14]

The type of capsulotomy employed during hip arthroscopy may also play a role in determining what the need for capsular repair is. In a double-blind, randomized control trial of 30 hips undergoing bilateral hip arthroscopy with a small, less than 3 cm, interportal capsulotomy, Strickland and colleagues noted no difference in capsular healing at 24 weeks postoperatively between repaired and unrepaired capsules on MRI.[38] These findings suggest that a very limited capsulotomy has the capacity to heal on its own due to minimal disruption and no violation of the zona orbicularis. Although these findings are applicable to small interportal capsulotomies, most evidence suggests that larger capsulotomies, particularly T-capsulotomies that violate the zona orbicularis, necessitate routine capsular closure. In an investigation by Abrams, an unrepaired T-capsulotomy or large capsulectomy significantly increased the native external rotation of a cadaveric hip compared to the intact or interportal capsulotomy states.[1]

At the present time, most authors agree that routine capsular closure is generally recommended, except in situations with adhesive capsulitis or limited range of motion of the hip. Capsular plication, a procedure in which the capsule's screw home mechanism is augmented, is recommended in situations with borderline dysplasia, elevated joint laxity, capsular redundancy, or impaired dynamic stability of the hip.[16]

CAPSULAR PRESERVATION STRATEGIES

Optimal management of the capsule starts with preserving it appropriately throughout the procedure. The most important aspect of this involves protecting the proximal leaflet during pincer and subspine decompression. The use of electrocautery for pincer exposure, instead of aggressive shaver use during this step, may better preserve the proximal leaflet, making it easier to repair at the end of the case. Additionally, capsular suspension sutures have been described as a means for capsular preservation during hip arthroscopy.[17]

With regard to the extent and type of capsulotomy, the least amount of capsular disruption is advised. If possible, it is important to try to avoid

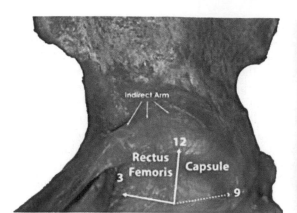

Figure 27.5 The rectus tendon is intimately associated with the anterior hip capsule and generally should be gently separated with electrocautery in order to avoid postoperative irritation from entrapment during capsular repair.

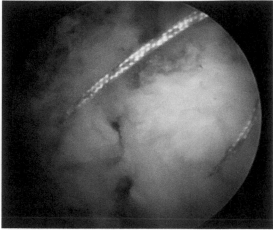

Figure 27.6 An example of a partially completed capsular closure of an interportal capsulotomy. Sutures should be tied in no more than 15° flexion to avoid excessive tightening and to reduce the risk that the repair will be under undue tension in the immediate postoperative phase.

excessively medializing the interportal capsulotomy beyond 2 o'clock to limit the exposure of the iliopsoas. Although the capsulotomy has to be large enough to adequately perform femoral osteoplasty, pincer and labral work, as previously noted, the smaller the capsulotomy, the less repair is required.[1]

Once the procedure is completed, it is imperative to mobilize the capsule, proximally and distally, in order to most optimally repair or plicate the capsule. The rectus tendon is intimately associated with the anterior hip capsule (Figure 27.5) and generally should be separated with electrocautery in order to avoid postoperative irritation from entrapment during capsular repair. Mobilization also allows the leaflets to be under reduced tension, thereby reducing the risk of suture pullout postoperatively.

In order to pass the sutures for capsular repair, the camera is typically placed in the anterolateral portal and sutures are passed with the hip in 45° of flexion with a self-passing suture device or suture lasso and penetrating grasper. If a T-capsulotomy is performed, the vertical limb should be closed first prior to the interportal capsulotomy. Typically, 2–4 sutures are used to close the vertical limb of the T-capsulotomy and 2–3 sutures are used to close the interportal or transverse limb. If a plication is desired, the distal sutures of the interportal capsulotomy can be passed more laterally to result in a shift of the distal leaflet, thereby accentuating the screw home mechanism.[14] Sutures should be tied in no more than 15° flexion to avoid excessive

tightening and to reduce the risk that the repair will be under undue tension in the immediate postoperative phase (Figure 27.6).

Postoperatively, patients are limited from performing hip extension beyond neutral for 2 weeks. Some authors advocate the limitation of external rotation beyond neutral as well for 14–21 days.

CONCLUSION

Labral reconstruction provides an alternative treatment option for challenging intra-articular hip problems. Labral reconstruction provides several biomechanical advantages compared to labral debridement as a treatment option for labral pathology, including improved fluid pressurization, stabilization of the hip to distractive forces, and reduced contact pressure in the hip joint.[32] The authors' indications for labral reconstruction include irreparable labral tears or insufficient labral tissue in a primary setting, and previous labral debridements or failed repairs with poor quality tissue in a revision setting. Currently, given the lack of mid- and long-term outcomes and associated risk with labral reconstruction, in patients with a labral tear and adequate labral tissue, primary labral repair remains the standard of care.

REFERENCES

1. Abrams GD, Hart MA, Takami K et al. Biomechanical evaluation of capsulotomy, capsulectomy, and capsular repair on hip rotation. *Arthroscopy* 2015; 31(8): 1511–7.

2. Alzaharani A, Bali K, Gudena R et al. The innervation of the human acetabular labrum and hip joint: an anatomic study. *BMC Musculoskelet Disord* 2014; 15(1): 1–8.

3. Bedi A, Galano G, Walsh C, Kelly BT. Capsular management during hip arthroscopy: From femoroacetabular impingement to instability. *Arthroscopy* 2011; 27(12): 1720–31.

4. Bhatia S, Chahla J, Dean CS, Ellman MB. Hip labral reconstruction: The "Kite Technique" for improved efficiency and graft control. *Arthrosc Tech* 2016; 5(2): e337–42.

5. Bhatia S, Ellman MB, Nho S et al. Bilateral hip arthroscopy: Direct comparison of primary acetabular labral repair and primary acetabular labral reconstruction. *Arthroscopy* 2018; 34(6): 1748–51.

6. Boykin RE, Patterson D, Briggs KK, Dee A. Results of arthroscopic labral reconstruction of the hip in elite athletes. *Am J Sports Med* 2013; 41(10): 2296–301.

7. Byrd J. Labral lesions: An elusive source of hip pain case reports and literature review. *Arthroscopy* 1996; 12(5): 603–12.

8. Cadet ER, Chan AK, Vorys GC, Gardner T, Yin B. Investigation of the preservation of the fluid seal effect in the repaired, partially resected, and reconstructed acetabular labrum in a cadaveric hip model. *Am J Sports Med* 2012; 40(10): 2218–23.

9. Chahla J, Soares E, Bhatia S, Mitchell JJ, Philippon MJ. Arthroscopic technique for acetabular labral reconstruction using iliotibial band autograft. *Arthrosc Tech* 2016; 5(3): e671–7.

10. Chandrasekaran S, Darwish N, Close MR, Lodhia P, Suarez-Ahedo C, Domb BG. Arthroscopic reconstruction of segmental defects of the hip labrum: Results in 22 patients with mean 2-year follow-up. *Arthroscopy* 2017; 33(9): 1685–93.

11. Cvetanovich GL, Weber AE, Kuhns BD et al. Hip arthroscopic surgery for femoroacetabular impingement with capsular management: Factors associated with achieving clinically significant outcomes. *Am J Sports Med* 2017; 46(2): 288–96.

12. Youm T. Editorial commentary: Wanted dead or alive: Primary allograft labral reconstruction of the hip is as successful, if not more successful, than primary labral repair. *Arthroscopy* 2018; 34(2): 441–3.

13. Domb BG, Hartigan DE, Perets I. Decision making for labral treatment in the hip. *J Am Acad Orthop Surg* 2017; 25(3): e53–62.

14. Domb BG, Philippon MJ, Giordano BD. Arthroscopic capsulotomy, capsular repair, and capsular plication of the hip: Relation to atraumatic instability. *Arthroscopy* 2013; 29(1): 162–73.

15. Domb BG, Stake CE, Finley ZJ, Chen T. Influence of capsular repair versus unrepaired capsulotomy on 2-year clinical outcomes after arthroscopic hip preservation surgery. *Arthroscopy* 2015; 31(4): 643–50.

16. Domb BG, Stake CE, Lindner D, El-Bitar Y, Jackson TJ. Arthroscopic capsular plication and labral preservation in borderline hip dysplasia two-year clinical outcomes of a surgical approach to a challenging problem. *Am J Sports Med* 2013; 41(11): 2591–8.

17. Federer AE, Karas V, Nho S, Coleman SH, Mather RC. Capsular suspension technique for hip arthroscopy. *XATS* 2015; 4(4): e317–22.

18. Ferguson SJ, Bryant JT, Ganz R, Ito K. An *in vitro* investigation of the acetabular labral seal in hip joint mechanics. *J Biomech* 2003; 36(2): 171–8.

19. Geyer MR, Philippon MJ, Fagrelius TS. Acetabular labral reconstruction with an iliotibial band autograft outcome and survivorship analysis at minimum 3-year follow-up. *Am J Sports Med* 2013; 41(8): 1750–6.

20. Griffin DR, Dickenson EJ, O'Donnell J et al. The Warwick Agreement on femoroacetabular impingement syndrome (FAI syndrome): An international consensus statement. *Br J Sports Med* 2016; 50(19): 1169–76.

21. Harris JD, McCormick FM, Abrams GD et al. Complications and reoperations during and after hip arthroscopy: A systematic review of 92 studies and more than 6,000 patients. *Arthroscopy* 2013; 29(3): 589–95.

22. Harris JD, Slikker W III, Gupta AK, McCormick FM, Nho SJ. Routine complete capsular closure during hip arthroscopy. *Arthrosc Tech* 2013; 2(2): e89–94.

23. Kalisvaart MM, Safran MR. Microinstability of the hip – It does exist: Etiology, diagnosis and treatment. *J Hip Preserv Surg* 2015; 2(2): 123–35.

24. Wylie JD, Beckmann JT, Maak TG, Aoki SK. Arthroscopic capsular repair for symptomatic hip instability after previous hip arthroscopic surgery. *Am J Sports Med* 2016; 44(1): 39–45.

25. Larson CM, Giveans MR, Stone RM. Arthroscopic debridement versus refixation of the acetabular labrum associated with femoroacetabular impingement mean 3.5-year follow-up. *Am J Sports Med* 2012; 40(5): 1015–21.

26. Larson CM, Giveans MR. Arthroscopic debridement versus refixation of the acetabular labrum associated with femoroacetabular impingement. *Arthroscopy* 2009; 25(4): 369–76.

27. Larson CM, Giveans MR. Arthroscopic management of femoroacetabular impingement: Early outcomes measures. *Arthroscopy* 2008; 24(5): 540–6.

28. Lee S, Wuerz TH, Shewman E et al. Labral reconstruction with iliotibial band autografts and semitendinosus allografts improves hip joint contact area and contact pressure: An *in vitro* analysis. *Am J Sports Med* 2015; 43(1): 98–104.

29. McCormick F, Slikker W III, Harris JD, Gupta AK. Evidence of capsular defect following hip arthroscopy. *Knee Surgery* 2014; 22(4): 902–5.

30. Menge TJ, Bhatia S, McNamara SC, Briggs KK, Philippon MJ. Femoroacetabular impingement in professional football players: Return to play and predictors of career length after hip arthroscopy. *Am J Sports Med* 2017; 45(8): 1740–4.

31. Moya E, Natera LG, Cardenas C, Astarita E, Bellotti V, Ribas M. Reconstruction of massive posterior nonrepairable acetabular labral tears with peroneus brevis tendon allograft: Arthroscopy-assisted mini-open approach. *Arthrosc Tech* 2016; 5(5): e1015–22.

32. Nepple JJ, Philippon MJ, Campbell KJ et al. The hip fluid seal – Part II: The effect of an acetabular labral tear, repair, resection, and reconstruction on hip stability to distraction. *Knee Surg Sports Traumatol Arthrosc* 2014; 22(4): 730–6.

33. Newman JT, Briggs KK, McNamara SC, Philippon MJ. Revision hip arthroscopy: A matched-cohort study comparing revision to primary arthroscopy patients. *Am J Sports Med* 2016; 44(10): 2499–504.

34. Philippon M, Schenker M, Briggs K, Kuppersmith D. Femoroacetabular impingement in 45 professional athletes: Associated pathologies and return to sport following arthroscopic decompression. *Knee Surg Sports Traumatol Arthrosc* 2007; 15(7): 908–14.

35. Philippon MJ, Briggs KK, Hay CJ, Kuppersmith DA, Dewing CB, Huang MJ. Arthroscopic labral reconstruction in the hip using iliotibial band autograft: Technique and early outcomes. *Arthroscopy* 2010; 26(6): 750–6.

36. Philippon MJ, Nepple JJ, Campbell KJ et al. The hip fluid seal – Part I: The effect of an acetabular labral tear, repair, resection, and reconstruction on hip fluid pressurization. *Knee Surg Sports Traumatol Arthrosc* 2014; 22(4): 722–9.

37. Register B, Pennock AT, Ho CP, Strickland CD, Lawand A, Philippon MJ. Prevalence of abnormal hip findings in asymptomatic participants. *Am J Sports Med* 2012; 40(12): 2720–4.

38. Strickland CD, Kraeutler MJ, Brick MJ et al. MRI evaluation of repaired versus unrepaired interportal capsulotomy in simultaneous bilateral hip arthroscopy. *J Bone Joint Surg* 2018; 100(2): 91–8.

39. Tibor LM, Sekiya JK. Differential diagnosis of pain around the hip joint. *Arthroscopy* 2008; 24(12): 1407–21.

40. Tresch F, Dietrich TJ, Pfirrmann CWA, Sutter R. Hip MRI: Prevalence of articular cartilage defects and labral tears in asymptomatic volunteers. A comparison with a matched population of patients with femoroacetabular impingement. *J Magn Reson Imaging* 2016; 46(2): 440–51.

41. White BJ, Herzog MM. Arthroscopic labral reconstruction of the hip using iliotibial band allograft and front-to-back fixation technique. *Arthrosc Tech* 2016; 5(1): e89–97.

42. White BJ, Herzog MM. Labral reconstruction: When to perform and how. *Front Surg* 2015; 2: 27.

43. White BJ, Patterson J, Herzog MM. Bilateral hip arthroscopy: Direct comparison of primary acetabular labral repair and primary acetabular labral reconstruction. *Arthroscopy* 2018; 34(2): 433–40.

44. White BJ, Patterson J, Herzog MM. Bilateral hip arthroscopy: Direct comparison of primary acetabular labral repair and primary acetabular labral reconstruction. *Arthroscopy* 2018; 34(2): 433–40.

45. White BJ, Patterson J, Herzog MM. Revision arthroscopic acetabular labral treatment: Repair or reconstruct? *Arthroscopy* 2016; 32(12): 2513–20.

46. White BJ, Stapleford AB, Hawkes TK, Finger MJ, Herzog MM. Allograft use in arthroscopic labral reconstruction of the hip with front-to-back fixation technique: Minimum 2-year follow-up. *Arthroscopy* 2016; 32(1): 26–32.

28

The anterior approach to the hip for a minimally invasive prosthesis

ALESSANDRO GERACI AND ALBERTO RICCIARDI

INTRODUCTION

When orthopedic surgeons discuss the direct anterior approach (DAA) to the hip, they talk about a surgical approach that has a history of more than a hundred years. Hueter described this approach 150 years ago, and since then, the development of surgical techniques and prosthetic technology has had important and advanced innovation. However, this surgical method has been abandoned for many years to make room for wider and more destructive surgical approaches. In the last decades of the twentieth century, the majority of orthopedic surgeons denigrated "small approaches," defining minimally invasive surgery as "keyhole surgery."

The DAA, which exploits the transition between the sartorius muscle and the tensor fasciae latae muscle to reach the hip joint, has initially experienced a long phase of abandonment following the advent of other approaches with a broader view of the anatomy: direct lateral (DLA) and posterior (PLA) approaches.

Today, the DAA is returning to be the protagonist, due to the mini-invasive surgery that entails muscle tissue savings and less blood loss. These features involve a better clinical recovery of the patient and reduction of hospitalization costs.

THE HISTORY OF THE ANTERIOR SURGICAL APPROACH TO THE HIP

The first published description of anterior access to the hip was carried out by the German surgeon Carl Hueter, born in 1838 in Marburg.[1] He graduated in medicine in 1858 and worked with Virchow and Langenbeck. Also, other surgeons, like Bernhard Bardenheuer (1839–1913) and Otto Gerhard Karl Sprengel (1852–1915), have been indicated as possible fathers of the DAA, but in his *Compendium of Surgery*,[2] published in 1881, Hueter first described the DAA, still known today.

In 1917, Marius N. Smith-Petersen (1886–1953), an American surgeon born in Norway, spread the knowledge of this surgical approach in the Anglo-Saxon world[3] and in 1949 applied this approach to treat the inborn dysplasia of the hip and the anterior fractures of the acetabulum.[4] In 1950, Judet theorized about the possibility to perform the DAA for prosthetic replacement.[5] However, despite the theoretical bases and anatomical evidence, the majority of orthopedic surgeons believed that the DAA was inadequate to obtain a good vision and exposure of the acetabulum. When Charnley published positive data on the trochanteric approach, the DAA was underestimated and devalued. In 1985, Judet described a procedure for implanting hip replacement using an DAA with a traction bed,[6] a concept taken from Matta with the advent of minimally invasive surgery.[7] Recently, Frédéric Laude, a pupil of Robert Judet, has developed the concept of DAA respecting the joint capsule and devising a traction bed to better position the lower limb, and the surgical instruments to make this surgical approach simple: anterior minimally invasive surgery (AMIS).[8]

In recent years, different variants of surgical techniques have been described with direct mini-invasive approaches to the hip that do not require a traction bed and with cosmetically beneficial skin incisions.

ANTERIOR MINIMALLY INVASIVE SURGERY

A DAA is a method of inserting the artificial joint through the front (i.e. anterior) without cutting any muscles or damaging nerves. Recently, there has been an increase interest in performing hip replacement surgery by less invasive means and by smaller incisions. AMIS is a surgical technique used in total hip replacement procedures that follows an intermuscular and internervous plane to reduce the risk of injury to muscles, tendons, vessels, and nerves. By respecting the nerves and because no muscles are cut, this aids in rapid recovery for patients following surgery.

The first steps before embarking on the surgical procedure are: patient selection, preoperative planning, and choice of surgical instruments.

Patient selection

Patient selection is certainly the first step for every surgeon. There are no specific contraindications in the anterior approach to the hip, except for the surgeon's experience. The surgeon is an expert who can use this surgical procedure even in very difficult cases, such as severe hip dysplasia. The ideal patient chosen by the neophyte surgeon is a patient with arthritis of the hip, female, lean, and not muscular. This is because muscular and fat patients give more difficulty during exposure of the femur, even using an appropriate traction bed. Moreover, in the first selected cases, patients should be chosen with a long femoral neck because it improves the femoral exposure. In some cases AMIS can be contraindicated. For example, if there was a prior approach, it is helpful and logical to use the existing scar. A severe deformity of the acetabulum or femoral neck should be performed by an experienced surgeon.

In obese patients, it is essential to pay attention to abdominal fat, which can obstruct surgical access. It is essential to use skin adhesives that keep the patient's fat in a right position (Figure 28.1).

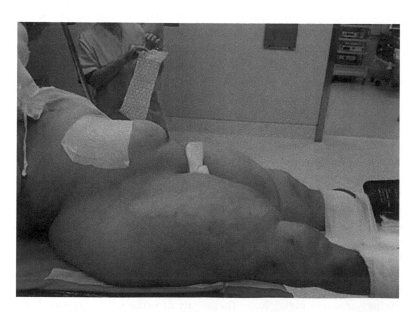

Figure 28.1 Obese patient placed on the traction bed, pulling belly fat with a dermal adhesive.

Preoperative planning

Preoperative planning is of paramount importance to obtain reproducible results in modern hip arthroplasty. Planning helps the surgeon to visualize the operation after careful review of the clinical and radiographic findings.[9] Hip replacement surgery requires preoperative planning, a process in which the surgeon assesses the hip joint and determines the best-sized components for the hip replacement. In this procedure, the position of the acetabular component (socket) and femoral component (stem) can be predicted from imaging. Radiological evaluation is used in order to choose the appropriate implant to restore normal joint geometry. Indeed, the leg length can be altered in hip replacement surgery and often the leg is slightly short due to wear of the articular cartilage in the joint. The aim is to obtain the correct leg length so that the patient may have a correct gait without proprioceptive disorder.

The x-ray examination must be performed in the entire pelvis and serves to create precise anatomical landmarks of the pelvis and the femur. These exams are printed on film or presented on digital media. Using a marker or a digital pen, the lines joining the small trochanter can be drawn with the pelvis of both hips to verify possible dysmetries (Figure 28.2) and restore the correct length in the operative area (Figure 28.3).

Imaging intraoperatively for hip replacement surgery is not commonly performed with a conventional approach. However, with the anterior approach, the patient is placed lying face up on the operating table. Therefore, there are no bulky clamps around the hip and it is easy to see the bony anatomy of the pelvis, hip, and upper part of the femur. This allows an assessment of intraoperative leg length to optimize leg length.

After marking the anatomical landmarks, evaluating the quality of the radiograph, and defining the mechanical references, a fitting implant size is chosen for both the acetabular and the femoral component. In most cases the aim will be to restore the original hip anatomy and biomechanics. However, in some cases this will not be possible or advisable, and compensations for failing to do so will have to be considered.[10] The measurements

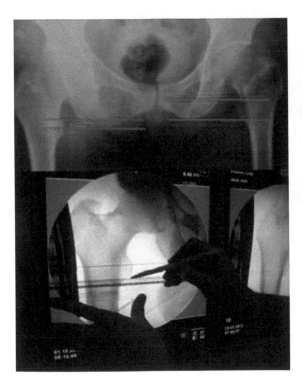

Figure 28.2 Example of preoperative planning to verify the length of the limbs before a hip replacement surgery.

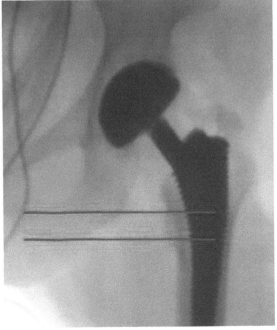

Figure 28.3 X-ray performed during the hip surgery to evaluate the success of the desired length.

of the prosthetic components and the levels of bone cuts can be calculated using appropriate computer programs or x-ray templates (Figure 28.4).

It is important to remember that the control of the limbs' dysmetry is also performed by viewing the height of the patellae, placed on the dedicated traction bed (Figure 28.5).

Choice of surgical instruments

MOBILE LEG POSITIONER

This surgical method can be performed either on a normal operating bed or using dedicated devices to reduce the fatigue of the surgeon and number of surgeons, and speed up the procedure. In our experience, the OPT 80 or OPT 100 surgical bed is used. Slightly dedicated traction is applied to this operative limb (Figure 28.6).

This bed called mobile leg positioner (MLP) is used all over the world, and the main feature is to fit with any surgical bed through special adapters (Figure 28.7).

There are various models of such traction beds, and we usually use the AMIS MLP. The shoe on which the foot is inserted allows movement outside the surgical field. Moreover, the limb movement

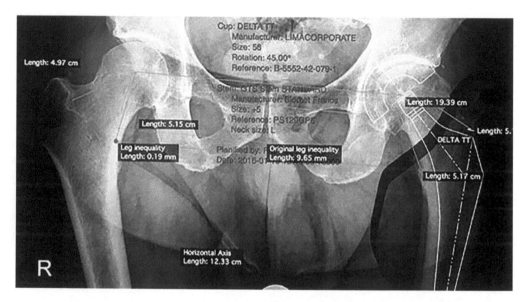

Figure 28.4 Example of preoperative planning for the choice of prosthetic components.

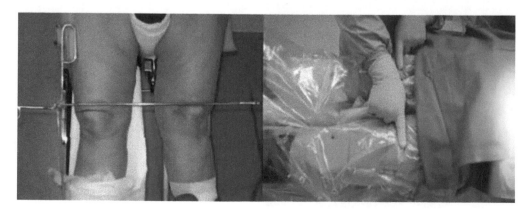

Figure 28.5 The measurement of possible limb dysmetry can be assessed using visual findings, such as the height of the patellae.

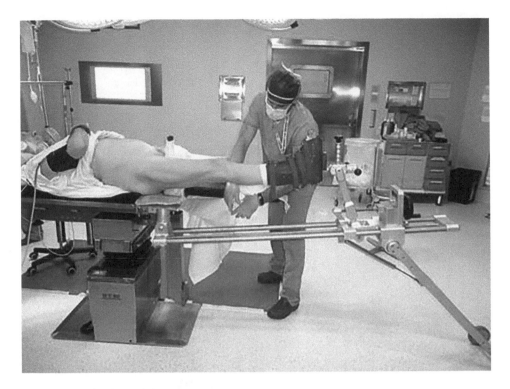

Figure 28.6 Traction bed used during surgery.

can be done in intrarotation, extrarotation, flexion, adduction, and abduction to facilitate the observation of the joint components during the surgical act (Figure 28.8).

A vertical padded cylinder works as a perineal counterthrust and is positioned on the pubis (Figure 28.9).

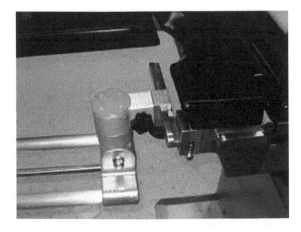

Figure 28.7 The mobile leg positioner adapter.

DEDICATED SURGICAL INSTRUMENTS

Tissue-sparing surgery is a surgical strategy aimed to reduce tissue damage in joint replacement. This can be achieved by reducing soft tissue trauma, performing minimally invasive access routes, and limiting bone removal with implantation of conservative prostheses. In order to facilitate mini-anterior approaches, special instrumentation was developed to avoid impingement of the soft tissues and provide an easier and more correct placement of the components.[11] The dedicated instruments for minimally invasive techniques are used to improve the surgical exposure of the joint in conditions of limited exposure influenced by the dimensions of the wound. The main difficulties in this type of surgery are the poor visualization of the anatomic structures and the troublesome preparation, and positioning of prosthetic components.[12] Hohmann retractors with long handles and various angulations have been developed so that the assistant's hands are distanced from the operative field. The reamers for the preparation of the acetabulum have also been modified. In offset reamers, an angled handle is provided to avoid impingement of

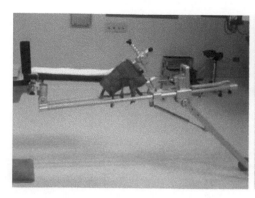
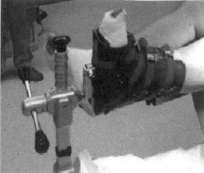

Figure 28.8 The mobile leg positioner allows numerous movements, and the shoe can be maneuvered out of the surgical field.

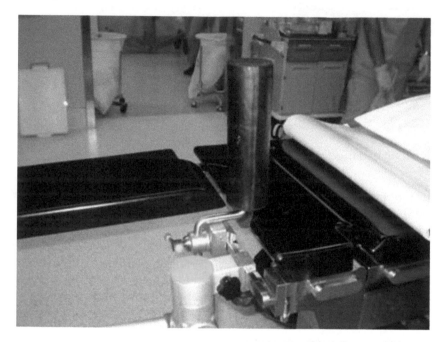

Figure 28.9 A vertical padded cylinder acts as a perineal counterthrust and is positioned on the pubis.

the soft tissues and avoid eccentric reaming. The choice of the femoral broach handle, either straight or angled, depends on the surgical approach, while in AMIS femoral preparation generally is easier with curved broach handles (Figure 28.10).

SURGICAL DESCRIPTION

The anterior minimally invasive approach consists of a modification from the classic method described by Carl Heuter in 1881.[2] The patient is first placed in a supine position on the operating table, and a folded towel is placed under the operative hemipelvis. This

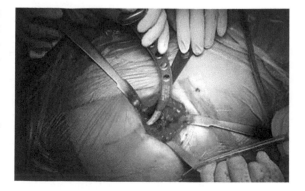

Figure 28.10 Femoral broach handle.

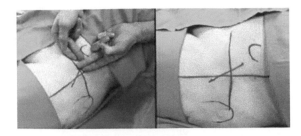

Figure 28.11 Landmarks for skin incision. The incision is 6–8 centimeters long and runs 1–2 fingerbreadths lateral to a line connecting the anterior superior ilian spine to the Gerdy's tubercle. The locations of the iliac crest, greater trochanter, and anterior superior iliac spine will be marked.

allows the pelvis to be brought forward for easier access. The incision is 6–8 centimeters (cm) long and runs 1–2 fingerbreadths lateral to a line connecting the anterior superior iliac spine to the Gerdy's tubercle. Subsequently, the locations of the iliac crest, greater trochanter, and anterior superior iliac spine will be marked (Figure 28.11).

The incision will be made approximately 3 cm lateral and 1 cm distal to the ASIS, and carried on a posterior and distal direction toward the anterior border of the femur. The incision will be 6–8 cm and parallel with the fibers of the tensor fascia lata muscle (Figure 28.12a).

The location of the lateral femoral cutaneous nerve must be taken into consideration in this approach in order to preserve lateral thigh sensation. It is located about 1 cm medial and below the anterior superior iliac, and passes over the sartorius. The incision is extended straight to the superficial aponeurosis of the tensor fascia lata (Figure 28.12b and c).

This aponeurosis is incised to expose the muscle fibers of the tensor, which run downward (Figure 28.12d).

The medial aponeurosis is lifted with a finger or clamp. Now, we are looking for the space between the fascia lata muscle and the sartorius muscle. The medial side of the muscle is retracted laterally, sparing the aponeurosis of the sartorius (Figure 28.12e).

Digital mobilization is easy, so the tensor fascia lata can be pushed laterally. It is important that the split in the aponeurosis of this muscle be carried well proximally and distally beneath the skin, so that the retractors will not damage the muscle. A Beckmann retractor is inserted to hold the tensor, and the aponeurosis covering the rectus femoris is visualized. The rectus femoris muscle can be seen below its aponeurosis. It is possible to see three colors that identify different areas: white, red, and yellow areas representing the aponeurosis, muscle, and fat above the joint capsule, respectively. The thin aponeurosis covering the red area is incised. Here again, some hemostasis is often required. It is now possible to retract the muscle medially using the Beckmann retractor. Furthermore, placing this retractor between the lateral side of the rectus femoris and the medial side of the tensor fascia lata, an unnamed pearly aponeurosis is seen, which represents the only structure standing in the way of the capsule (Figure 28.12f).

Below this aponeurosis, and rather in the distal part, the anterior circumflex arteriovenous bundle is seen. Most of the time, at the upper part, this aponeurosis is thin or even absent. The capsule is palpated with a finger. The aponeurosis is thicker at the distal part of the approach, and should be incised with great caution in order to not injure the circumflex vessels. After the aponeurosis has been opened, the circumflex vessels are easily isolated with a Lambotte rasp and cut between two ligatures. These relatively big vessels are directly connected to the femoral artery, and simple coagulation does not seem safe to us. Proximally, the reflected tendon of the rectus femoris is isolated from front to rear with the Lambotte rasp. After resecting the fatty tissue in front of the capsule, the muscles around the capsule are exposed, and these should not be touched. Proximally and on laterally, it is possible to see some fibers of the gluteus minimus, and, on the medial side, the iliocapsularis. On the lateral side, the tensor fascia lata retracted by the Beckmann retractor is seen, and more distal, the fibers of the vastus lateralis that follow the inferior insertion of the capsule on the anterior intertrochanteric line are also visible. The capsule is opened precisely and a flap is detached (Figure 28.12g).

The capsula flap should be conserved and closed at the end, or remove it. The joint capsule is incised following the iliocapsularis muscle edge from distally to proximally. At the top, the incision ends at the anterior edge of the acetabulum, but may follow very slightly the edge of the acetabulum outward. Distally, the incision runs to the inferomedial

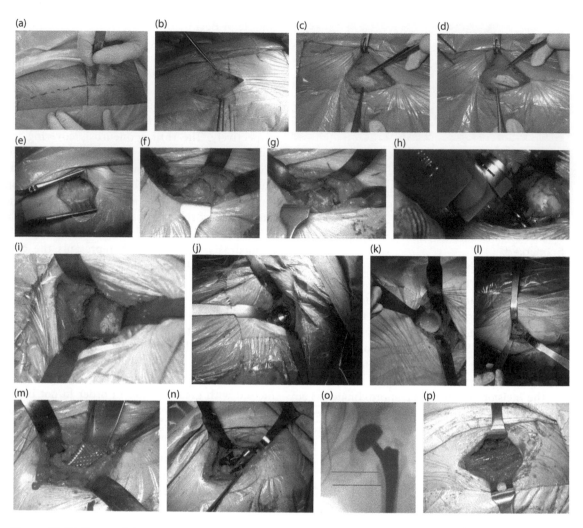

Figure 28.12 Steps of the anterior approach to the hip. (a) Skin incision. (b) The incision is extended straight to the superficial aponeurosis of the tensor fascia lata. (c) The aponeurosis is incised. (d) The muscle fibers of the tensor run downward. (e) The medial aponeurosis is lifted with a finger or clamp. Now, we look for the space between the fascia lata muscle and sartorius muscle. The medial side of the muscle is retracted laterally, sparing the aponeurosis of the sartorius. (f) The hip capsule is visible. (g) The capsule is opened precisely and a flap is detached. (h) Perform the femoral neck cut. (i) The cup is perfectly visible. (j) A hemispherical-shaped reamer can be easily inserted into the acetabulum. (k) After the acetabulum has been prepared, the cup is inserted. (l) Femoral preparation can begin by opening the medullary channel using a starter rasp. (m) The femur is prepared with rasps of various sizes. (n) The femoral stem is inserted and a femoral head is selected. (o) An x-ray is performed to check the anatomical references seen in the preoperative planning. (p) After reduction of the prosthetic implant, retractors are removed and spontaneous closure of the intermuscular space between the sartorius and the tendor fasciae latae muscle is observed.

insertion of the capsule, then laterally following the intertrochanteric line, along the vastus lateralis fibers. Release the flap laterally until the pertrochanteric tubercle is visualized. Now it is possible to place two Hohmann retractors between the neck and capsule. It is necessary to continue to release the capsule up to its insertions to expose the femoral neck around the greater trochanter and in the lower part toward the lesser trochanter. By freeing the capsule this way, the anterior neck will be better visualized. Before performing the femoral neck cut, increase traction about 1–1.5 cm. The cut is made with the head *in situ*, using an oscillating saw (Figure 28.12h).

It starts from the most external part of the neck, at the junction with the greater trochanter, and runs toward the femoral neck. The best anatomic landmark is the pertrochanteric tubercle. The cut is made at an angle of 45° to the horizontal plane just over the upper fiber of the vastus laterali. The saw blade is perpendicular to the floor. Before cutting the neck, the position of lower limb should be checked by palpating the patella. The saw must be fine and long. It is important to be gentle and careful and not go too far posteriorly, to prevent injury to the posterior circumflex artery. To facilitate the extraction of the femoral head, the surgeon can perform a second osteotomy proximally to the first to allow the removal of a bone cylinder with a thickness of 5–10 millimeters ("wafer technique"). The femoral head appears more easily removable with the appropriate extractor. Now it is possible to place three Hohmann retractors on the anterior, posterior (here you can use a retractor muller) and proximal cortical of the acetabulum. Now the cup is perfectly visible (Figure 28.12i).

The labrum and round ligament are excised, the acetabular fossa is identified, and the transverse ligament can be cut on its anterior edge to prevent excessive bleeding. A hemispherical-shaped reamer can be easily inserted into the acetabulum. After the acetabulum has been prepared, the cup is inserted (Figure 28.12j and k).

Our experience is to use hemispherical and noncemented acetabular prosthesis with a very rough surface. We usually resort to ceramic-ceramic or polyethylene-ceramic coupling. Once the acetabulum has been prepared and the acetabular component is in place, attention should be turned to the femoral side. Hohmann retractors are now extracted. The iliofemoral and ischiofemoral capsular components should be dissected near the femur with the cautious and superficial use of the electrosurgical unit, following the superomedial profile of the great trochanter. Thanks to this release, the movements of the femur can now be performed. With the help of the MLP, the limb is externally extended by 90° and lowered by about 50°. These movements must be helped by the surgeon who acts on the knee accompanying the movements and avoiding rotating only the foot through the shoe, at the risk of fracturing or damaging capsular ligaments. It is necessary to place

a Hohmann retractor above the summit of the greater trochanter. Another Hohmann retractor is placed superolaterally at the apex of the great trochanter in order to move the tissues and free the field for the femoral preparation. The surgeon stands against the patient's thigh and accentuates the adduction effect with his/her own thigh pushing the limb in further adduction. In the great majority of cases, femoral preparation can begin by opening the medullary channel using a starter rasp (Figure 28.12l), without the need for touching the capsule or the lateral rotator group muscles. With broaches dedicated to this surgical approach, the femur is prepared (Figure 28.12m).

This preparation is considered complete when the last inserted broach reaches the preoperatively planned level. A basic landmark is usually palpation of the lesser trochanter. The surgeon should not modify the physiological anteversion of the femur in order to decrease posterior dislocation, as posterior dislocation is potentially reduced with the anterior approach.[13,14] A trial prosthetic stem is inserted with the prosthetic femoral head. The joint is reduced to perform a test. After a stability test performed with trial components, the stem is inserted and a femoral head is selected (Figure 28.12n).

Its neck length depends on the position of the implant with respect to the preoperative templating. To perform stability and range-of-motion tests, it is possible to disconnect the traction shoe from the MLP, but care should be taken to keep the surgical field sterile. Also, we prefer to perform an x-ray to check the anatomical references seen in the preoperative planning. If the trial implant is satisfactory, it is replaced with the definitive femoral prosthesis (Figure 28.12o).

After reduction of the prosthetic implant, retractors are removed and spontaneous closure of the intermuscular space between the sartorius and the tendor fasciae latae muscle is observed (Figure 28.12p).

The superficial aponeurosis of the fascia lata is closed with a running suture, taking care not to catch a branch of the femoral cutaneous nerve.

ADVANTAGES AND DISADVANTAGES OF ANTERIOR HIP REPLACEMENT

Kennon and Keggi performed the largest and most established case study of 2132 patients who underwent total hip replacement using an anterior approach.[15] They observed no damage to the sciatic nerve, 28 dislocations, 7 infections, 21 diaphyseal femoral fractures, 24 fractures of the great trochanter, 2 fractures of the small trochanter, 37 fractures of the calcar, and 5 lesions of the lateral femoral cutaneous nerve. The authors conclude that the complication rate is flat and that the blood losses were very low. Petis et al. declare that the anterior approach to the hip has gained significant popularity recently, and can be a valuable technique for hip replacement in most patients. Although it has been associated with a steep learning curve, overall complication rates in the available literature do not appear to exceed those of other approaches to the hip. The growing desire for less invasive arthroplasty with improvement in functional results makes this approach an attractive choice.[16] Lloyd exalts the anterior approach because its use in hip replacement has also been accompanied by improvements to clinical pathways and the adoption of fast-track protocols.[17] Kelly et al. show that thoughtful perioperative and postoperative rehabilitation after hip preservation surgery may help minimize the morbidity of a more invasive surgical procedure while optimizing functional recovery.[18] The differences between the "traditional" surgical techniques and the anterior approach boil down to the amount of unavoidable muscle, nerve, and tendon damage the patient experiences during the surgery. Traditional approaches to the hip invariably cut through muscle, nerves, and possibly tendons before entering the hip joint to perform the replacement.[19] The anterior approach passes between muscles and tendons from the front of the hip. By accessing the hip joint through an internervous/intermuscular plane, the surgeon can avoid injury to the same muscles and tendons that once would have been cut. The difference between the anterior approach and the other surgical approaches is clear. DLA requires the removal of tendons to allow access to the hip and then their reattachment following the procedure with the possibility that they may not heal properly. Gait abnormalities are more common with the DLA, which involves the removal of part of the abductor medius and abductor minimus tendons, which are very important in stabilizing the hip joint when walking. The PLA involves detachment of smaller muscles from the top of the femur to allow access to the hip. This approach has been associated with an increased rate of dislocation,

which in some cases may require reoperation. The anterior approach does not require any muscles to be detached to allow access to the hip joint capsule. A window is made in the hip joint capsule to allow exposure of the joints and following surgery being performed. The advantage of the anterior approach is that the normal gait is not dependent on tendon healing since no tendons have been removed and repaired, as they have in the DLA and PLA.[19] Therefore, it is possible to discourse about "tissue-sparing surgery." This is not a particular technique but a "surgical philosophy," consisting of a maximum respect for soft tissues and bone, including reduction of operative invasiveness and use of minimally invasive surgical solutions.[20] This entails a rapid recovery of joint function and a decreased loss of blood, as amply demonstrated by the literature.[21–23] Anterior minimally invasive hip replacement surgery has a number of potential advantages over the standard approaches, such as: smaller scar, reduced blood loss, decreased postoperative pain, early mobilization, shorter hospital stay, and fast return to daily activities. However, we cannot fail to mention the possible complications, which, although few have been registered (in 2%–4% of cases), are related to the learning curve.[24,25] Using a small surgical wound can cause bruising due to the instruments that touch the skin. The lateral cutaneous femoral nerve can be traumatized by the use of retractors, while the tensor fasciae latae muscle can be damaged by incorrect use of retractors. Abnormal hematomas can occur at an incorrect ligation of the circumflex vessels. Fracture of the femoral diaphysis or great trochanter can occur during limb movement maneuvers. The dislocation of the new joint can occur due to poor positioning of the prosthetic components. Some authors claim that this surgical method is not indicated in obese subjects;[26,27] in our study, we have shown how the anterior approach to the hip is mainly indicated in obese patients.[28] The particular aspect of anterior approach is to act on the hip front portion where there is less adipose tissue. Small-incision surgery of obese patients through the anterior approach is possible partly because the subcutaneous fat over the anterolateral proximal thigh does not increase in thickness as dramatically as it does posteriorly or laterally. DAA meets the needs of the orthopedic surgeon who wants to implant a hip prosthesis in the obese patient, eliminating the difficulties caused by the fat.

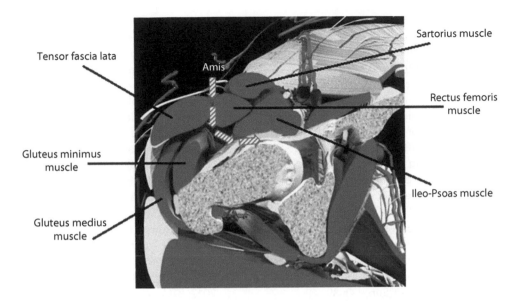

Figure 28.13 The AMIS is internervous and does not include the dissection of the muscles and tendons. The surgeon crosses the space between the tensor fascia lata and the sartorius muscle, the space between the gluteus medius and the rectus femoris muscle.

CONCLUSIONS

AMIS, DLA, and PLA can be used for hip replacement. In the literature, the advantages and disadvantages of each surgical approach have been documented and which approach will be chosen depends on the experience of the surgeon. The AMIS is internervous and does not include dissection of the muscles and tendons (Figure 28.13), allowing a saving of tissues and a quick recovery of the patient. The use of dedicated instruments and MLP have made the surgical approach simple and allow ever-smaller skin incisions.

REFERENCES

1. Rachbauer F, Kain MS, Leunig M. The history of the anterior approach to the hip. *Orthop Clin North Am* 2009; 40: 311–20.
2. Hueter C. Fünfte abtheilung: Die verletzung und krankheiten des hüftgelenkes, neunundzwanzigstes capitel. In: Hueter C, editor. *Grundriss der chirurgie*. 2nd ed., Leipzig: FCW Vogel; 1883. pp. 129–200.
3. Smith-Petersen MN. A new supra-articular subperiosteal approach to the hip joint. *J Bone Joint Surg Am* 1917; s2-15: 592–5.
4. Smith-Peterson MN. Approach to and exposure of the hip joint for mold arthroplasty. *J Bone Joint Surg Am* 1949; 31: 40–6.
5. Judet J, Judet R. The use of an artificial femoral head for arthroplasty of the hip joint. *J Bone Joint Surg Br* 1950; 32-B: 166–73.
6. Judet J, Judet H. Voie d'abord anterieure dans l'arthroplastie totale de la hanche. *Presse Med* 1985; 14: 1031–3.
7. Matta JM, Shahrdar C, Ferguson T. Single-incision anterior approach for total hip arthroplasty on an orthopaedic table. *Clin Orthop Relat Res* 2005; 441: 115–24.
8. Mast NH, Laude F. Revision total hip arthroplasty performed through the Hueter interval. *J Bone Joint Surg Am* 2011; 93(Suppl 2): 143–8.
9. Della Valle AG, Padgett DE, Salvati EA. Preoperative planning for primary total hip arthroplasty. *J Am Acad Orthop Surg* 2005; 13(7): 455–62.
10. Scheerlinck T. Primary hip arthroplasty templating on standard radiographs. A stepwise approach. *Acta Orthop Belg* 2010; 76(4): 432–42.
11. Capone A, Podda D, Civinini R, Gusso MI. The role of dedicated instrumentation in total hip arthroplasty. *J Orthop Traumatol* 2008; 9(2): 109–15.

12. Howell JR, Masri BA, Duncan CP. Minimally invasive versus standard incision anterolateral hip replacement: A comparative study. *Orthop Clin North Am* 2004; 35(2): 153–62.

13. Miller LE, Gondusky JS, Kamath AF, Boettner F, Wright J, Bhattacharyya S. Influence of surgical approach on complication risk in primary total hip. Arthroplasty. *Acta Orthop* 2018; 89(3): 289–94.

14. Müller DA, Zingg PO, Dora C. Anterior minimally invasive approach for total hip replacement: Five-year survivorship and learning curve. *Hip Int* 2014; 24(3): 277–83.

15. Kennon RE, Keggi JM, Wetmore RS, Zatorski LE, Huo MH, Keggi KJ. Total hip arthroplasty through a minimally invasive anterior surgical approach. *J Bone Joint Surg Am* 2003; 85-A(Suppl 4): 39–48.

16. Petis S, Howard JL, Lanting BL, Vasarhelyi EM. Surgical approach in primary total hip arthroplasty: Anatomy, technique and clinical outcomes. *Can J Surg* 2015; 58(2): 128–39.

17. Lloyd JM, Wainwright T, Middleton RG. What is the role of minimally invasive surgery in a fast track hip and knee replacement pathway? *Ann R Coll Surg Engl* 2012; 94(3): 148–51.

18. Adler KL, Cook PC, Geisler PR, Yen YM, Giordano BD. Current concepts in hip preservation surgery: Part II – rehabilitation. *Sports Health* 2016; 8(1): 57–64.

19. Lindgren V, Garellick G, Kärrholm J, Wretenberg P. The type of surgical approach influences the risk of revision in total hip arthroplasty: A study from the Swedish Hip Arthroplasty Register of 90,662 total hip replacements with 3 different cemented prostheses. *Acta Orthop* 2012; 83(6): 559–65.

20. Pipino, F. Tissue-sparing surgery (T.S.S.) in hip and knee arthroplasty. *J Orthopaed Traumatol* 2006; 7: 33.

21. Regis D, Residori A, Rossi N, Bartolozzi P. Tissue-sparing surgery in total hip arthroplasty: Sensible approaches and tested evidence. *J Orthop Traumatol* 2007; 8(4): 199–201.

22. Reichert JC, Volkmann MR, Koppmair M, Rackwitz L, Lüdemann M, Rudert M, Nöth U. Comparative retrospective study of the direct anterior and transgluteal approaches for primary total hip arthroplasty. *Int Orthop* 2015; 39: 2309–13.

23. Faldini C, Perna F, Mazzotti A, Stefanini N, Panciera A, Geraci G, Mora P, Traina F. Direct anterior approach versus posterolateral approach in total hip arthroplasty: Effects on early post-operative rehabilitation period. *J Biol Regul Homeost Agents* 2017; 31(4 suppl 1): 75–81.

24. Seng BE, Berend KR, Ajluni AF, Lombardi AV Jr. Anterior-supine minimally invasive total hip arthroplasty: Defining the learning curve. *Orthop Clin North Am* 2009; 40(3): 343–50.

25. De Geest T, Vansintjan P, De Loore G. Direct anterior total hip arthroplasty: Complications and early outcome in a series of 300 cases. *Acta Orthop Belg* 2013; 79(2): 166–73.

26. Obalum DC, Fiberesima F, Eyesan SU, Ogo CN, Nzew C, Mijinyawa M. A review of obesity and orthopaedic surgery: The critical issues. *Niger Postgrad Med J* 2012; 19(3): 175–80.

27. Horan F. Obesity and joint replacement. *J Bone Joint Surg Br* 2006; 88(10): 1269–71.

28. Ricciardi A, Geraci A. Anterior minimally invasive surgery for hip replacement in obese patients. *Minerva Ortopedica e Traumatologica* 2017; 68(3): 131–8.

29

Digital templating in total hip arthroplasty

SHALIN SHAUNAK AND WASIM KHAN

INTRODUCTION

The major aims of hip arthroplasty are to provide good long-term survival of the implants and good functional outcomes and to avoid both impingement and dislocation as well as leg length discrepancy. In order to attain these ideals, it is essential that the normal biomechanics of the hip be restored by proper implant positioning. Furthermore, use of the wrong-sized implant can lead to periprosthetic fractures or failure of ingrowth in uncemented implants. One method of effectively and consistently achieving this is preoperative templating. This process also encourages the surgeon to think of the hip in three dimensions as well as allowing for preoperative checking of inventory prior to the procedure. It also allows for planning for any potential complications intraoperatively.

Charnley himself espoused the use of radiographic studies to choose the correct implant size and to restore offset. Muller also reported that templating "forces the surgeon to think in three dimensions, greatly improves the precision of surgery, shortens the length of the procedure, and greatly reduces the incidence of complications." It is also important to restore leg length as well as the center of rotation of the hip. This was traditionally achieved through the use of hard-copy radiographs and acetate templates supplied by the implant manufacturer. This has now been superseded, in the majority of cases, by digital radiography and consequently digital templating. Templating itself has become more important given the advent of a great number of different prosthesis designs and sizes in the current era of arthroplasty surgery.

Templating should follow a stepwise process, i.e. replicating the steps intraoperatively. Each piece of software has its own idiosyncrasies; however, it is the aim of this chapter to discuss the combined and essential steps regardless of software choice.

DIGITAL VERSUS CONVENTIONAL TEMPLATING

The vast majority of hospitals have moved their radiography onto digital systems, such as picture archiving and communication (PACS). This adds a limitation and difficulty to obtaining hard-copy radiographs for use in conventional templating. A hybrid approach, wherein printed digital images templated using analogue templating methods, correctly selected the prosthetic selection 69% of the time. The use of a fully digital system should, in theory, eliminate errors associated with manual manipulation of the acetate templates and printing process. It also eliminates variations in magnification; acetate templates rely on a fixed magnification, whereas digital templating allows modification based on the reference magnification. This is most reproducible where a scaling marker is used.

In real terms, however, there remains little difference, in terms of accuracy, between the methods used. Both have an accuracy of approximately 65–80% in predicting acetabular and femoral component sizes. With this in mind, the advantages of preoperative digital templating must be considered. These include an absence of the requirement to produce hard copies of the radiograph, creation of a permanent record of the template, and the advent of software that takes the novel user through a stepwise approach to templating the hip, with replicable results. It also allows the user to have a bank of different prostheses without having to provide a plethora of different acetate templates.

THE PREOPERATIVE RADIOGRAPH

Most radiographs are magnified in the region of 110–125%. With quite a broad range, prone to variations within a single department due to human error, it is essential to know the precise magnification. The most precise method of doing so, at present, is the use of a radio-opaque marker. This is set at a predetermined size (usually 28 or 30 mm) and held at the level of the hips by the patient during the application of the x-ray beam. The method requires the marker to be placed at the same distance from the cassette as the center of rotation of the hip. This allows us to use this in a way almost akin to a scale on a map.

In terms of technical aspects of the radiograph, it is essential to obtain a true anteroposterior (AP) of the pelvis, showing both hips, proximal femurs, and acetabulae. This should be centered over the pubic symphysis. An AP of the operative hip should also be taken with approximately 10–15° of internal rotation. This places the femoral neck parallel to the cassette; external rotation will lead to falsely decreased offset, creating a valgus-appearing femoral neck as well as falsely decreasing the diameter of the femoral canal.

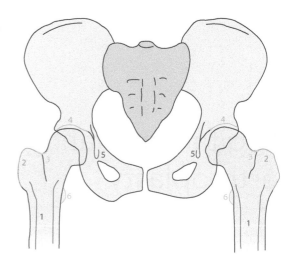

Figure 29.1 Anatomical landmarks: (1) proximal femoral canal; (2) greater trochanter; (3) saddle; (4) superior acetabular rim; (5) "teardrop"; (6) lesser trochanter.

This should be of sufficient penetration as well as avoiding undue rotation. Once the overall quality of the radiograph has been confirmed, it is essential to ensure that the anatomical references are present and well aligned. Once this is completed, we can proceed to templating in earnest (Figure 29.1).

LIMB-LENGTH DISCREPANCY AND CENTER OF HIP ROTATION

All of this should be closely examined in reference to the preoperative examination of the patient for both true and apparent limb-length discrepancy. To begin, start with the AP pelvis radiograph. A horizontal line should be drawn connecting both teardrops at their bases, while ensuring the line extends bilaterally beyond the medial femoral cortices. Alternatively, a line can be drawn along the two ischial tuberosities instead. A second line should be drawn at a predetermined and reproducible area on the lesser trochanters (usually the most proximal point). Following this, the distance between both the two lesser trochanter lines and the teardrop line should be measured. Any discrepancy should point to a limb-length discrepancy.

At this point, the center of rotation of the hip should also be marked and compared to the contralateral hip. This is the point at which all hip movement occurs. This is best marked by drawing a circle fitted to both the femoral head and acetabular roof and medial wall and finding the center. In cases of deformity, the original center of rotation should be found by drawing these circles separately, using the intact proportions of the femur and acetabulum and then fitting both rotational centers together. The contralateral hip can be used as a reference.

FEMORAL, ACETABULAR, AND COMBINED OFFSET

Femoral offset is defined as the distance between the center of rotation of the femoral head and the longitudinal axis of the femur. The center of rotation has been discussed above. The best means of denoting the longitudinal axis is by drawing a line in the middle of the femoral canal and projecting this upward. The distance between the center of rotation and this line is the femoral offset. This is an important factor, as failure to restore the offset can lead to excessive wear, limping, and instability. Increasing the offset overly can lead to overloading of the femoral component and micromotion with increased risk of implant loosening or, indeed, failure of ingrowth. It can also lead to overtensioning of the abductor musculature and consequent pain, tightness, and impingement.

Acetabular offset is the distance between the center of rotation of the acetabulum (where this varies from the femoral center) and a line drawn perpendicular to our interteardrop line. Decrement of this, through excessive medialization of the cup, can lead to instability or limping, with overtly increasing it leading to excessive loading and wear of the cup as well as tightness.

The combined offset is the sum of the femoral and acetabular offsets and is very important in determining abductor muscle tension, as it directly demonstrates the distance between the greater trochanter and pelvis, i.e. the trajectory of these muscles (Figure 29.2).

ACETABULAR TEMPLATING

Placement of the acetabular component precedes that of the femoral component preoperatively and as such should be templated first. Correct placement is paramount to obtaining stability of the replacement. The horizontal interteardrop line should be used in order to represent the level of the true floor of the acetabulum. Also, the ilioischial line and

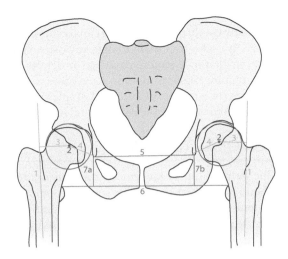

Figure 29.2 Mechanical landmarks: (1) longitudinal axis of proximal femur; (2) hip rotation center; (3) femoral offset; (4) acetabular offset; (5) interteardrop line; (6) intertrochanteric line; (7) "leg-length discrepancy" calculated as the difference between 7a and 7b.

superolateral margin of the acetabulum should also be marked on the preoperative radiograph.

If the anatomy of the hip is largely preserved, the operative hip can be used. In cases of severe deformity, it is often better practice to template the contralateral "normal" side. The cup should consequently be sized so that it lies in approximately 45° of abduction and the medial border approximates the ilioischial line. The abduction angle should be defined according to the angle between the longest axis of the cup and the interteardrop line. The inferior border should lie along that of the teardrop line and there should be sufficient lateral coverage as per the superolateral acetabular margin. It is also important to ensure that a uniform 2–3 mm gap is left for cemented implants. It is of utmost importance that the acetabular offset be maintained; this can be compared to the contralateral "healthy" hip as a reference, where available.

Any hip dysplasia, protrusio acetabuli, or overly lateralized acetabulum should be noted by looking at the acetabular offset and comparing it to the contralateral side. In protrusion acetabuli, i.e. where the femoral head projects medially from Kohler's line, it is often necessary to graft the medial wall and lateralize the cup, thereby restoring the acetabular rotational center. In dysplastic hips, lack of superolateral cover may require bone grafting or augmentation in order to avoid inadvertently overly medializing the cup to obtain coverage. It is also important to note any osteophytes or cysts that may require curettage or defects that may require augmentation. In some cases, such as with severe bone loss of ipsilateral dysplasia, it can be useful to template the contralateral hip.

FEMORAL TEMPLATING

The overall aims of the femoral component are to obtain the correct size for the femoral component, restoration of femoral offset, and optimization of limb length, all of which have been discussed above.

The stem size should be approximated first, given the variation in offset between sizes in some prostheses. In cemented stems, a uniform margin of 2–3 mm should be left to allow for the cement mantle. In cementless prostheses, the stem should obtain endosteal contact either proximally or in the diaphysius, dependent on stem design.

To anatomically align the level of the center of rotation of the implanted head, a perpendicular line can be drawn from the center of the femoral shaft at the level of the greater trochanter. This will approximate the height of the center of rotation. In coxa vara or coxa valgus hips, this can lie below and above the true center of rotation of the hip; therefore, exercise caution in these cases. The distance between the center of rotation of the implanted head and that of the center of rotation of the acetabular component will demonstrate the degree of lengthening or shortening that will take place with this implant. The stem can be translated proximally or distally until the selected limb length is attained.

Finally, it is time to template the implant to restore the femoral offset of the "normal" hip. This can depend on the stem size, in some implants. It can be altered by up- or downsizing the implant in such cases, while ensuring there is either an adequate cement mantle or bony contact in cementless implants. It can also be altered by use of a standard or offset stem, choosing a stem with a different neck-shaft angle, altering the height of the neck cut, or using a femoral head with minus or plus size options.

A coxa vara–type stem, i.e. one that decreases the neck-shaft angle, will increase offset but also reduce limb length. This would consequently need to be altered by using a femoral head with a longer neck or by cutting the neck higher up. A coxa valga stem, on the other hand, will decrease offset but lengthen the limb. Using a femoral head with a longer neck will increase both the offset and limb length and vice versa. It is often useful to try a combination of the above techniques until the appropriate limb length and offset are obtained.

Finally, the neck cut should be marked. After the templating process is complete, it is often useful to look at the lateral of the hip in order to assess and plan the opening of the femur, femoral bow, and also the AP diameter, as well as excessive native femoral anteversion.

ADDITIONAL INFORMATION

In cases where the original anatomy cannot be restored, the mainstays of treatment are to restore both combined offset and limb length. When anatomical constraints result in overmedialization of the cup, it is often necessary to increase the femoral offset to restore the distance between the pelvis and greater trochanter. Wherein the femoral offset is reduced, the cup can be lateralized to obtain the same effect. It may also become necessary while lengthening the limb to decrease the offset by medializing the cup or using a low-offset stem in order to avoid overtensioning the soft tissues. The opposite is true when shortening a limb, with increasing the offset to allow for adequate tension.

In valgus hips, the reduction in combined offset needs to be maintained to avoid overtensioning the soft tissues. This is best attained by medializing the cup, as this reduces the tension on the acetabular fixation and also allows preservation of the femoral offset, allowing for optimized abductor lever arms.

In varus hips, there is excessive femoral offset. This can be restored by using a high offset stem, often with a lower neck cut to avoid overlengthening the limb. The cup can also be lateralized to increase the combined offset; however, this places a greater strain on the cup and should be avoided unless absolutely necessary.

CONCLUSION

With the advent of newer and varied options within hip arthroplasty surgery, the need for templating is at its greatest. It not only encourages preoperative thought and planning, but helps selection of the correct prostheses and the planned approach and also ensures that adequate prosthesis sizes are available prior to proceeding. With the advent of schemes such as "The Getting It Right First Time (GIRFT) programme" and increased patient expectations, it is essential that we, as surgeons, employ any means that improve outcomes, reduce operative time, and also increase the survivorship of the implants, while removing only enough native bone as necessary to allow for revision surgery in the future.

BIBLIOGRAPHY

Berstock JR, Webb JC, Spencer RF. A comparison of digital and manual templating using PACS images. *Ann R Coll Surg Engl* 2010; 92(1): 73–4.

Blackley HR, Howell GE, Rorabeck CH. Planning and management of the difficult primary hip replacement: Preoperative planning and technical considerations. *Instr Course Lect* 2000; 49: 3–11.

Capello WN. Preoperative planning of total hip arthroplasty. *Instr Course Lect* 1986; 35: 249–57.

Carter LW, Stovall DO, Young TR. Determination of accuracy of preoperative templating of noncemented femoral prostheses. *J Arthroplasty* 1995; 10: 507–13.

Charnley J. Low friction principle. In: *Low Friction Arthroplasty of the Hip*. Springer, Berlin, Heidelberg, 1979.

Conn KS, Clarke MT, Hallett JP. A simple guide to determine the magnification of radiographs and to improve the accuracy of preoperative templating. *J Bone Joint Surg* 2002; 84-B: 269–72.

Crooijmans HJ, Laumen AM, van Pul C, van Mourik JB. A new digital preoperative planning method for total hip arthroplasties. *Clin Orthop Relat Res* 2009; 467(4): 909–16.

Cucker JM. Limb length and stability in total hip replacement. *Orthopaedics* 2005; 28(9): 951–3.

Della Valle AG, Padgett DE, Salvati EA. Preoperative planning for primary total hip arthroplasty. *J Am Acad Orthop Surg* 2006; 13(17): 455–62.

Della Valle AG, Comba F, Taveras N et al. The utility and precision of analogue and digital preoperative planning for total hip arthroplasty. *Int Orthop* 2008; 32: 289–94.

Eckrich SG, Noble PC, Tullos HS. Effect of rotation on the radiographic appearance of the femoral canal. *J Arthroplasty* 1994; 9: 419–26.

Efe T, El Zayat BF, Heyse TJ, Timmesfeld N, Fuchs-Winkelmann S, Schmitt J. Precision of preoperative digital templating in total hip arthroplasty. *Acta Orthop Belg* 2011; 77(5): 616–2.

Eggli S, Pisan M, Müller ME. The value of preoperative planning for total hip arthroplasty. *J Bone Joint Surg Br* 1998; 80(3): 382–90.

Hofmann AA, Bolognesi M, Lahav A, Kurtin S. Minimizing leg-length inequality in total hip arthroplasty: Use of preoperative templating and an intraoperative x-ray. *Am J Orthop (Belle Mead NJ)* 2008; 37(1): 18–23.

Knight JL, Atwater RD. Preoperative planning for total hip arthroplasty. Quantitating its utility and precision. *J Arthroplasty* 1992; 42: 455–61.

Kosashvili Y, Shasha N, Olschewski E, Safir O, White L, Gross A, Backstein D. Digital versus conventional templating techniques in preoperative planning for total hip arthroplasty. *Can J Surg* 2009; 52(1): 6–11.

Müller ME. Lessons of 30 years of total hip arthroplasty. *Clin Orthop Relat Res* 1992; 274: 12–21.

Oddy MJ, Jones MJ, Pendegrass CJ, Pilling JR, Wimhurst JA. Assessment of reproducibility and accuracy in templating hybrid total hip arthroplasty using digital radiographs. *J Bone Joint Surg Br* 2006 May; 88(5): 581–5.

Scheerlinck T. Primary hip arthroplasty templating on standard radiographs. A stepwise approach. *Acta Orthop Belg* 2010; 76(4): 432–42.

The B, Diercks RL, van Ooijen PM, Van Horn JR. Comparison of analog and digital preoperative planning in total hip and knee arthroplasties. A prospective study of 173 hips and 65 total knees. *Acta Orthop* 2005; 76: 78–84.

Whiddon DR, Bono JV, Lang JE, Smith EL, Salyapongse AK. Accuracy of digital templating in total hip arthroplasty. *Am J Orthop (Belle Mead NJ)* 2011; 40(8): 395–8.

White SP, Bainbridge J, Smith EJ. Assessment of magnification of digital pelvic radiographs in total hip arthroplasty using templating software. *Ann R Coll Surg Engl* 2008; 90(7): 592–6.

30

Safe surgical dislocation for hip joint preservation surgery

MILIND M. CHAUDHARY

INTRODUCTION

Femoroacetabular impingement is an important cause of pain and limitation of movement in the hip.[1,2] It is now recognized as an important cause leading to osteoarthritis of the hip joint.[3]

Cam impingement is caused by an insufficient femoral head–neck offset in the anterior and anterolateral zone, which causes excessive pressure against the labrum and chondrolabral junction in flexion adduction and internal rotation (Figure 30.1).[4] It may be caused by a developmental anomaly of the hip joint. It can also be caused by any disease or condition that deforms the femoral head, like Perthes disease, dysplasia, or avascular necrosis.

Partial destruction of the femoral head due to septic arthritis in childhood is an important cause of a misshapen femoral head. Avascular necrosis may give rise to extrusion of the femoral head beyond the acetabular rim. Pressure under the weight-bearing lip of the acetabulum may dent or damage the central part of the femoral head. Pincer impingement is caused by acetabular retroversion and overcoverage (Figure 30.2). Despite advances in total hip arthroplasty (THA), all efforts must be made to preserve the hip joint in young people and postpone replacement arthroplasty for as long as possible.

CLINICAL PRESENTATION

Patients present with pain in the groin, especially on prolonged sitting, especially on low chairs. Indian women, in their thirties complain of pain on floor sitting and squatting for the toilet. The pain may be a dull ache or sharp and cutting. It is usually poorly localized, and differentiation from pain of lumbar origin can be confusing. It may go undetected for several years and be mistaken for a lumbar pathology. It is not uncommon to have patients come in with MRI scans of the lumbar spine when they have a hip pathology. Occasionally, patients may point to the groin with a curved index and middle finger, hence the name "C-sign."[5] The patient may be asked to point to the most painful area with a single finger. A history of trauma leading to avascular necrosis or treatment of Perthes disease in childhood may be present. A history of minor trauma may be present, with initial intense pain that subsided after a few days and has increased since then. The patient may present

(a)

(b)

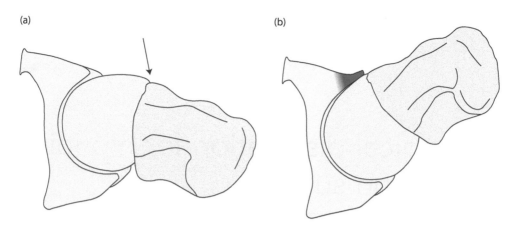

Figure 30.1 Cam impingement: There is no normal femoral head–neck offset due to which the "cam" or bulging part of the femoral head–neck causes friction with the acetabular rim and labrum in flexion.

(a)

(b)

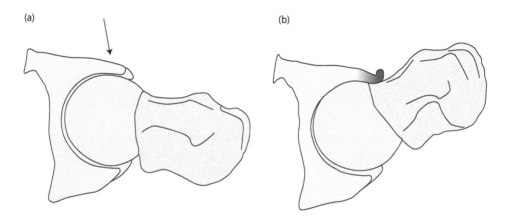

Figure 30.2 Pincer impingement: There is overcoverage of the femoral head which leads to excessive friction at the acetabular rim and labrum against the normal femoral head. This causes wear and tear of the chondro-labral junction and initiates arthritis of the hip joint.

with limb length discrepancy, which frequently accompanies a dysplastic hip.

CLINICAL EXAMINATION

Examining the gait as the patient walks in may reveal pointers to a hip pathology. A limp may be caused by a painful, irritable hip. The limp may also be due to true limb length discrepancy. The lumbar spine is examined briefly to rule out any pathology or radiculopathy.

Limb lengths are measured from Anterior Superior Iliac Spine (ASIS) to medial malleolus. Thigh girth is measured 10–15 cm below the ASIS. The hip range of motion is examined with the patient supine, prone, and on the side. Restriction

of full range of motion in the hip in any direction is a pointer to underlying hip pathology. In structural abnormalities of the hip with a cam femoroacetabular impingement, pain is elicited on hip flexion, adduction, and internal rotation (FADDIR test). A restriction of abduction denotes the presence of a deformed femoral head, as in Perthes or avascular necrosis.

The logroll test gently rolls the lower limb with knee extended in supine position in external and internal rotation and is positive for any intra-articular hip pathology.

The FABER test with the limb in flexion abduction external rotation helps distinguish sacroiliac joint pain. A snapping iliopsoas tendon is diagnosed when the hip comes down against resistance from the Faber position into adduction-internal rotation and extension.

RADIOLOGICAL INVESTIGATION

Plain x-ray imaging

Over the last 15 years, a greater understanding of subtle features seen on seemingly normal hip x-rays has helped identify various types of femoroacetabular impingement. A standard pelvis with both hips AP x-ray (PBH) can yield sufficient information. X-rays convert three-dimensional anatomy into two-dimensional. The pelvis must be controlled for rotation and tilt. Rotation is proper when the coccyx lines up with the symphysis pubis. Tilt of the pelvis is deemed appropriate when distance between the symphysis and coccyx is around 2 cm.

A cam deformity is seen on the AP x-ray of the hip as a pistol grip deformity of the femoral head, as the sagging rope sign, or by the presence

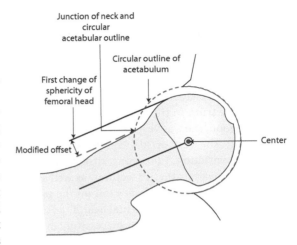

Figure 30.4 Offset measurement: Normally the offset is measured by a line that joins the centre of the femoral head to the first aspherical point of the femoral head–neck junction. The modified method measures this as a vertical distance between the extended circle of the acetabular cavity and its junction of the femoral neck. The circular outline of the femoral head is extended distally. The distance between the two lines gives the offset.

of anterolateral extrusion of the femoral head. The false profile and modified Dunn view show the loss of femoral head–neck offset or the presence of a bump at the anterior head–neck junction. This is quantified by the alpha angle (Figure 30.3), which measures the location of loss of sphericity of the femoral head contour. A normal angle may be around 50°, whereas a cam may create an angle closer to 80° or more. Though originally described for radial MRI cuts, it can also be appreciated on plain AP and modified Dunn views.

The modified offset (Figure 30.4) can quantify the amount by which the offset between the head and neck contours has changed. Pincer impingement is caused by acetabular retroversion and overcoverage. This is easily seen on an AP x-ray of the hip as the crossover sign and prominence of the ischial spine.[6]

ALTERNATIVE TO TOTAL HIP ARTHROPLASTY

Total hip arthroplasty is often considered "the operation of the twentieth century,"[7] and it undoubtedly holds pride of place in the armamentarium of the orthopedic surgeon for treating hip arthritis and

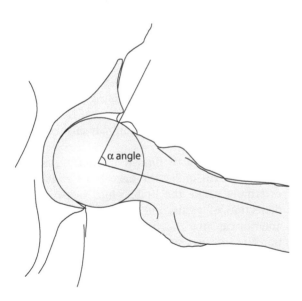

Figure 30.3 Alpha angle: Though this was initially calculated only on radial MRI cuts, it can be measured on AP, modified Dunn and cross table lateral views. The axis of the neck is drawn center. A line from center is drawn towards the first point of loss of sphericity of the femoral head. Normally this angle is around 50°. In a pistol grip deformity or in presence of a bump at the anterior edge of the femoral head it may be as high as 80–85°. A higher angle points to increased impingement on hip movement.

pathologies that cripple the old. Better instrumentation, and improved tribology have improved the longevity of hip arthroplasty. However, THA carries with it a high price economically and in terms of infrastructure necessary to enable its consistent success. Many have discovered to their chagrin and dismay the truth in this Longfellow poem. "When she was good, she was very very good, but when she was bad … she was horrid." Complications of THA can be devastating. Loosening, dislocation, instability, and periprosthetic fractures, as well as deep infection, can extract a heavy toll on the patient's economic, physical, and mental health.

The prostheses needed to successfully maintain long-term function in the young are expensive, and long-term results are few and far between. With the advent of THA, many useful operations that helped preserve and improve the function of diseased hips fell by the wayside and lie forgotten. Various osteotomies that helped redirect the femoral head and reduce loading on the hip are almost extinct. The Varus, Valgus, medial displacement and pelvic support osteotomy are rarely performed. Joint Preservation of the young hip has been neglected in favor of total hip arthroplasty.

In this scenario, two surgical procedures have emerged that revive hope for preserving damaged hips in the young patient. One is arthroscopy of the hip with its special long instruments and steep learning curve, which can help sportspersons and others recover from many pathologies, through small incisions and less time. All pathologies cannot be tackled satisfactorily.

The second and most useful surgical technique to emerge in the last two decades has been the safe surgical dislocation of the hip discovered by Reinhold Ganz. This enables the general orthopedic surgeon to access to the hip by surgical dislocation without fear of adding vascular insult. The approach enables complete anterior dislocation of the femoral head to gain 360° visualization of the femoral head and acetabulum. This enables performance of many intra-articular procedures, including those that will correct femoroacetabular impingement.

The instruments needed to perform this surgery are routine and inexpensive, including the operation tables. The surgical approach is a minor variation in common hip surgeries performed and is hence capable of being done by every orthopedic surgeon.

SURGICAL TECHNIQUE

Safe surgical dislocation has been described in detail.[8] It is easy to follow the technique without making any modifications. The patient is placed in a lateral decubitus after regional anesthesia. After a 15–20 cm long skin incision, we find the Gibson's interval and retract the Tensor Fascia Lata (TFL) anteriorly and gluteus maximus posteriorly. Instead of dissecting through the gluteus medius, we first retract it anteriorly and locate the piriformis muscle and tendon. We delineate the interval between the piriformis and gluteus minimus by blunt dissection. Next, we turn our attention to the trochanteric flip osteotomy. Here we make the two sloping cuts with broad osteotomes or oscillating saw blades parallel to each other; with the proximal cut being posterior and distal cut anterior. The interval between the two is connected with a 5-mm or 1/4″ osteotome. This step helps in secure fixation of the trochanteric osteotomy. The thickness of the trochanteric osteotomy is 15 mm and it contains the insertions of the gluteus medius and vastus lateralis. The trochanteric flip fragment may become trigastric, having the insertion of the gluteus minimus tendon, or at times a part of the insertion of the piriformis as well. The depth of cut can be difficult to determine in dysplastic hips. Orienting the osteotome or saw blade parallel to direction of the leg, held in 15–20° of internal rotation may ensure proper depth of cut.

The trochanter is flipped anteriorly. An assistant's forearm under the knee helps abduct and externally rotate the limb, which helps anterior dissection of vastus intermedius origin and the anterior capsule. The limb is taken back in adduction and internal rotation, which helps to perform the posterior soft tissue dissection.

The external rotators are not detached. The main blood supply to the femoral head comes from the deep branch of the medial circumflex femoral artery (MCFA).[9] This artery is constant in its extra-articular portion. The deep branch of the MCFA gives a trochanteric branch at the proximal border of the quadratus femoris. The level of this small artery denotes the location of the tendon of obturator externus behind which runs the deep branch of the MCFA. It ascends anterior to the tendons of the short external rotators and enters the hip capsule at the gemellus superior.

The anastomotic branch of the inferior gluteal artery runs along the inferior border of the piriformis muscle and provides additional supply to the femoral head. Hence, the insertion of the piriformis and all the short external rotators are kept intact and dissection is maintained between the superior part of the piriformis and gluteus minimus. This serves as double insurance for protecting femoral head blood supply.

The gluteus minimus is elevated with the medius to expose the hip capsule. A z-shaped capsulotomy extends postero-superiorly, preserving the labrum. The extremity is externally rotated to dislocate the head and the leg is placed in a sterile drape bag on the opposite side of table. An osteotome is used to recreate the femoral head–neck offset. The extreme medial and posterolateral aspects of the head–neck junction are not interfered with. The exposed femoral head is kept moist during the entire duration that it remains dislocated. Care is taken to ensure that the head is not separated from the acetabulum for more than 11 cm so as not to stretch the retinacular vessels.

At the end of the procedure, the femoral head is relocated and the capsule sutured. The mobile trochanteric fragment is relocated and fixed with two oblique screws going down to the lesser trochanter.

Procedures that can be performed after surgical dislocation of the hip:

1. Osteochondroplasty to recreate the head–neck junction offset for cam femoroacetabular impingement
2. Acetabular rim resection to reduce effect of retroversion and pincer impingement
3. Labral resuturing, repair, or reconstruction with fascia lata
4. Evaluation of acetabular floor reduction in acetabular fractures
5. Extended retinacular release in modified Dunn osteotomy for SCFE
6. Synovectomy, loose body removal, exostosis removal
7. Relative neck lengthening in coxa breva with trochanteric advancement
8. Femoral head reduction osteotomy for recreating an almost-spherical femoral head
9. Debridement of dead bone in and bone grafting in AVN with "light-bulb" technique
10. Any of the above procedures along with a subtrochanteric osteotomy[10]

Osteochondroplasty[11,12] to improve offset of the femoral head–neck junction is performed in the vast majority of cases of cam femoroacetabular impingement (Figure 30.5).

A curved osteotome or burr is used to recreate the femoral head–neck offset. Except for the posterolateral corner, the femoral head may be reshaped in its entire circumference. Punctate bleeding from the raw bony surfaces confirms the intact vascularity. An impingement test is performed intraoperatively to ensure adequacy of excision. If the neck is thinned inadvertently, one or two screws may be inserted up the neck to protect it against fracture.

Osteochondroplasty is needed in dysplastic hips as well, where there is extrusion of the hip anteriorly and laterally. It is commonly needed in post-fracture neck femur avascular necrosis where a bump has formed in the anterior and lateral quadrant during the avascular phase of AVN.[13] With revascularization, the head survives but the excrescence of the femoral head creates severe friction at the acetabular labrum and causes chondrolabral erosion.

Relative neck lengthening[14,15] is useful in coxa breva. It is performed by a subperiosteal dissection using a thin sharp osteotome to preserve the extended retinacular flap. Bony resection at the inferolateral corner of neck is performed along with distalization of the trochanter. The extent of distalization is no more than 15 mm. Relative neck lengthening can be combined with a modified Dunn procedure (Figure 30.6) for slipped capital femoral epiphysis. The posteriorly displaced capital epiphysis is relocated on top of the femoral neck after resecting the bump that forms on the anterior surface of the neck. Fixation of the head fragment is done with one or two screws. This gives far better results compared to in-situ screw fixation in SCFE and preserves the femoral head as well due to the low rate of AVN.

A subtrochanteric osteotomy can be performed simultaneously along with intra-articular procedures and fixed with a locking plate or an external fixator like the Ilizarov.[16] Medial displacement may be performed to help reduce the loads on the hip. A valgus or varus angulation may be given to redirect the femoral head as necessary. A distal neutralizing and lengthening osteotomy can be performed as well.

Intra-articular osteotomy to reshape the femoral head[17] is possible in deformity of the femoral

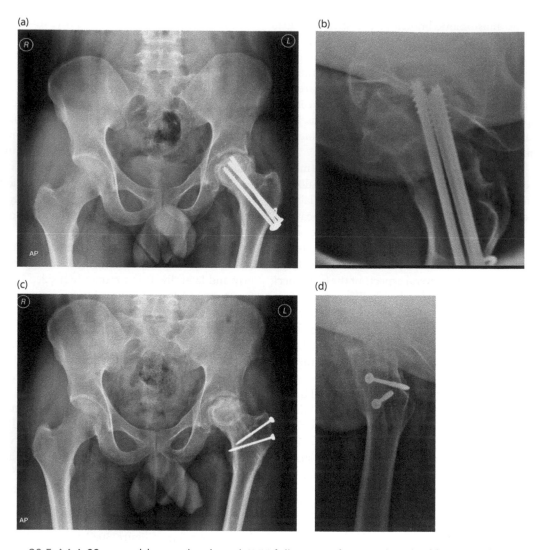

Figure 30.5 **(a)** A 23-year-old man, developed AVN following a fractured neck of femur. Softening of the femoral head caused extrusion of the femoral head with a visible bump anterolaterally on AP x-ray. He had significant pain on sitting in a low chair and on flexion-adduction-internal rotation. **(b)** A cross-table lateral x-ray shows the large bump present anterior to the femoral head. **(c,d)** After safe surgical dislocation, the femoral head–neck offset is restored after osteochondroplasty. There is no more impingement, and hip movements have become free.

head caused by Perthes disease or avascular necrosis. The femoral head may be grossly deformed with a saddle-shaped deformity with the depression in the femoral head under the lip of the acetabulum. The central depressed zone of the femoral head is excised (Figure 30.7).

The extruded lateral portion may have reasonably good articular cartilage and so may the medial portion of the femoral head. These are brought together and fixed with two countersunk screws. This creates a femoral head contour that is reasonably spherical and a distinct improvement from the preoperative status. Bleeding from the cut edges of the osteotomy is noted during surgery.

Retroversion of the acetabulum is defined as a posterior orientation of the acetabular opening in the sagittal plane. It can be detected on plain radiographs by the crossover sign and the posterior wall sign. The crossover sign is seen when the anterior wall shadow passes horizontally and medially and

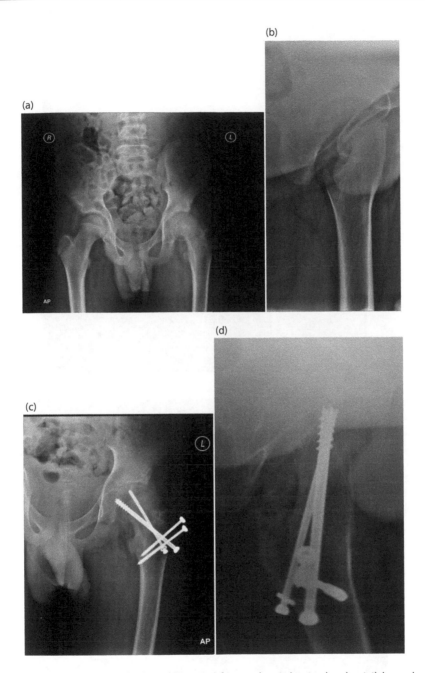

Figure 30.6 **(a,b)** A 15-year-old with slipped capital femoral epiphysis clearly visible on lateral x-rays with the posterior slip, with a history of 3 months. **(c,d)** After surgical dislocation of hip and extended retinacular flap, the capital femoral epiphysis is reduced over the femoral neck and the bump is excised. Two cross screws fix the epiphysis and two screws fix the trochanteric osteotomy.

crosses the more vertical outline of the posterior wall. Normally these do not cross on a proper pelvis AP radiograph (which shows a distance of 2–5 cm between symphysis pubis and coccyx). The posterior wall sign is positive when the outline of

the posterior wall lies medial to the center of the femoral head. CT scans show this well in horizontal acetabular cross-sections.

Acetabular retroversion causes a "pincer" impingement where the anterolateral aspect of the

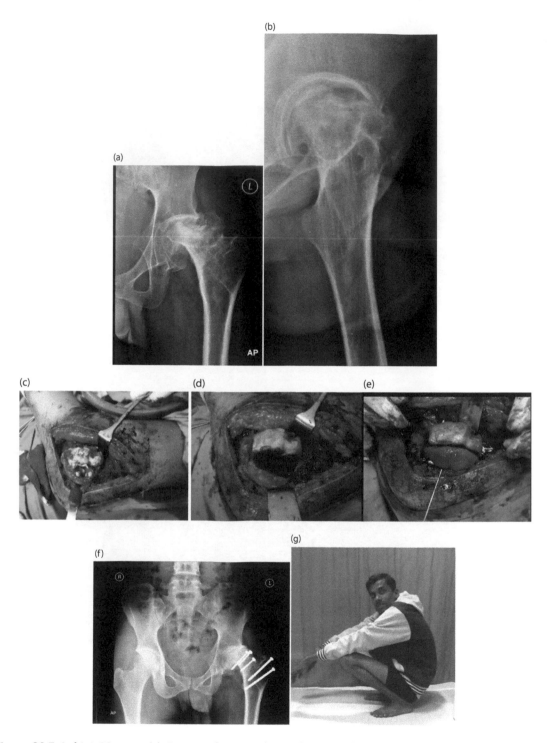

Figure 30.7 **(a,b)** A 22-year-old, 3 years after AVN hip with severe destruction of the femoral head with a saddle-shaped trough defect in the center under the lip of the acetabulum. Patient cannot walk at all and HHS < 30. **(c–e)** Surgical dislocation of the hip showing the severe damage to femoral head in the center. The central portion is excised **(d)** and the lateral and medial ends coapted together with screws to recreate a semblance of sphericity of the femoral head. **(f,g)** Seven years after surgery, the femoral head is well maintained and he has almost full flexion in the hip, though external rotation is still restricted. There is no pain, he can walk at least 6 km at a stretch, and his HHS is more than 90.

acetabulum impinges on the femoral head–neck junction, especially if it has a poor head–neck offset. This is apparent with the FADDIR test in which the flexion-adduction-internal rotation will clearly cause the patient to wince in pain.

In many instances, both cam and pincer impingement are present. With repeated impingement, the acetabular labrum starts getting worn and this may progress to acetabular cartilage damage over time.

Acetabular retroversion can be treated either by trimming the acetabular rim (especially anteriorly and laterally) or by a redirectional periacetabular osteotomy. This chapter will focus on surgical dislocation of the hip to either perform femoral head surgery or at the acetabular rim.

We can perform an acetabular rim trim with refixation of the labrum[18] with anchor sutures. If the acetabular labrum is badly frayed or deficient, reconstruction of the labrum may be attempted with a rolled portion of the fascia lata.

Pipkin-type femoral head fracture can be reduced and fixed nicely with this approach.[19]

In a case with a large exostosis of the femoral neck caused by hereditary multiple exostosis, the exposure with this method enables us to perform almost circumferential excision of the exostosis, dramatically improve the range of motion, and prevent arthritis.

COMPLICATIONS

General complications like wound infection, Deep Vein Thrombosis (DVT), and pulmonary embolism are possible, and routine precautions are needed. Nonunion of the greater trochanter flip fragment is possible. The step cut osteotomy helps in better fixation and can avoid the problem.

Heterotopic ossification around the tip of the trochanter can develop. Routine prophylaxis using indomethacin may or may not be used depending on extent of muscle handling and damage.

Excessive excision of the head–neck junction may lead to weakening of the neck and fracture. Notching at the femoral head–neck junction may result in early degeneration of the femoral head. Careless technique or excessive anterior displacement may lead to iatrogenic avascular necrosis, though its rates are not found to be high. Laser Doppler flowmetry[20] probes can be implanted to ascertain femoral head blood flow.

CONCLUSION

Safe surgical dislocation of the hip gives complete access to the hip joint. Surgeries to correct femoroacetabular impingement caused by common conditions like AVN, post Perthes, and dysplastic hips can be done. The approach offers possibility of performing intra-articular surgeries to overcome impingement and prolong the life of these hips in the short to medium term.

REFERENCES

1. Notzli HP et al. The contour of the femoral head–neck junction as a predictor for the risk of anterior impingement. *J Bone Joint Surg Br* 2002; 84: 556–60.
2. Ito K et al. Femoroacetabular impingement and the cam-effect. A MRI-based quantitative anatomical study of the femoral head neck offset. *J Bone Joint Surg Br* 2001; 83: 171–6.
3. Ganz R et al. Femoroacetabular impingement: A cause for osteoarthritis of the hip. *Clin Orthop Relat Res* 2003; 417: 112–20.
4. Lavigne M, Parvizi J, Beck M, Siebenrock KA, Ganz R, Leunig M. Anterior femoroacetabular impingement: Part I. Techniques of joint preserving surgery. *Clin Orthop Relat Res* 2004; (418): 61–6.
5. Byrd JW. Evaluation of the hip: History and physical examination. *N Am J Sports Phys Ther* 2007; 2(4): 231–40.
6. Clohisy JC, Carlisle JC, Beaule PE, Kim Y-J, Trousdale RT, Sierra RJ. A systematic approach to the plain radiographic evaluation of the young adult hip. *J Bone Joint Surg [Am]* 2008; 90(Suppl. 4): 47–66.
7. Learmouth Ian D, Young C, Rorabeck C. The operation of the century: Total hip replacement. *Lancet* 2007; 370(9597): 1508–19.
8. Ganz R, Gill TJ, Gautier E, Ganz K, Krugel N, Berlemann U. Surgical dislocation of the adult hip: A technique with full access to the femoral head and acetabulum without the risk of avascular necrosis. *J Bone Joint Surg Br* 2001; 83(8): 1119–24.
9. Gautier E, Ganz K, Krugel N, Gill T, Ganz R. Anatomy of the medial femoral circumflex artery and its surgical implications. *J Bone Joint Surg [Br]* 2000; 82-B: 679–83.

10. Chaudhary MM, Chaudhary IM, Vikas K, KoKo A, Zaw T, Siddhartha A. Surgical hip dislocation for treatment of cam femoro-acetabular impingement. *Indian J Orthop* 2015; 49: 496–501.

11. Peters CL, Erickson JA. Treatment of femoro-acetabular impingement with surgical dislocation and debridement in young adults. *J Bone Joint Surg Am* 2006; 88: 1735–41.

12. Beaulé PE, Le Duff MJ, Zaragoza E. Quality of life following femoral head–neck osteochondroplasty for femoroacetabular impingement. *J Bone Joint Surg Am* 2007; 89: 773–9.

13. Mont M, Jones L, Hungerford D. Current concepts review: Nontraumatic osteonecrosis of the femoral head: Ten years later. *J Bone Joint Surg Am* 2006; (88-A): 1117–32.

14. Leunig M, Ganz R. Relative neck lengthening and intracapital osteotomy for severe Perthes and Perthes-like deformities. *Bull NYU Hosp Jt Dis* 2011; 69(Suppl 1): S62–7.

15. Leunig M, Ganz R, Huff TW. Extended retinacular soft tissue flap for intra-articular hip surgery: surgical technique, indications, and results of application. *AAOS-Instructional Course Lectures* 2009; 58.

16. Ilizarov GA. *Transosseous Osteosynthesis. Theoretical and Clinical Aspects of Regeneration and Growth of Tissue.* Berlin: Springer, 1992.

17. Paley D. The treatment of femoral head deformity and coxa magna by the Ganz femoral head reduction osteotomy. *Ortho Clin North Am* 2011; 42(3): 389–99.

18. Espinosa N, Rothenfluh DA, Beck M, Ganz R, Leunig M. Treatment of femoro-acetabular impingement: Preliminary results of labral refixation. *J Bone Joint Surg Am* 2006; (88-A): 925–35.

19. Swiontkowski MF, Thorpe M, Seiler JG, Hansen ST. Operative management of displaced femoral head fractures: Case matched comparison of anterior versus posterior approaches for Pipkin I and Pipkin II fractures. *J Orthop Trauma* 1992; 6: 437–42.

20. Nötzli HP, Siebenrock KA, Hempfing A, Ramseier LE, Ganz R. Perfusion of the femoral head during surgical dislocation of the hip monitoring by laser Doppler flowmetry. *J Bone Joint Surg [Br]* 2002; 84-B: 300–4.

31

Endoscopic shelf acetabuloplasty for the treatment of patients in the setting of hip dysplasia

SOSHI UCHIDA, DEAN K. MATSUDA, AND AKINORI SAKAI

One of the authors (S.U.) is a consultant for Smith & Nephew and Zimmer-Biomet and received research funds from Smith & Nephew, Pfizer, and Johnson & Johnson. This article is unrelated to any funds. The authors report no other conflicts of interest to disclose that may affect the information and recommendations presented in the manuscript.

Each author certifies that he or she has no commercial associations (e.g., consultancies, stock ownership, equity interest, patent/licensing arrangements, etc.) that might pose a conflict of interest in connection with the submitted article. Informed consent has been obtained from the patient. The patient approved the use of her data for the publication of this manuscript.

INTRODUCTION

Hip dysplasia is one of the most common causes of hip pain in athletes in the Asian population.[1] Athletes with hip dysplasia typically present with groin and lateral hip pain, which is associated with intra-articular pathologies, including labral tear and cartilage damage. Numerous studies have demonstrated that the anterosuperior and superolateral shallow acetabulum can cause repetitive overloading, resulting in labral tearing, cartilage damage, and sometimes rim stress fracture, which predispose them to osteoarthritis. In addition, many patients with hip dysplasia also present with groin and lateral hip pain that can result from chronic fatigue overload of the periarticular musculotendon structures, including the gluteus maximus, Ilio Tibial (IT) band, rectus femoris, and ilopsoas tendon snapping issues. Hip dysplasia has been better defined as being closely linked with hypermobile sports activities such as rhythmic gymnastics, figure skating, and ballet.[2] Another study has shown that throwing athletes (baseball players) also have hip dysplasia in 7.9% and borderline hip dysplasia in 15.9%.[3] Recent studies have emerged indicating that cam deformities often coexist with developmental dysplasia of hip (DDH).[4]

Previous studies have established hip arthroscopy as a beneficial procedure for treating borderline and mild DDH; however, the recent literature reports a high reoperation rate and progressing osteoarthritis with conversion to total hip arthroplasty. Our study advises against performing hip arthroscopy for DDH when patients have a broken Shenton line, a femoral neck shaft angle greater than 140°, and lateral center edge angle less than 19°. Some recent studies have shown that patients in the setting of borderline DDH (BDDH) can respond favorably to hip arthroscopic labral preservation and capsular plication surgery.[5] Furthermore, our recent study also counsels against performing hip arthroscopic labral preservation for BDDH when patients have a broken Shenton line, age older than 42 years, vertical center anterior angle less than 13°, acetabular inclination greater than 17°, and severe cartilage damage at the time of the surgery.[6] There are several reports looking at the effectiveness of various surgical procedures to address hip dysplasia. In this chapter, we describe how to manage hip dysplasia in athletes.

PURPOSE

The purpose of this chapter is to demonstrate surgical technique and effectiveness of endoscopic shelf acetabuloplasty in the treatment of patients in the setting of hip dysplasia.

INDICATIONS

Indications for endoscopic shelf acetabuloplasty must include all of the following: (1) symptomatic borderline, mild to moderate DDH (5° < LCEA < 25°, 5° < VCA < 25°); (2) Tonnis grade 0 or 1; (3) young active patients; (4) age younger than 45 years old; and (5) femoral neck shaft angle less than 140° and no severe femoral deformity.

CONTRAINDICATIONS

This procedure should not be recommended for severe dysplasia (broken Shenton line and LCEA <5°) and progressive osteoarthritis, including severe chondral damage.

Patients older than 50 years old are relatively contraindicated for this procedure.

If femoral anteversion is greater than 40°, femoral derotational osteotomy should be considered at the same time.

Preoperative radiographic evaluation

Plain radiographs are widely available and give us a good visualization of the overall morphology of the pelvis and the proximal femur. They can also serve as the basis for surgical decision-making in joint-preservation surgery including hip arthroscopy or endoscopic shelf acetabuloplasty.

An anterior posterior pelvis view at supine and standing positions should be performed. Lateral center edge angle, Tonnis angle, femoral neck shaft angle, and Shenton line can be assessed[7] (Figure 31.1a).

The false profile view of Lequesne is performed to evaluate the anterior acetabular coverage or anterosuperior subluxation of the femoral head, which is of particular interest in DDH.[8] The ventral center anterior (VCA) angle should be measured (Figure 31.1b). Modified Dunn view is performed to evaluate cam deformity at femoral head–neck junction which is high-frequently associated with DDH (Figure 31.1c).

Preoperative three-dimensional imaging and CT scanning are really invaluable to evaluate the head–neck junction, acetabular coverage, acetabular version and femoral version. If you get additional cuts through the distal femoral condyles, you can also look at femoral neck angle to evaluate femoral anteversion[9] (Figure 31.1d).

Femoral anteversion is correlated with acetabular version in DDH patients with anterior and global shallow socket.[10] Increased femoral anteversion is most likely to be associated with osteoarthritis.[11]

SURGICAL TECHNIQUE

Supine hip arthroscopy is performed on a traction table under general anesthesia. Anterolateral, midanterior and proximal midanterior portals (ALP, MAP, and PMAP) are created. Interportal capsulotomy is performed. Intra-articular pathologies, including acetabular chondrolabral damage and femoral head chondral damage, are assessed and documented (Figure 31.2a).

Microfracture chondroplasty is performed if ICRS grade III or IV chondral defects are present. Next, unstable labral tears are addressed with midsubstance repair following conservative rim trimming using a motorized burr to create a bleeding bone surface. Midsubstance labral repair is performed using bioabsorbable suture anchors (OsteoRaptor, Smith & Nephew, Andover, MA) with knots tied on the capsular side of the labrum (Figure 31.2b).

Arthroscopic dynamic examination is performed to assess for cam impingement. When necessary, cam osteochondroplasty using a motorized round burr is performed (Figure 31.2c).

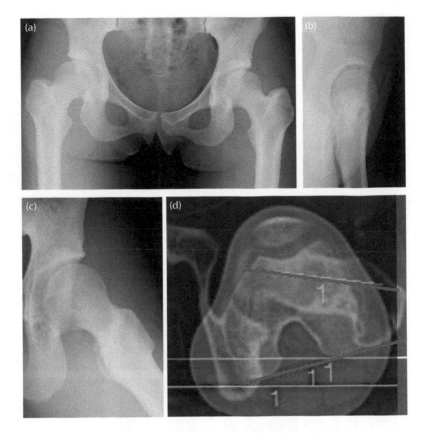

Figure 31.1 (a) A 19-year-old female rhythmic gymnast with developmental dysplasia of the hip presented to us with a 6-month history of right hip pain. Diagnostic preoperative pelvic AP radiograph shows DDH. The center edge angle was 14° and the Sharp angle was 50°. (b) Preoperative false profile view also shows anterior shallowness of acetabulum. The vertical-center-anterior (VCA) angle was 14°. (c) A modified Dunn view showing aspherical shape of the femoral head and alpha angle is 55, suggesting cam lesion. (d) A computed tomography with additional cut of distal femur showing femoral version is 28°.

Following cam impingement evaluation and reshaping, shoelace capsular closure is performed using Ultratape (Smith & Nephew, Andover, MA) with the hip at 40° of flexion via the MAP and PMAP (Figure 31.2d).[12]

Endoscopic shelf acetabuloplasty is then performed as described previously.[1] A 30° arthroscope is positioned into the extracapsular space under fluoroscopic guidance. After identifying the straight and reflected heads of the rectus femoris and debriding the latter with a shaver and radiofrequency ablator, two parallel 2.4-mm guide wires are introduced using the drill guide through the MAP, along the anterior acetabular rim adjacent to the capsule (Figure 31.2e).

The slot is enlarged with the use of 10-mm osteotome to measure approximately 5 to 6 mm in height, 25 mm in width, and at least 20 mm in depth (Figure 31.2f).

The optimum width and depth are confirmed using a custom-made dilator. Autologous tricortical bone graft (tricortical) is harvested from the ipsilateral iliac crest (Figure 31.2g).

Two 1.5-mm Kirschner wires are introduced in 1.8-mm-diameter drill holes, helping to control the graft position during endoscopic insertion into the aforementioned anterolateral periacetabular slot (Figure 31.2h). Finally, the free bone graft is secured into the appropriate position, with the cortical surface facing the femoral head in intimate contact with the intervening capsule, using a press-fit technique with a cannulated bone tamp (Smith & Nephew, Japan) (Figure 31.2i).

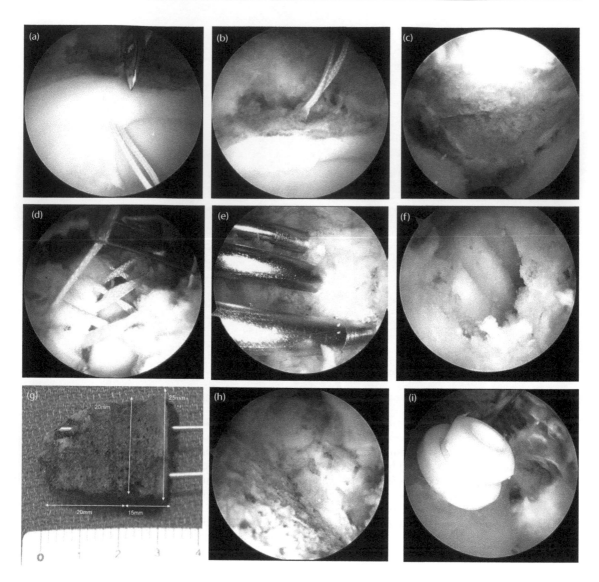

Figure 31.2 Endoscopic shelf acetabuloplasty. (a) Supine arthroscopic view from the anterolateral portal (ALP) showing an anterior superior labral tear, and suture anchors was placed at the acetabulum. (b) Labral repair with suture anchor is visualized from the ALP. (c) Arthroscopic view from the midanterior portal (MAP) showing cam osteoplasty. (d) Shoelace capsular closure using Ultratape via the midanterior portal (MAP) and the proximal midanterior portal (PMAP) viewing from the ALP. (e) Three 2.4-mm guide wires were introduced through the MAP under fluoroscopy. (f) Cannulated drill is used through the guide wires to make the shelf slot. (g) A free bone graft harvested from ipsilateral iliac crest, with two parallel 1.5-mm Kirschner wires. (h) A free bone autograft is inserted into the slot through the guide wires with press-fit fixation. (i) An additional cortical bone graft is inserted above the new shelf and fixed with hydroxyapatite PLLA screw and washer to support shelf graft under endoscopic guidance[1].

Postoperative rehabilitation

Patients are instructed to use flat foot weight bearing for the first 3 weeks. If microfracture is performed, weight-bearing limitations are extended to 6–8 weeks. Patients are placed in a brace (U hip brace; Sigmax) for 2–3 weeks to protect the hip and limit flexion (0~120°), abduction (0~45°), and rotation (external rotation 0°). Gentle, passive range of motion (ROM) exercise is initiated during the first week, under supervision of a physiotherapist. Circumduction is performed at 70° of hip

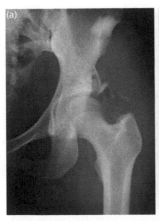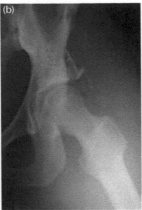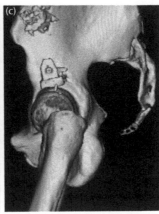

Figure 31.3 **(a, b)** A pelvic AP and modified Dunn radiographs showing improved coverage of the acetabulum with a shelf graft just after surgery. LCE angle was 41°. **(c)** A 3D-CT showing proper location of the shelf graft.

flexion and neutral hip flexion for the first 2 weeks. Then, continuous passive motion (CPM) is used to avoid adhesive capsulitis by applying 0–90° of hip flexion for up to 4 hours a day for 2 weeks.

During Phase II (weeks 6–12), patients improve their mobility, stability, and proprioception activity. Endurance strengthening is commenced only after range of motion is maximized and after a good stability in gait and movement is demonstrated.

Patients are allowed to progress to Phase III (weeks 12–16) only if passive ROM is symmetric pain free, with a normal gait patter. Aerobic conditioning is advanced using an elliptical machine with a goal of 30 min of continuous exercise at a low to moderate intensity.

Patients are allowed to progress to physical activity only if passive ROM is symmetric and pain free, with a normal gait pattern. The goal of Phase IV is to allow safe and gentle sports drills to prepare the patients to return to play or work activities. Gentle sports-specific or work agility exercises are initiated.[13]

Postoperative radiographs (AP and modified Dunn view) show the improvement of lateral center-edge angle (LCEA) and femoral head–neck offset. The three-dimensional CT shows a shelf graft was inserted in the anterosuperior aspect of the hip joint (Figure 31.3a–c).

Outcomes of shelf

Our recent study described in a series of 32 active patients undergoing endoscopic shelf acetabuloplasty combined with labral repair that the mean PRO scores (modified Harris hip score, nonarthrithis hip score, and iHot) significantly improved from preoperatively to postoperatively.

We demonstrated 90% of patients returned to sports-related activity within a mean period of 9 months, and UCLA activity score also significantly improved.[1]

Recent technical notes have shown that endoscopic shelf acetabuloplasty can address hip dysplasia athletes with large bone cysts as well as rim stress fracture.[14,15]

Take-home message

Preoperative patient evaluation and planning is paramount for successful treatment.

Patient's history, examination, and imaging studies are helpful to understand the existing pathology and offer the best treatment option.

The patient's view and expectations should not be neglected.

Educate your patients about their disease and discuss the importance of compliance with postoperative rehabilitation.

REFERENCES

1. Uchida S et al. Endoscopic shelf acetabuloplasty can improve clinical outcomes and achieve return to sports-related activity in active patients with hip dysplasia. *Knee Surg Sports Traumatol Arthrosc* 2018; 26(10): 3165–77.

2. Charbonnier C et al. Assessment of congruence and impingement of the hip joint in professional ballet dancers: A motion capture study. *Am J Sports Med* 2011; 39(3): 557–66.

3. Fukushima K et al. Prevalence of radiological findings related to femoroacetabular impingement in professional baseball players in Japan. *J Orthop Sci* 2016; 21(6): 821–5.

4. Uchida S et al. Clinical and radiographic predictors for worsened clinical outcomes after hip arthroscopic labral preservation and capsular closure in developmental dysplasia of the hip. *Am J Sports Med* 2016; 44(1): 28–38.

5. Domb BG, Chaharbakhshi EO, Perets I, Yuen LC, Walsh JP, Ashberg L. Hip arthroscopic surgery with labral preservation and capsular plication in patients with borderline hip dysplasia: Minimum 5-year patient-reported outcomes. *Am J Sports Med* 2018; 46(2): 305–13.

6. Hatakeyama A et al. Predictors of poor clinical outcome following arthroscopic labral preservation, capsular plication and cam osteoplasty in the setting of borderline hip dysplasia. *Am J Sports Med* 2017; 46(1): 135–43.

7. Wiberg G. The anatomy and roentgenographic appearance of a normal hip joint. *Acta Chir Scand* 1939; 83(Suppl 58): 7–38.

8. Chosa E, Tajima N. Anterior acetabular head index of the hip on false-profile views. New index of anterior acetabular cover. *J Bone Joint Surg Br* 2003; 85(6): 826–9.

9. Boster IR, Ozoude GC, Martin DE, Siddiqi AJ, Kuppuswami SK, Domb BG. Femoral anteversion in the hip: Comparison of measurement by computed tomography, magnetic resonance imaging, and physical examination. *Arthroscopy* 2012; 28(5): 619–27.

10. Akiyama M et al. Femoral anteversion is correlated with acetabular version and coverage in Asian women with anterior and global deficient subgroups of hip dysplasia: A CT study. *Skeletal Radiol* 2012; 41(11): 1411–8.

11. Tonnis D, Heinecke A. Acetabular and femoral anteversion: Relationship with osteoarthritis of the hip. *J Bone Joint Surg Am* 1999; 81(12): 1747–70.

12. Uchida S et al. Arthroscopic shoelace capsular closure technique in the hip using Ultratape. *Arthrosc Tech* 2017; 6(1): e157–61.

13. Spencer-Gardner L, Eischen JJ, Levy BA, Sierra RJ, Engasser WM, Krych AJ. A comprehensive five-phase rehabilitation programme after hip arthroscopy for femoroacetabular impingement. *Knee Surg Sports Traumatol Arthrosc* 2014; 22(4): 848–59.

14. Uchida S, Shimizu Y, Yukizawa Y, Suzuki H, Pascual-Garrido C, Sakai A. Arthroscopic management for acetabular rim stress fracture and osteochondritis dissecans in the athlete with hip dysplasia. *Arthrosc Tech* 2018; 7(5): e533–9.

15. Yamada K, Matsuda DK, Suzuki H, Sakai A, Uchida S. Endoscopic shelf acetabuloplasty for treating acetabular large bone cyst in patient with dysplasia. *Arthrosc Tech* 2018; 7.

32

Osteotomy to correct unstable intertrochanteric fractures

MUHAMMAD ZAHID SAEED

INTRODUCTION

The art of osteotomy has been practiced in the management of unstable intertrochanteric hip fractures in order to increase the stability of fracture fragments and improve load sharing between them.[1] The reported incidence of loss of fixation of intertrochanteric fractures is 4–12%, most commonly witnessed with unstable fracture patterns.[2]

Intertrochanteric fractures occur in the region between the greater and lesser trochanters of the proximal femur. The intertrochanteric region consists of dense trabecular cancellous bone with an abundant blood supply. As a consequence, nonunion and osteonecrosis (avascular necrosis) are less challenging than in femoral neck fractures.[2]

An unstable intertrochanteric fracture of the hip is a challenging situation for the patient and the surgeon. The fracture has characteristics that predispose it to displace even after satisfactory reduction and fixation have been accomplished. Severe displacement and an unstable fracture pattern, however, can result in malunion, nonunion, and failure of the fixation device.[3]

Osteotomies are rarely used as salvage procedures to treat malunion and nonunion following fixation of unstable intertrochanteric fractures.[4]

ANATOMY

The intertrochanteric area exists between greater and lesser trochanters. The calcar femorale consists of the vertical wall of dense bone that extends from the posteromedial aspect of the femoral shaft to the posterior portion of the femoral neck. It helps determine stable versus unstable fracture patterns.[1-5]

The muscle forces usually produce shortening, external rotation, and varus deformity at the fracture site as follows:[1-5]

- Hip abductors cause the greater trochanter to displace laterally and proximally.
- The iliopsoas causes the lesser trochanter to displace medially and proximally.
- The hip flexors, extensors, and adductors cause the distal fragment to move proximally.

DEFINITION OF UNSTABLE FRACTURES

Early identification of the instability is imperative.[3] The posteromedial bony contact, which acts as a buttress against fracture collapse, has been historically used to determine fracture stability.[2] Reverse oblique intertrochanteric fractures are unstable fractures and are described by an oblique fracture line extending from the medial cortex proximally to the lateral cortex distally. The reverse oblique fracture configuration is inherently unstable because of the tendency for medial displacement of the femoral shaft.[1-3]

Intertrochanteric hip fractures are defined as unstable by the presence of one or more of the following:[1]

- Four-part fractures[1]
- Fractures with posteromedial cortical commination[2]
- Fractures with reverse obliquity of the main fracture line[3]
- Fractures with large and separate posterior trochanteric fragment[4]
- Fractures with subtrochanteric extension[5]

CLINICAL ASSESSMENT

Unstable intertrochanteric fractures can sometimes be predicted during the physical examination.[2,3] An unstable intertrochanteric fracture may present with an internally rotated or severely shortened painful limb.[3] Radiographs are likely to show marked displacement, commination, or reverse obliquity in unstable fracture patterns. An anteroposterior (AP) view of the pelvis (Figure 32.1) and an AP and cross-table lateral view of the involved proximal femur are helpful in making the diagnosis.[2]

A internal rotation view of the injured hip may be helpful to elucidate the fracture configuration further.[2]

Magnetic resonance imaging (MRI) is currently the investigation of choice in delineating displaced or occult fractures that are not clearly seen on plain

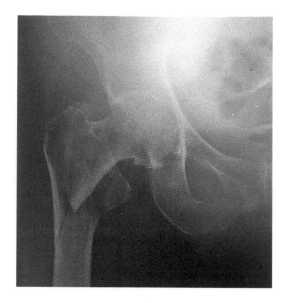

Figure 32.1 Unstable intertrochanteric fracture with posteromedial commination. (From Royal Free Hospital data.)

radiographs. Bone scans or computed tomography (CT) scanning is helpful for those who have contraindications to MRI scan.[2,5] Preoperative diagnosis of the unstable intertrochanteric hip fracture helps the surgeon to select the treatment that most reduces the risks of malunion, nonunion, and failure of the fixation device.[3,5]

PRINCIPLES OF FIXATION OF UNSTABLE FRACTURE

The basic principles of fracture fixation are identical to fracture fixation elsewhere in the body.[2,3,5,6]

A. Accurate fracture reduction to restore anatomical relationships: Accurate approximation of the medial cortices of the two major fragments of an intertrochanteric fracture greatly enhances the effectiveness of the fixation provided by the internal fixation. Failure to achieve such reduction or disruption of the medial cortex results in complications, the most common being superior migration of compression lag screw.

B. Stable fracture fixation as guided by the "personality" of fracture, patient, and injury requires: Stability of fracture fixation depends on the bone quality, fracture pattern, fracture reduction, implant design, and implant placement. There is sufficient evidence that surgery should be performed in a timely manner once the patient has been medically stabilized.

A surgeon should avoid a varus malreduction and obtain stable fixation of the proximal fragment to elude failure of fixation. Additionally, the surgeon must bypass the most distal shaft stress riser by two diaphysis diameters (about 6 cm).

Fixation into the femoral head, whether associated with a side plate or a nail, should be centered in both planes. The "tip to apex" distance has been designated as a method to quantify a deep and central position of the lag screw in the femoral head, and should be used as a guideline in these cases.[6,7]

C. Preservation of blood supply to soft tissues and bone.

D. Early and safe mobilization of the injured part and the patient as a whole: The objective is stable internal fixation to permit early mobilization and full weight-bearing ambulation.

CHOICE OF IMPLANTS

Historically, the dynamic hip screw (DHS) has been the most frequently used device for both stable and unstable fracture patterns. It is available in plate angles from 130° to 150°.

Plates with 95° blades are very beneficial because they are placed in the bone in the inferior portion of the femoral head, which typically has not been violated before by fixation devices.

Intramedullary fixation can be used:

- Where the lateral femoral wall is fractured
- In fractures with reverse obliquity configuration
- In fractures with subtrochanteric extension
- In fractures with large posteromedial fragments[2–5]

Intramedullary hip screw nail

This implant is designed with the features of a dynamic hip screw and intramedullary nail (IMN).

Prosthetic replacement is reserved for cases when the unstable fractures are not amenable for surgical fixation due to severely comminuted and poor quality of bone, mainly due to osteoporosis.

External fixation is rarely used today.

ROLE OF OSTEOTOMIES

In the past, Dimon and Hughston osteotomies and the medial displacement osteotomy have been promoted as a means of increasing resistance to varus displacement.[8] Sarmiento developed a valgus osteotomy technique to decrease bending forces at the fracture site and achieve stable configuration to facilitate fracture healing.

DIMON AND HUGHSTON OSTEOTOMY

It is an established fact that restoration of medial continuity is crucial to successful internal fixation of three- and four-part intertrochanteric fractures. Dimon and Hughston described techniques of osteotomy in the trochanteric region with valgus lag screw placement and medial displacement to improve stability.

Surgical technique

The surgical procedure is carried out with the patient in the supine position on a radiolucent fracture table with c-arm fluoroscopy, which is used throughout the procedure to check the position of wire, screws, and plate (Figures 32.2 and 32.3). The limb is held by the foot support (boot). A straight lateral incision is made approximately two fingerbreadths below the vastus ridge to a point

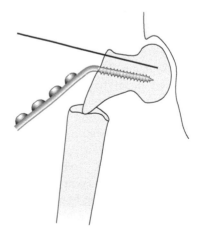

Figure 32.2 Dimon and Hughston described techniques of osteotomy in the trochanteric area with valgus lag screw placement and medial displacement to improve stability.

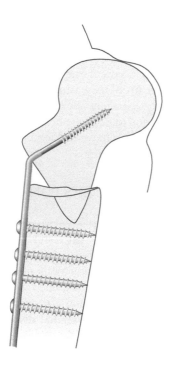

Figure 32.3 Dimon and Hughston osteotomy: The lag compression screw is inserted over a guide wire, the calcar spike (proximal fragment) is placed into the medially displaced distal fragment, and a 135° angle side plate is fixed to the femoral shaft with four screws.

5–7 cm distally. The greater trochanteric fragment is returned superiorly for exposure if required. A transverse osteotomy is created at a level approximately 2 cm below the lesser trochanter. A pin or k wire is inserted into the superior third of the femoral head (Figure 32.2). A large towel clip can be inserted onto the superior portion of neck segment in order to control rotation. The calcar spike (proximal fragment) is positioned into the medially displaced distal fragment (Figure 32.2). A guide wire is placed into the lower half of femoral head. This wire position must ensure a more valgus orientation of femoral neck once the screw and side plate have been applied. Measure the appropriate screw length. The bone is reamed with triple reamer. Insert lag compression screw over the guide wire. Abduct leg to bring the reduction into valgus. Apply the side plate, which consists of 135° angles with short or long barrel segments (Figure 32.3). Release traction, and apply the standard or locking screws though the 135° angle plate. Consider reattaching the trochanteric fragment if necessary. Check the final position with c-arm

fluoroscopy. Close the wound in layers and apply surgical dressing. Postoperatively, the patient should be advised to mobilize full weight bearing as tolerated to reduce the complications associated with immobility, i.e. DVT, PE, pressure sores, and chest infection.

SARMIENTO OSTEOTOMY FOR INTERTROCHANTERIC FRACTURES

Sarmiento developed a valgus osteotomy technique (Figures 32.4 and 32.5) for the treatment of unstable intertrochanteric fractures. It involves creating an oblique osteotomy of the distal fragment (valgus osteotomy) to obtain stability in unstable intertrochanteric fractures. The osteotomy changes the fracture plane from vertical to near horizontal and approximates the cortical surfaces of the two major fragments and medial and posterior cortex of proximal and distal fragments, and places the neck of the femur in a valgus position. The goal is to obtain posteromedial stability. The advantage of this valgus osteotomy is that valgus realignment of proximal fragment makes up for less of the length at the ostetomy site so that limb lengths remain equal.[9]

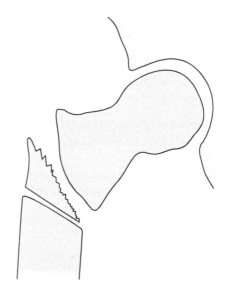

Figure 32.4 An oblique osteotomy of the distal fragment is made, starting proximally and laterally slightly below the flare of the grouter trochanter and extending distally and medially to a point approximately 1 cm below the apex of the fracture.

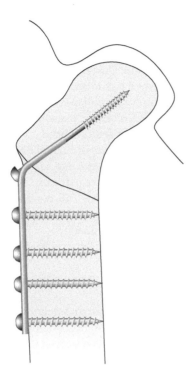

Figure 32.5 A lag compression screw is placed over the wire in the femoral head. Abduct the leg to bring the distal fragment in contact with the plate, appose the medial cortices, and apply four-hole 135° angle plate.

Surgical technique

The surgical procedure is carried out with the patient in the supine position on a fracture table; the limb is placed in the foot piece in approximately 10° of internal rotation. Through a lateral incision, which at its proximal end curves slightly forward toward the anterior superior spine of the ilium, the shaft of the femur is exposed. At this time, an attempt must be made to reduce the fracture.

An oblique osteotomy of the distal fragment is fashioned, starting proximally and laterally slightly below the flare of the grouter trochanter and extending distally and medially to a point approximately 1 cm below the apex of the fracture (Figure 32.4). Before starting the osteotomy, drill holes are made through the distal fragment, with special care being taken to drill through the medial cortex of the bone to prevent its shattering as the osteotomy is finalized with a sharp osteotome. Once the osteotomy is accomplished,

the resulting wedge-shaped fragment is retracted laterally (Figure 32.5) to expose the medullary canal of the proximal fragment. Then a guide wire is placed into the proximal end or the femur parallel to the anterior cortex and at approximately 90° to the plane of the fracture line. In patients in whom the plane of the fracture is more vertical, the wire should be inclined distally so that the inferior angle of entry of the guide wire with respect to the plane of the fracture is less than 90°. Make sure the distance of the entry point from the medial cortex essentially is equal to the medial-to-lateral width of the osteotomized surface of the distal fragment. However, to allow for the width of the nail/lag screw, the guide wire should be placed 0.5 cm higher than the measured point of insertion. Once accurate placement of the wire has been confirmed under the image intensifier, a lag compression screw is placed over the wire in the femoral head.

Abduct the leg to bring the distal fragment in contact with the plate. This maneuver will appose the medial cortices accurately (Figure 32.5).

In fractures with severe damage to the postero-medial cortex of the femur, the contact surface may be too small to provide adequate stability. Any bone on the lateral and proximal portion of the distal fragment that obstructs the proper contact of the metallic plate and the lateral surface of the femoral shaft must be taken away with a rongeur. Once the fragments have been approximated, the plate portion of the lag screw is fixed to the shaft with four standard or locking screws (Figure 32.5).

Internal rotation of the distal fragment during the entire surgical procedure is essential because during the insertion of the lag screw, the proximal fragment is lifted and therefore internally rotated. If a similar degree of internal rotation is not given to the distal fragment, there will be an external rotation deformity of the limb at the conclusion of the surgical procedure. No effort is made to reapproximate the trochanter to the femur. Nonunion of the loose trochanter has not resulted from this procedure.

The shortening of the extremity would be anticipated after fixation as the osteotomy is fashioned below the surface of the fracture. However, the valgus deformity of the proximal fragment counterbalances for the loss of length with the result that in most cases the extremities are of equal length. Check the final position of fractured bones and fixation with c-arm fluoroscopy. Close the wound in layers and apply surgical dressing. Full weight bearing as tolerated is advised to reduce the complications associated with immobility, i.e. DVT, PE, chest infection, and pressure sores.

PLACEMENT OF CALCAR SPIKE (PROXIMAL FRAGMENT) INTO THE MEDIALLY DISPLACED DISTAL FRAGMENT WITHOUT OSTEOTOMY

In fractures with severe commination, the operating surgeon can place the calcar spike (proximal fragment) into the medially displaced distal fragment without osteotomy. It helps to convert the unstable fracture configuration into the stable fracture pattern, and excellent results can be achieved with fixation of the fracture with a dynamic hip screw (Figure 32.6).

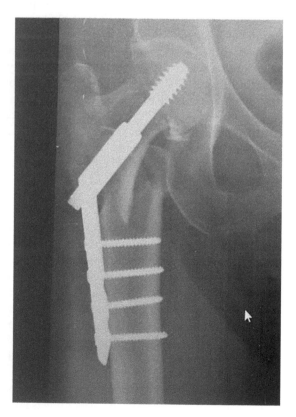

Figure 32.6 Placement of calcar spike (proximal fragment) into the medially displaced distal fragment without osteotomy. (From Royal Free Hospital data.)

COMPLICATIONS OF SURGICAL FIXATION

A. *Loss of fixation*: Unstable fracture pattern is an established risk factor. It most frequently results from varus collapse of the proximal fragment and eccentric placement of the lag screw within the femoral head.
B. *Nonunion*: It is a rare occurrence and is seen in less than 2% of patients, especially in patients with unstable fracture patterns.
C. *Malrotation deformity*: This results from excessive internal rotation of the distal fragment at the time of internal fixation.
D. Osteonecrosis of the femoral head is rarely seen.
E. Deep vein thrombosis and pulmonary embolism are rare.
F. Mortality risk is approximately 20%–30% in the first year following the fracture. A decrease in 1-year mortality is observed if surgery is performed within 48 hours.

SALVAGE OF FIXATION FAILURE

For young patients with unstable intertrochanteric fracture fixation failures, repeat Open Reduction and Internal Fixation (ORIF) is preferred. It is recommended to support the inferior femoral head bone with a fixed angle device, such as a blade plate. In older osteoporotic patients with intertrochanteric fracture fixation failures, total hip replacement or hip hemiarthroplasty remains the best option. The lag screw cut-out has typically happened and little proximal bone remains. Hemiarthroplasty or total hip replacement can both be effective, depending on the status of the acetabular articular surface. Femoral reconstruction in such scenarios highlights multiple challenges, including stress risers, bone loss, and greater trochanteric malunion. Careful consideration of indications, techniques, and circumventing common pitfalls is vital for a logical, effective salvage strategy.

DISCUSSION

Early recognition of an unstable intertrochanteric fracture and planning a treatment strategy are vital. In the past, medial displacement osteotomy has been advocated as a means of increasing resistance to varus displacement. It did not, however, prove to be more useful than an accurate anatomic reduction. Reducing the fracture into varus or valgus was endorsed to decrease the incidence of device failure, but biomechanical studies have showed no improvement in stability with these procedures. Valgus osteotomy was originally thought to decrease bending forces at the fracture site, but has largely been abandoned today, as the evidence in literature did not support the idea.[3,10]

A biomechanical study by Chang et al. noted that an anatomic reduction of a four-part fracture and fixation with sliding hip screw provided more compression across the fracture site than observed with the medial displacement osteotomy. The other disadvantages of osteotomy were increased blood loss and operative time. With the advent of modern sliding hip screws, medial displacement osteotomy is infrequently indicated for unstable intertrochanteric fractures. If the fracture is anatomically reduced and the fixation device is fixed accurately, the rate of fixation failures will be low.[11]

Rao et al.[12] also discovered no advantage of medial displacement osteotomy in a retrospective study of 39 patients, but Harrington and Johnston,[13] in another retrospective study, found the medial displacement osteotomy useful with a sliding hip screw. Clark and Ribbans,[14] after a prospective study, recommended that accurate anatomical reduction and fixation without osteotomy was the treatment of choice.

CONCLUSION

Early identification of the instability is imperative. Preoperative reorganization of the unstable intertrochanteric hip fracture pattern allows the surgeon to select the treatment that most reduces the risks of loss of reduction and fixation. Unstable intertrochanteric fracture fixation has a potential for failure, so anatomical reduction and stable fixation are vital. If a fracture is reduced to an accurate anatomical position and fixed with appropriate implants, it is very unlikely that the fixation will fail.[5,6,10,15]

However, more recent studies have indicated that anatomical reduction allows greater load shearing than does a medium displacement

osteotomy or valgus osteotomy. With the advent of modern sliding hip screws, medial displacement osteotomy is rarely indicated for unstable intertrochanteric fractures, but the knowledge of these techniques is important. In some extremely comminuted unstable intertrochanteric fractures, in which anatomical reduction is not feasible, the practice of these techniques will be required.[5,6,10,15]

REFERENCES

1. Gargan MF, Gundle R, Simpson AH. How effective are osteotomies for unstable intertrochanteric fractures? *J Bone Joint Surg Br* 1994; 76(5): 789–92.
2. Egol KA, Koval KJ, Zuckerman JD. Chapter 30. In: *Handbook of fractures* (5th edn). Wolters Kluwer Health; 2015.
3. Lichtblau S. The unstable intertrochanteric hip fracture. *Orthopedics* 2008; 31(8).
4. Petrie J, Sassoon A, Haidukewych GJ. When femoral fracture fixation fails salvage options. *Bone Joint J* 2013; 95-B(Supple A): 7–10.
5. https://www.orthobullets.com/trauma/1038/intertrochanteric-fractures (last visited 09 May 2018)
6. https://aotrauma.aofoundation.org/(last visited 09 May 2018)
7. Baumgaertner MR, Solberg BD. Awareness of tip-apex distance reduces failure of fixation of trochanteric fractures of the hip. *J Bone Joint Surg [Br]* 1997; 79-B: 969–71. Done in the text at appropriate places.
8. Dimon JH, Hughston JC. Unstable intertrochanteric fractures of the hip. *J Bone Joint Surg Am* 1967; 49(3): 440–50.
9. Sarmiento A, Williams EM. The unstable intertrochanteric fracture: treatment with a valgus osteotomy and I-beam nail-plate. A preliminary report of one hundred cases. *J Bone Joint Surg Am* 1970; 52(7): 1309–18.
10. Sarathy MP, Madhavan P, Ravichandran KM. Nonunion of intertrochanteric fractures of the femur. Treatment by modified medial displacement and valgus osteotomy. *J Bone Joint Surg Br* 1995; 77(1): 90–2.
11. Chang WS, Zuckerman JD, Kummer FJ, Frankel VH. Biomechanical evaluation of anatomic reduction versus medial

displacement osteotomy in unstable intertrochanteric fractures. *Clin Orthop Relat
Res* 1987; 466(225): 141–6.

12. Rao JP, Banzon MT, Weiss AB, Rayhack J.
    Treatment of unstable intertrochanteric
    fractures with anatomic reduction and
    compression hip screw fixation. *Clin Orthop
    Relat Res* 1983; 24(175): 65–71.

13. Harrington KD, Johnston JO. The manage-
    ment of comminuted unstable intertrochan-
    teric fractures. *J Bone Joint Surg Am* 1973;
    55(7): 1367–76.

14. Clark DW, Ribbans WJ. Treatment of unsta-
    ble intertrochanteric fractures of the femur:
    A prospective trial comparing anatomical
    reduction and valgus osteotomy. *Injury*
    1990; 21(2): 84–8.

15. Desjardins AL, Roy A, Paiement G, Newman
    N, Pedlow F, Desloges D, Turcotte RE.
    Unstable intertrochanteric fracture of the
    femur. A prospective randomised study
    comparing anatomical reduction and medial
    displacement osteotomy. *J Bone Joint Surg Br*
    1993; 75(3): 445–7.

Index

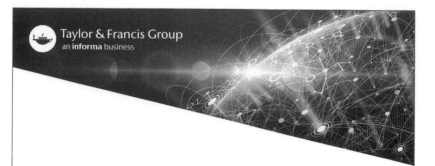

Taylor & Francis Group
an **informa** business

Taylor & Francis eBooks

www.taylorfrancis.com

A single destination for eBooks from Taylor & Francis
with increased functionality and an improved user
experience to meet the needs of our customers.

90,000+ eBooks of award-winning academic content in
Humanities, Social Science, Science, Technology, Engineering,
and Medical written by a global network of editors and authors.

TAYLOR & FRANCIS EBOOKS OFFERS:

A streamlined
experience for
our library
customers

A single point
of discovery
for all of our
eBook content

Improved
search and
discovery of
content at both
book and
chapter level

REQUEST A FREE TRIAL
support@taylorfrancis.com

 Routledge
Taylor & Francis Group

 CRC Press
Taylor & Francis Group